A·N·N·U·A·L   E·D·I·T·I·O·N·S

Health

Twenty-Seventh Edition

06/07

EDITOR

Eileen L. Daniel

SUNY at Brockport

Eileen Daniel, a registered dietitian and licensed nutritionist, is a Professor in the Department of Health Science and Associate Dean of Professions at the State University of New York at Brockport. She received a B.S. in Nutrition and Dietetics from the Rochester Institute of Technology in 1977, an M.S. in Community Health Education from SUNY at Brockport in 1987, and a Ph.D. in Health Education from the University of Oregon in 1986. A member of the American Dietetics Association, and other professional and community organizations, Dr. Daniel has published more than 40 journal articles on issues of health, nutrition, and health education. She is the editor of *Taking Sides: Clashing Views on Controversial Issues in Health and Society, 6th edition,* (Contemporary Learning Series, 2004).

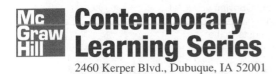

Contemporary Learning Series

2460 Kerper Blvd., Dubuque, IA 52001

Visit us on the Internet
http://www.mhcls.com

Credits

1. **Promoting Healthy Behavior Change**
   Unit photo—© McGraw-Hill Companies/Maggie Lytle.
2. **Stress and Mental Health**
   Unit photo—© Getty Images/Ryan McVay.
3. **Nutritional Health**
   Unit photo—© Corbis/Royalty-Free
4. **Exercise and Weight Management**
   Unit photo—© by Cleo Freelance Photography.
5. **Drugs and Health**
   Unit photo—© Getty Images/Keith Brofsky
6. **Sexuality and Relationships**
   Unit photo—© Getty Images/Jonnie Miles.
7. **Preventing and Fighting Disease**
   Unit photo—© Getty Images/Jason Reed
8. **Health Care and the Health Care System**
   Unit photo—© Getty Images/Photodisc Collection.
9. **Consumer Health**
   Unit photo—© Getty Images/Don Farrall
10. **Contemporary Health Hazards**
    Unit photo—© Getty Images/Nick Rowe.

Copyright

Cataloging in Publication Data
Main entry under title: Annual Editions: Health. 2006/2007.
1. Health—Periodicals. I. Daniel, Eileen L., *comp.* II. Title: Health.
ISBN 0–07–320966–X   658'.05   ISSN 0278–4653

Twenty-Seventh Edition

Cover image © Keith Brofsky/Maggie Lytle
Printed in the United States of America   1234567890QPDQPD98765   Printed on Recycled Paper

Preface

In publishing ANNUAL EDITIONS we recognize the enormous role played by the magazines, newspapers, and journals of the public press in providing current, first-rate educational information in a broad spectrum of interest areas. Many of these articles are appropriate for students, researchers, and professionals seeking accurate, current material to help bridge the gap between principles and theories and the real world. These articles, however, become more useful for study when those of lasting value are carefully collected, organized, indexed, and reproduced in a low-cost format, which provides easy and permanent access when the material is needed. That is the role played by ANNUAL EDITIONS.

America is in the midst of a revolution that is changing the way millions of Americans view their health. Traditionally, most people delegated responsibility for their health to their physicians and hoped that medical science would be able to cure whatever ailed them. This approach to health care emphasized the role of medical technology and funneled billions of dollars into medical research. The net result of all this spending is the most technically advanced and expensive health care system in the world. In an attempt to rein in health care costs, the health care delivery system has moved from privatized health care coverage to what is termed "managed care." While managed care has turned the tide regarding the rising cost of health care, it has done so by limiting reimbursement for many cutting edge technologies. Unfortunately, many people also feel that it has lowered the overall quality of care that is being given. Perhaps the saving grace is that we live at a time in which chronic illnesses rather than acute illnesses are our number one health threat, and many of these illnesses can be prevented or controlled by our lifestyle choices. The net result of these changes has prompted millions of individuals to assume more personal responsibility for safeguarding their own health. Evidence of this change in attitude can be seen in the growing interest in nutrition, physical fitness, dietary supplements, and stress management. If we as a nation are to capitalize on this new health consciousness, we must devote more time and energy to educating Americans in the health sciences so that they will be better able to make informed choices about their health.

Health is a complex and dynamic subject, and it is practically impossible for anyone to stay abreast of all the current research findings. In the past, most of us have relied on books, newspapers, magazines, and television as our primary sources for medical/health information, but today, with the widespread use of personal computers connected to the World Wide Web, it is possible to access vast amounts of health information any time of the day without ever leaving one's home. Unfortunately, quantity and availability does not necessarily translate into quality, and this is particularly true in the area of medical/health information. Just as the Internet is a great source for reliable timely information, it is also a vehicle for the dissemination of misleading and fraudulent information. Currently there are no standards or regulations regarding the posting of health content on the Internet, and this has led to a plethora of misinformation and quackery in the medical/health arena.

Given this vast amount of health information, our task as health educators is twofold: (1) To provide our students with the most up-to-date and accurate information available on major health issues of our time and (2) to teach our students the skills that will enable them to sort out fact from fiction in order to become informed consumers. *Annual Editions: Health 06/07* was designed to aid in this task. It offers a sampling of quality articles that represent the latest thinking on a variety of health issues, and it also serves as a tool for developing critical thinking skills.

The articles in this volume were carefully chosen on the basis of their quality and timeliness. Because this book is revised and updated annually, it contains information that is not generally available in any standard textbook. As such, it serves as a valuable resource for both teachers and students. This edition of *Annual Editions: Health* has been updated to reflect the latest thinking on a variety of contemporary health issues. We hope that you find this edition to be a helpful learning tool filled with information and presented in a user-friendly format. The 10 topical areas presented in this edition mirror those that are normally covered in introductory health courses: Promoting Healthy Behavior Change, Stress and Mental Health, Nutritional Health, Exercise and Weight Management, Drugs and Health, Sexuality and Relationships, Preventing and Fighting Disease, Health Care and the Health Care System, Consumer Health, and Contemporary Health Hazards. Because of the interdependence of the various elements that constitute health, the articles selected were written by authors with diverse educational backgrounds and expertise including naturalists, environmentalists, psychologists, economists, sociologists, nutritionists, consumer advocates, and traditional health practitioners.

Annual Editions: Health 06/07 was designed to be one of the most useful and up-to-date publications currently available in the area of health. Please let us know what you think of it by filling out and returning the postage paid *article rating form* on the last page of this book. Any anthology can be improved. This one will be—annually.

Eileen L. Daniel
Editor

Contents

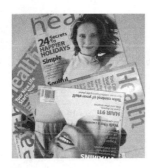

UNIT 1
Promoting Healthy Behavior Change

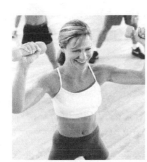

UNIT 2
Stress and Mental Health

The concepts in bold italics are developed in the article. For further expansion, please refer to the Topic Guide and the Index.

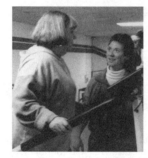

UNIT 3
Nutritional Health

UNIT 4
Exercise and Weight Management

The concepts in bold italics are developed in the article. For further expansion, please refer to the Topic Guide and the Index.

UNIT 5
Drugs and Health

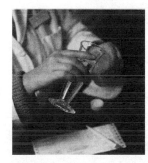

UNIT 6
Sexuality and Relationships

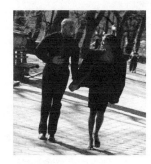

The concepts in bold italics are developed in the article. For further expansion, please refer to the Topic Guide and the Index.

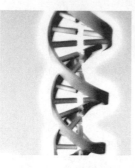

UNIT 7
Preventing and Fighting Disease

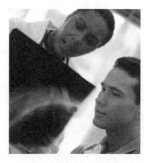

UNIT 8
Health Care and the Health Care System

The concepts in bold italics are developed in the article. For further expansion, please refer to the Topic Guide and the Index.

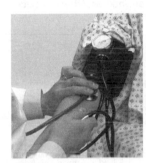

UNIT 9
Consumer Health

The concepts in bold italics are developed in the article. For further expansion, please refer to the Topic Guide and the Index.

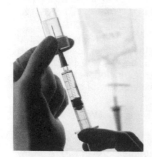

UNIT 10
Contemporary Health Hazards

The concepts in bold italics are developed in the article. For further expansion, please refer to the Topic Guide and the Index.

Topic Guide

This topic guide suggests how the selections in this book relate to the subjects covered in your course. You may want to use the topics listed on these pages to search the Web more easily.

On the following pages a number of Web sites have been gathered specifically for this book. They are arranged to reflect the units of this *Annual Edition.* You can link to these sites by going to the student online support site at *http://www.mhcls.com/online/.*

ALL THE ARTICLES THAT RELATE TO EACH TOPIC ARE LISTED BELOW THE BOLD-FACED TERM.

Internet References

The following internet sites have been carefully researched and selected to support the articles found in this reader. The easiest way to access these selected sites is to go to our student online support site at *http://www.mhcls.com/online/*.

AE: Health 06/07

The following sites were available at the time of publication. Visit our Web site—we update our student online support site regularly to reflect any changes.

General Sources

National Institute on Aging (NIA)
http://www.nia.nih.gov/

The NIA, one of the institutes of the U.S. National Institutes of Health, presents this home page to lead you to a variety of resources on health and lifestyle issues on aging.

U.S. Department of Agriculture (USDA)/Food and Nutrition Information Center (FNIC)
http://www.nal.usda.gov/fnic/

Use this site to find nutrition information provided by various USDA agencies, to find links to food and nutrition resources on the Internet, and to access FNIC publications and databases.

U.S. Department of Health and Human Services
http://www.os.dhhs.gov

This site has extensive links to information on such topics as the health benefits of exercise, weight control, and prudent lifestyle choices.

U.S. National Institutes of Health (NIH)
http://www.nih.gov

Consult this site for links to extensive health information and scientific resources. Comprising 24 separate institutes, centers, and divisions, the NIH is one of eight health agencies of the Public Health Service, which, in turn, is part of the U.S. Department of Health and Human Services.

U.S. National Library of Medicine
http://www.nlm.nih.gov

This huge site permits a search of a number of databases and electronic information sources such as MEDLINE. You can learn about research projects and programs and peruse the national network of medical libraries here.

World Health Organization
http://www.who.int/en

This home page of the World Health Organization will provide links to a wealth of statistical and analytical information about health around the world.

UNIT 1: Promoting Healthy Behavior Change

Ask Dr. Weil
http://www.drweil.com/u/Home/index.html

Dr. Weil, a Harvard-trained physician, is director of the Center for Integrative Medicine at the University of Arizona. He offers a comprehensive Web site that addresses alternative medicine. Look for research, FAQs, and links to related sites.

Columbia University's Go Ask Alice!
http://www.goaskalice.columbia.edu/index.html

This interactive site provides discussion and insight into a number of personal issues of interest to college-age people and those younger and older. Many questions about physical and emotional health and well-being are answered.

The Society of Behavioral Medicine
http://www.sbm.org/

This site provides listings of major, general health institutes and organizations as well as discipline-specific links and resources in medicine, psychology, and public health.

UNIT 2: Stress and Mental Health

The American Institute of Stress
http://www.stress.org

This site provides comprehensive information on stress: its dangers, the beliefs that build helpful techniques for overcoming stress, and so on. This easy-to-navigate site has good links to information on anxiety and related topics.

National Mental Health Association (NMHA)
http://www.nmha.org/index.html

The NMHA is a citizen volunteer advocacy organization that works to improve the mental health of all individuals. The site provides access to guidelines that individuals can use to reduce stress and improve their lives in small yet tangible ways.

Self-Help Magazine
http://www.selfhelpmagazine.com/index.html

Reach lots of links to self-help resources on the Net at this site, including resources on stress, anxiety, fears, and more.

UNIT 3: Nutritional Health

The American Dietetic Association
http://www.eatright.org

This organization, along with its National Center of Nutrition and Dietetics, promotes optimal nutrition, health, and well-being. This easy-to-navigate site presents FAQs about nutrition and dieting, nutrition resources, and career and member information.

Center for Science in the Public Interest (CSPI)
http://www.cspinet.org/

CSPI is a nonprofit education and advocacy organization that focuses on improving the safety and nutritional quality of our food supply and on reducing the health problems caused by alcohol. This agency also evaluates the nutritional composition of fast foods, movie popcorn, and chain restaurants. There are also good links to related sites.

Tufts University Nutrition Navigator
http://www.navigator.tufts.edu

The *Tufts University Nutrition Navigator* is the first online rating and review guide for those seeking nutrition information on the Web. It is designed to help sort out the useful, accurate, and trustworthy information from the large volume of information on the Web.

UNIT 4: Exercise and Weight Management

American Society of Exercise Physiologists (ASEP)
http://www.asep.org

The ASEP is devoted to promoting people's health and physical fitness. This extensive site provides links to publications related to exercise and career opportunities in exercise physiology.

Cyberdiet
http://www.cyberdiet.com/reg/index.html

This site, maintained by a registred dietician, offers CyberDiet's interactive nutritional profile, food facts, menus and meal plans, and exercise and food-related sites.

National Eating Disorders Association
http://www.nationaleatingdisorders.org

This site offers information on eating disorders, including suggestions for families and friends of sufferers, details for professionals, and general information on eating disorders for the interested public.

Shape Up America!
http://www.shapeup.org

At the Shape Up America! Web site you will find the latest information about safe weight management, healthy eating, and physical fitness.

UNIT 5: Drugs and Health

Food and Drug Administration (FDA)
http://www.fda.gov/

This site includes FDA news, information on drugs, and drug toxicology facts.

National Institute on Drug Abuse (NIDA)
http://165.112.78.61

Use this site index for access to NIDA publications and communications, information on drugs of abuse, and links to other related Web sites.

Prescription Drugs: The Issue
http://www.opensecrets.org/news/drug/

This site offers information on a variety of prescription drugs, including interactions, side effects, and related material.

UNIT 6: Sexuality and Relationships

Planned Parenthood
http://www.plannedparenthood.org/

This home page provides links to information on contraceptives (including outercourse and abstinence) and to discussions of other topics related to sexual health.

Sexuality Information and Education Council of the United States (SIECUS)
http://www.siecus.org/

Siecus is a nonprofit private advocacy group that affirms that sexuality is a natural and healthy part of living. This home page offers publications, what's new, descriptions of programs, and a listing of international sexuality education initiatives.

UNIT 7: Preventing and Fighting Disease

American Cancer Society
http://www.cancer.org

Open this site and its various links to learn the concerns and lifestyle advice of the American Cancer Society. It provides information on tobacco and alternative cancer therapies.

American Heart Association
http://www.amhrt.org

This award-winning comprehensive site of the American Heart Association offers information on heart disease, prevention, patient facts, eating plans, what's new, nutrition, smoking cessation, and FAQs.

National Institute of Allergy and Infectious Diseases (NIAID)
http://www.niaid.gov

Open this site and its various links to learn the concerns and lifestyle advice of the National Institute of Allergy and Infectious Diseases.

UNIT 8: Health Care and the Health Care System

American Medical Association (AMA)
http://www.ama-assn.org

The AMA offers this site to find up-to-date medical information, peer-review resources, discussions of such topics as HIV/AIDS and women's health, examination of issues related to managed care, and important publications.

MedScape: The Online Resource for Better Patient Care
http://www.medscape.com

For health professionals and interested consumers, this site offers peer-reviewed articles, self-assessment features, medical news, and annotated links to Internet resources. It also contains the *Morbidity & Mortality Weekly Report,* which is a publication of the Centers for Disease Control and Prevention.

UNIT 9: Consumer Health

FDA Consumer Magazine
http://www.fda.gov/fdac/796?toc.html

This site offers articles and information that appears in the *FDA Consumer Magazine.*

Global Vaccine Awareness League
http://www.gval.com

This site addresses side effects related to vaccination. Its many links are geared to provide copious information.

UNIT 10: Contemporary Health Hazards

Centers for Disease Control: Flu
http://www.cdc.gov/flu

This CDC site provides updates, information, key facts, questions and answers, and ways to prevent influenza (the flu). Updated regularly during the flu season.

Center for the Study of Autism
http://www.autism.org

This site provides resources for both professionals and family members of individuals with autism. The site includes interventions, family support, and stories of persons with the condition.

Noise Pollution Clearinghouse
http://www.nonoise.org

The Noise Pollution Clearinghouse is a national non-profit organization with extensive online noise related resources. The Noise Pollution Clearinghouse seeks to: Raise awareness about noise pollution, create, collect, and distribute information and resources reqarding noise pollution, strengthen laws and governmental efforts to control noise pollution, establish networks among environmental, professional, medical, governmental, and activist groups working on noise pollution issues, and assist activists working against noise pollution.

www.mhcls.com/online/

Food and Drug Administration Mad Cow Disease Page
http://www.fda.gov/oc/opacom/hottopics/bse.html
   This Food and Drug Administration page includes information,
   articles, and updates about Bovine Spongiform Encephalopathy
   (BSE) also known as "Mad Cow Disease."

Environmental Protection Agency
http://www.epa.gov
   Use this site to find environmental health information provided by
   various EPA agencies.

We highly recommend that you review our Web site for expanded information and our
other product lines. We are continually updating and adding links to our Web site in order
to offer you the most usable and useful information that will support and expand the value
of your Annual Editions. You can reach us at: *http://www.mhcls.com/annualeditions/*.

UNIT 1

Promoting Healthy Behavior Change

Unit Selections

1. **How To Live To Be 100**, Richard Corliss and Michael D. Lemonick
2. **Putting a Premium on Health**, John Dorschner
3. **Why the Rich Live Longer**, Dan Seligman

Key Points to Consider

- Why do you think that people continue to engage in negative health behaviors when they know that these behaviors will have a negative impact on their health? Have you ever done so? If so, why?

- What is the relationship between health behaviors and longevity?

- What behaviors do you wish you could undo?

- What factors contribute to successful lifestyle change?

- What personal health behaviors would you like to improve? What prevents you from making these changes? How can you overcome these obstacles?

- Should companies charge employees more for health insurance if they continue to engage in unhealthy behaviors?

Student Website

www.mhcls.com/online

Internet References

Further information regarding these websites may be found in this book's preface or online.

Ask Dr. Weil
   http://www.drweil.com/u/Home/index.html
Columbia University's Go Ask Alice!
   http://www.goaskalice.columbia.edu/index.html
The Society of Behavioral Medicine
   http://www.sbm.org/

"**T**hose of us who protect our health daily and those of us who put our health in constant jeopardy have exactly the same mortality: 100 percent. The difference, of course, is the timing." This quotation from Elizabeth M. Whelan, Sc.D., M.P.H., reminds us that we must all face the fact that we are going to die sometime. The question that is decided by our behavior is when and, to a certain extent, how. This book and especially this unit are designed to assist students in the development of cognitive skills and knowledge that, when put to use, help make the moment of our death come as late as possible in our lives and to maintain our health as long as possible. While we cannot control many of the things that happen to us, we must all strive to accept personal responsibility for, and make informed decisions about, things that we can control. This is no minor task, but it is one in which the potential reward is life itself.

Perhaps the best way to start this process is by educating ourselves on the relative risks associated with the various behaviors and lifestyle choices we make. To minimize all risk to life and health would be to significantly limit the quality of our lives, and while this might be a choice that some would make, it certainly is not the goal of health education. A more logical approach to risk reduction would be to educate the public on the relative risk associated with various behaviors and lifestyle choices so that they are capable of making informed decisions. While it may seem obvious that certain behaviors, such as smoking, entail a high level of risk, the significance of others such as toxic waste sites and food additives are frequently blown out of proportion to the actual risks involved. The net result of this type of distortion is that many Americans tend to minimize the dangers of known hazards such as tobacco and alcohol and focus attention, instead, on potentially minor health hazards over which they have little or no control.

Educating the public on the relative risk of various health behaviors is only part of the job that health educators must tackle in order to assist individuals in making informed choices regarding their health. They also must teach the skills that will enable people to evaluate the validity and significance of new information as it becomes available. Just how important informed decision making is in our daily lives is evidenced by the numerous health-related media announcements and articles that fill our newspapers, magazines, and television broadcasts. Rather than inform and enlighten the public on significant new medical discoveries, many of these announcements do little more than add to the level of confusion or exaggerate or sensationalize health issues. Why is this so? While there is no simple explanation, there appear to be at least two major factors that contribute to the confusion. The first has to do with the primary goals and objectives of the media itself. One only has to scan the headlines on the cover pages of magazines or newspapers to realize that the primary goal of these publications is to entice the potential reader into purchasing their product. How better to capture the readers' attention than to sensationalize and exaggerate scientific discoveries. This is not to blame the media but rather to remind the reader that given the economic realities of the competitive world in which we live, sometimes the methodical plodding of the scientific method takes second place to the marketing needs of a publisher.

Let's assume for a minute that the scientific community is in general agreement that certain behaviors clearly promote our health while others damage our health. Given this information, are you likely to make adjustments to your lifestyle to comply with the findings? Logic would suggest that of course you would, but experience has taught us that information alone isn't enough to bring about behavioral change in many people. Why is it that so many people continue to make bad choices regarding their health behaviors when they are fully aware of the risks involved? There may be many reasons, but two possible explanations are presented in the articles "How to Live to be 100" and "Putting a Premium on Health." According to the authors of the first, Richard Corliss and Michael Lemonick, the underlying motivation behind many of our behavioral decisions is our desire to receive immediate gratification, and in their article they suggests a strategy that can be used to counter the psychological appeal of immediate gratification that can help us live to 100! John Dorschner's article suggests that we can empower ourselves to change our behavior and benefit both physically and financially. We can vow to make changes to try to undo or minimize negative health behaviors of our past. While strategies such as these may work for those who feel they are at risk, how do we help those who do not feel that they are at risk or those who feel that it is too late in their lives for the changes to matter?

While the goal of health education is to promote healthy behaviors that lead to healthy lifestyles, this objective will not be reached unless, or until, the public is armed with the knowledge and skills necessary to make informed decisions regarding their health. Even then, there is no guarantee that the information gleaned will serve as motivation. In a free society such as ours, the choice is, and must remain, up to the individual.

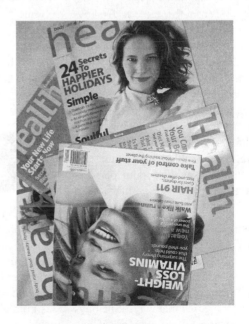

HOW TO LIVE TO BE
100

New research suggests that a long life is no accident. So what are the secrets of the world's centenarians?

By RICHARD CORLISS and MICHAEL D. LEMONICK

Margaret Dell is 96, but you'd need to check the birth date on her driver's license to believe it. Sporting a baseball cap with a Harley-Davidson logo on it, she is the designated driver for her seventysomething friends who no longer feel comfortable behind the wheel. Last winter a snowfall threatened to keep her from her appointed automotive rounds. She took a shovel and cleared a path to her car. Driving keeps Dell young. That and knitting. She constantly knits. She makes baby booties and caps and blankets for friends and family whenever a baby arrives—the newborn getting an early blessing from the ageless. And every month, she donates several blankets to a charity for unwed mothers. Driving, knitting … and tennis. She plays two or three times a week. She has a much younger doubles partner who "covers the court. I'm a little afraid to run too much because of the circulation in my legs," she explains. When she was in her 80s, she played in a doubles tournament that required that the ages of both partners add up to at least 100. Her partner was in his early 20s; they won the tournament.

A lifetime nonsmoker and nondrinker, Dell lives alone in a two-story house in Bethesda, Md., her bedroom on the second floor. "I could stay on the first floor, but I try to make myself walk up those stairs and keep going that way." She buys her own groceries; don't even ask if you can shop for her. At home she likes a chicken or turkey sandwich for lunch. If she eats at the country club after tennis, she usually finishes only half and saves the rest for dinner. (The doggie bag is the senior citizen's medical-supply kit.)

Driving, tennis, knitting … and eating chocolates. She keeps them in a drawer by her easy chair. "I am very bad about those Hershey Kisses," she confesses. "And I love those little Dove ice cream things. I take one before I go to bed." That's the only medication Dell will take without a fight. She's no fan of doctors. Some years back, she took a fall, and her doctor prescribed an MRI. "I just refused to go," she says. "They were having a party. It was my 90th birthday." And the party girl left his office. Fortunately, nothing was broken. But Dell knew that.

> **RACE: On average, white U.S. males live to be 75 vs. 68 for blacks; for women, the racial gap is 80 vs. 75.**

More than what she knows, it's how she glows that impresses people. "She has a light in her eyes that is very alive, alert and interested," says Carole Dell. "It radiates over her whole face. Her face is kind of timeless. It's deeply lined, but she's actually beautiful." Spoken like a proud daughter-in-law with 96 reasons to be proud. Ninety-six and counting.

How does science explain someone like Margaret Dell? How can a woman closing in on the start of her second century be so robustly, almost defiantly, healthy, while men and women decades younger are languishing feebly in nursing homes, plagued with failing bodies and failing minds and wishing they hadn't been so unlucky as to live so long?

For most of human history, a long and healthy life has been shrugged off as a gift from the gods—or maybe the undeserved reward for a lifetime of plain cussedness. But to gerontologists, the vagaries of aging have become the focus of intense scientific research.

Scientists are as obsessed with the question of why the superold survive and thrive as Ponce de León was to find the Fountain of Youth. They want to understand why the Japanese islands of Okinawa are home to the world's largest population of centenarians, with almost 600 of its 1.3 million inhabitants living into their second century—many of them active and looking decades younger than their actual years. Like weekend visitors on the summer ferry to Martha's Vineyard, scientists and sociologists clog the boats to Sardinia and Nova Scotia, Canada, to see why those craggy locales harbor outsize clusters of the superold. (Gerontologists are not so beguiled by the

Russian Caucasus, where exaggerated longevity claims sparked a series of Dannon yogurt commercials 30 years ago.)

As well as studying these populations intensively to unlock their secrets, scientists have also taken a hard look at the very old in the U.S., most notably in the New England Centenarian Study, led by Dr. Thomas Perls, a geriatrician at Boston University, and in a major study under way at the National Institute on Aging. While the very old are happy to offer homespun explanations for their longevity—"I never took a drink"; "I drank a shot of whiskey every day"—experts are trying to unravel and understand the biological factors that allow some people to reach 100 while others drop off in their 70s or 80s. Researchers are particularly interested in determining which factors allow up to 30% of those who reach 100 to do so in sufficient mental and physical health: a whopping 90% of centenarians, according to Perls, remain functionally independent up to age 92. "It's not 'the older you get, the sicker you get,' but 'the older you get, the healthier you've been,'" he says. "The advantage of living to 100 is not so much how you are at 100 but how you got there."

FAMILY: Married folk outlive singles (but men benefit more than women do); older siblings live longer than younger ones; mothers slightly outlive childless women

It's pretty obvious even to nonscientists that how you get there depends partly on the genes you are born with and partly on lifestyle—what and how much you eat, where you live and what types of stress and trauma you experience. How much depends on each factor, though, was unknown until Swedish scientists tackled the problem in 1998. They did it by looking at the only set of people who share genes but not lifestyle: identical twins who were separated at birth and reared apart. If genes were most important, you would expect the twins to die at about the same age. In fact, they don't, and the average difference convinced the scientists that only about 20% to 30% of how long we live is genetically determined. The dominant factor is lifestyle.

"You could have Mercedes-Benz genes," says Dr. Bradley Willcox, of the Pacific Health Research Institute in Honolulu, "but if you never change the oil, you are not going to last as long as a Ford Escort that you take good care of. Those who have healthier genes and live healthier lives—those guys really survive for a long time."

Studies of Seventh-Day Adventists in Utah support this finding. Those unusually clean-living Americans are genetically diverse, but they avoid alcohol, caffeine and tobacco—and they tend to live an average of eight years longer than their countrymen. All of this is good news, with a Surgeon General's warning attached: you can't change your genes, but you can change what you eat and how much you exercise. "The lesson is pretty clear from my point of view in terms of what the average person should be doing," says Perls. "I strongly believe that with some changes in health-related behavior, each of us can earn the right to have at least 25 years beyond the age of 60—years of healthy life at good function. The disappointing news is that it requires work and willpower."

At least that's true for many Americans, whose fat-and calorie packed diets and largely exercise-free lives are a prescription for heart disease and plenty of other ills. For Okinawans, by contrast, the traditional way of life seems tailor-made for living forever—one day at a time.

Each day, Seiryu Toguchi, 103, of Motobu, Okinawa, wakes at 6 a.m., in the house in which he was born, and opens the shutters. "It's a sign to my neighbors," he says, "that I am still alive." He does stretching exercises along with a radio broadcast, then eats breakfast: whole-grain rice and miso soup with vegetables. He puts in two hours of picking weeds in his 1,000-sq.-ft. field, whose crops are goya—a variety of bitter gourd—a reddish-purple sweet potato called imo, and okra. A fellow has to make a living, so Toguchi buys rice and meat with the profits from his produce.

Since his wife Kame's death seven years ago, at 93, he has done all the housework himself. He rejected his children's suggestion to come live with them because, he explains, "I enjoy my freedom." Although his doctors insist Toguchi is in excellent health, the farmer

ACHIEVEMENT: Americans with higher education live six years longer than high school dropouts; Oscar winners outlive unsuccessful nominees by four years; CEOs outlive corporate VPs.

takes no chances. "If he feels that something is wrong," says his daughter Sumiko Sakihara, 74, "even in the middle of the night, he calls a taxi and goes to the hospital." But he doesn't want the other villagers to worry, so, she says, "he writes a note explaining where he is and tapes it to the shutters."

At 12:30 Toguchi eats lunch: goya stir-fry with egg and tofu. He naps for an hour or so, then spends two more hours in his field. After dinner he plays traditional songs—a favorite is *Spring When I Was 19*—on the three-stringed *sanshin* and makes an entry in his diary, as he has every night for the past decade. "This way," he says, "I won't forget my Chinese characters. It's fun. It keeps my mind sharp." For a nightcap he may have a sip of the wine he makes from aloe, garlic and tumeric. And as he drifts off, he says, "my head is filled with all the things I want to do tomorrow."

Scientists working for the U.S. National Institutes of Health and Japan's Ministry of Health have been following oldsters like Toguchi since 1976 in the Okinawa Centenarian Study (OCS) and they've learned that he's typical. Elderly Okinawans tend to get plenty of physical and mental exercise. Their diets, moreover, are exemplary: low in fat and salt, and high in fruits and vegetables packed with fiber and antioxidant substances that protect against cancer, heart disease and stroke. They consume more soy than any other population on earth: 60–120 g a day, compared to 30–50 g for the average Japanese, 10 for Chinese and virtually 0 g for the average American. Soy is rich in flavonoids—antioxidants strongly linked to low rates of cancer. This may be one of many reasons why the annual death rate from cancer in Okinawa is far below the U.S. rate.

FAITH: The elderly who attend worship services weekly live longer than those who don't

3

DIET RESTRICTION

Eat Less, Live Longer?

A few years ago, Harvard researcher Dr. David Sinclair joined the growing ranks of scientists who believe that severely restricting calorie intake can slow down the aging process. Evidence for that surprising phenomenon emerged in the 1930s, when scientists learned that underfed rodents lived up to 40% longer than their well-fed counterparts. The results have since been duplicated in fruit flies, worms, monkeys and other lab animals. And preliminary research on humans suggests that some markers of aging—levels of blood glucose, blood pressure, cholesterol—improve on calorie-restriction (CR) diets.

So Sinclair put himself on the same sort of severe diet that members of the tiny but highly motivated Calorie Restriction Society, follow. He lasted a week. "It was too tough," he says. "My hat's off to the calorie restricters. Now I'm hoping to find drugs that can give people the benefits of CR without the diet."

Those drugs haven't been perfected yet, but Sinclair and other researchers are making progress by trying to understand at the molecular level what it is about CR that seems to slow aging. Sinclair has found, for example, that resveratrol, a chemical found in red wine, increases life-spans of yeast and fruit flies. It works by amplifying the action of a molecule called SIRT1, which is present in all life forms and is produced in response to stress. "It's like a cell's 911 center," says Sinclair, and resveratrol is like a false alarm.

That fits with one of the leading theories about why CR works in the first place: starving the body puts it under mild, constant stress, priming it to resist the more severe stresses that make cells age—a sort of self-vaccination against decline. "With resveratrol," says Sinclair, "we're tricking the body into thinking it's not getting enough calories." If he can create a form of resveratrol that's easily absorbed by human cells and can demonstrate that it works without dangerous side effects, Sinclair may eventually come up with what amounts to an antiaging pill.

At the University of California, San Francisco, meanwhile, molecular geneticist Cynthia Kenyon is taking a different approach to aging research, identifying a number of genes in roundworms that help stave off disease and extend life. One such gene directs the action of a receptor for insulin and an insulin-like hormone called IGF-1, and by manipulating it along with other genes, she can increase the worms' life-span sixfold. "It's not so much that they're just living longer she says. "What's remarkable about these worms is how healthy they are."

But the story is more complex: Kenyon has found that hormones in her long-lived worms actually regulate several unusual genes to increase life-span. One set of genes triggers the worms' cells to make antioxidants, which fight off the ravages of molecules called free radicals, which can damage DNA. Another set directs the creation of proteins called chaperones; they help other proteins fold into their proper shapes. They also detect and destroy improperly folded proteins that can cause such aging-related ailments as Huntington's disease. Other genes affect the transport of fat around the body—which may also have an effect on aging—and create proteins that kill invading microbes. "It's like an orchestra," says Kenyon. "The conductor is the hormones. You have the flutes as the antioxidant genes. The violins would be the chaperones, the cellos the metabolic genes. And maybe the drums would be the antimicrobial genes. So many different kinds of genes can have enormous effects on life and death, and each one on its own could potentially have an effect on human lifespan or disease.

At the University of Wisconsin at Madison, gerontologist Richard Weindruch studies deprivation, like Sinclair, but has a different idea about why calorie restriction works. He has been comparing calorie-restricted rhesus monkeys with unrestricted ones and has found striking differences. The CR monkeys have shown no evidence of diabetes, for example, while it affects about half of normal monkeys. Only four of his CR monkeys, moreover, have died from age-related diseases—half the rate of the control group. He believes the explanation lies in the complex activities of fat cells. The CR monkeys have much less body fat, and that—just as with slim vs. obese humans—seems to protect against a wide range of ills.

Calorie restriction has its downside, though, and it's not just hunger. Weindruch's monkeys experience changes in bone density, and other labs have reported changes in libido; menstrual cycles and body temperature in calorie-restricted monkeys. And Sinclair's worms and flies suffer from loss of appetite and fertility. Researchers hope to create drugs based on resveratrol or on the genetic research that would avoid those pitfalls.

In the meantime, members of the CR movement are proceeding with their personal experiments in consumption. Although early CR advocates tried extreme diets, hoping to live to 120 or beyond, most current practitioners take a more moderate approach and have the more modest goal of staving off illness. For the past five years, Andrea Tiktin-Fanti, 61, of Uhrichsville, Ohio, has been adhering to a l,200-calorie-a-day diet—about half what U.S. women typically eat. Diabetes killed both her parents in their 60s, but her diabetes is under control, thanks to her Spartan diet. "If I live to 85 or 90," she says, "I will have extended my lifespan, and I'll be real happy with that.

—By Michael D. Lemonick. Reported by Dan Cray/Los Angeles

But it's not just what Okinawans eat; it's how much. They practice a dietary philosophy known as *hara hachi bu*—literally, eight parts out of 10 full. Translation: they eat only to the point at which they are about 80% sated. That makes for a daily intake of no more than 1,800 calories, compared to the more than 2,500 that the average American man scarfs down. And as scientists have learned from lab animals, the simple act of calorie restriction can have significant effects on longevity (*see box*).

Aging Okinawans also have a much lower incidence of dementia—Alzheimer's or other forms of senility—than their U.S. and European counterparts do. Part of that may also owe to diet; it's high in vitamin E, which seems to protect the

LONGEVITY
Meet the Oldest American

Who is more qualified than Verona Johnston to expound on the secrets behind a long, healthy life? The retired Latin teacher, mother of four, grandmother of 13 and great-grandmother of 23 turned 114 on Aug. 6, which makes her the oldest documented person in the U.S. And there's plenty of life in her yet. "I can remember names pretty well," says Johnston, who lived on her own in an apartment until age 98 but now shares a house in Worthington, Ohio, with her daughter Julie Johnson, 81, and Julie's husband Bruce, 83. In fact, Johnston's mind is so sharp that she still solves word jumbles in her head; remembers joke punch lines; and, when she has trouble sleeping, runs through the names of her 36 grandchildren and great-grandchildren, rather than counting sheep.

Oh, sure, her vision is nearly gone, so she had to give up playing bridge at 110. She no longer travels solo to visit kin in Omaha, Neb., and San Diego, as she did at 100, and she relies on a cane to take steps, but Johnston can still hear fairly well, and she loves listening to books on tape. (Now it's *Lark Rise to Candleford*, about life at the end of the 19th century—a period otherwise known as her childhood.)

Johnston doesn't dwell on what age has taken away from her. "She's never been a complainer," says Julie. That attitude may have much to do with her prodigious longevity. Not to mention good genes and a whopping dose of good luck. Johnston's father, a Presbyterian minister, died at 69, her mother at 85. Her younger sister Vern died in 1997 at 105. Though Johnston had surgery for breast cancer in her 90s and a heart attack so minor she never noticed it, she has generally enjoyed superb health.

"I never had a special diet," she says. "I really like mashed potatoes and gravy." But Johnston has always been big on moderation. Even today, her daily snack consists of orange juice and exactly one cracker, one cinnamon-drop candy and one cashew. "That's enough," she insists.

Johnston, who graduated from Drake University in 1912, never smoked. This church-going minister's daughter never touched alcohol either, until she moved in with Julie and Bruce, who introduced her to Baileys Irish Cream, now part of an occasional family happy hour. As for exercise, it was just woven into an active schedule. Well into her 90s, she climbed up and down seven flights of stairs to her old apartment.

Johnston has certainly seen change in her life, and she rolls with it. "Electricity was the most important thing that happened to us," she reflects. The computer was intimidating, but she gave it a whirl: "I worked that mouse." And she's ready for more. "You can get too old to enjoy life," she says, adding slyly, "I never got that old."

—By Wendy Cole/Worthington

---

brain. But perhaps just as important is a sense of belonging and purpose that provides a strong foundation for staying mentally alert well into old age. Okinawans maintain a sense of community, ensuring that every member, from youngest to oldest, is paid proper respect and feels equally valued. Elderly women, for example, are considered the sacred keepers of a family's bond with the ancestors, maintaining the family altars and responsible for organizing festivals to honor them. OCS data show that elderly Okinawans express a high level of satisfaction with life, something that is not as true in Western societies, where rates of suicide and depression are high among the elderly.

Need convincing evidence that our modern lifestyle can shorten lives? Look what happens when Okinawans move permanently off the island. They pick up the diet and cultural behaviors of their adopted country—and within a generation, their life-spans decrease and their rates of cancer and heart attack zoom. Even on the island, young males are following the seductive, virulent American style and renouncing imo for hamburgers. "Okinawan male life expectancy used to be No. 1 in Japan," says Dr. Makoto Suzuki, leader of the study of Okinawan elders. "It started to decline 10 years ago and hit 26th out of 47 prefectures in the 2000 census. I expect it to decline even further in the next census."

HEALTH: Smoking typically costs you 10 years; obesity costs an average of 7.1 years for females, 5.8 years for males; those who sleep seven hours a night live longest; tall folk (6 ft. to 6 ft. 3 in. for men, 5 ft. 7 in. to 5 ft. 9 in. for women) average three more years than short people

Oldsters in Sardinia, another wellspring of longevity, have many similarities to their Okinawan counterparts—except that the Sardinian ratio of centenarians is about equal for men and women (in most societies, 100-plus females outnumber males by 3 or 4 to 1). They maintain very active lives and powerful social networks; extended family and friends are available to share troubles and take some of the emotional burden out of life. Says researcher Gianni Pes, part of a team from Sardinia's University of Sassari, which is studying the group: "The 100-year-olds are less depressed than average 60-year-olds."

That makes perfect sense to Leonard Poon, director of the University of Georgia Gerontology Center. Since 1988 he has studied American centenarians—he calls them "expert survivors"—and compared them to people in their 80s ("master survivors") and to relative youngsters in their 60s. Poon found that out of 16 personality traits, the experts exhibited four coping mechanisms. First, he says, "centenarians are more dominant. They want to have their way," and they are not easily pushed around. Many are characterized by "suspiciousness. They do not take information on the superficial level" but will question an issue and think it through. They tend to be practical rather than idealistic. And in their approach to life, they are likely to be more relaxed. In other words, they are strong but not inflexible characters.

Poon also determined that people whose age reaches three figures tend to have a high level of cognition, demonstrating skill in

HOW LONG WILL YOU LIVE?

An average person living in an industrialized nation has the genetic makeup and environment to enable him or her to live to the age of 87.

INSTRUCTIONS: Start with **87 years**. Depending on your answers to the questions below, add or subtract the appropriate number of years.

ATTITUDE: Are you optimistic? Do you generally approach life with good humor? Are you able to let go of things that are stressful?
If no, subtract five years

GENES: Do you have at least some family members who have lived into their 90s or later? Exceptional longevity runs strongly in families.
If yes, add 10 years

EXERCISE: Do you set aside at least 30 minutes a day, three days a week to exercise? Muscle-building exercises are particularly important.
If no, subtract five years

INTERESTS: Do you do things that are challenging to your brain regularly? It's important to take on activities that are novel and complex.
If yes, add five years

NUTRITION: do you have a diet that keeps you lean? carrying extra weight is not conducive to longevity.
If no, subtract seven years

GET RID OF SMOKING: Do you smoke?
If yes, subtract five years

TOTAL

Source: Adapted from Living to 100

everyday problem solving and learning. That's another reason exercise is important: to keep plenty of blood flowing to the brain as well as to stay in shape. Many of his subjects aren't rich; some of them have homes with mud floors. But they make good out of making do. "Many have their own gardens," he notes. "They can their own vegetables. They're living down to earth."

Like the Okinawans, Sardinians and Nova Scotians, the U.S. centenarians enjoy a strong social-support system. Few Americans live in a village anymore, but having outlived family and friends of the same age, the superold find new helpers and confidants among people younger by a generation or more. It might be someone to help with groceries or car trips or simply a sympathetic voice on the other end of the line. Maintaining a connection with the world, with younger people, keeps their outlook youthful.

With so much evidence that lifestyle is the key to healthy aging, it might be tempting to ignore the role of genes altogether. That would be a mistake. Brothers of centenarians are 17 times as likely to live to 100 as are people without 100-year-olds in the family, while sisters of centenarians are 8.5 times as likely to live into their second century. Given statistics like that, says Winifred Rossi, director of the National Institute on Aging's study on exceptional survival, "we are interested in looking for some kind of genetic component to longevity." Her approach is to look at family members, especially the children, of centenarians. Says Perls, who does similar research: "Kids of centenarians who are in their 70s and early 80s are very much following in the footsteps of their parents, with a 60% reduced risk of heart disease, stroke and diabetes. They are the model for successful aging and a great group to study."

Indeed, despite what the Swedish and Adventist studies suggest, there's evidence that in some families, at least, genes exert pretty powerful effects on life-span. The centenarians registered in the New England Centenarian Study, for example, showed no consistent patterns in diet, exercise or healthy habits that could explain their extended years. About 20% had smoked at some point in their lives, and some had eating habits that should have made them obese or unhealthy but somehow did not. At least 10% to 15% had a history of heart disease, stroke or diabetes for more than 20 years. Something in that group's genes was protecting them from succumbing to diseases that had felled the average American decades earlier. "These people still get to 100,"

says Perls. "They seem to have a functional reserve or adaptive capacity that allows them to get disease but not necessarily suffer from it. The key seems to be resilience."

Some of that resilience may be linked to human leukocyte antigen (HLA) genes, a group clustered on chromosome 6 that affects vulnerability to such autoimmune diseases as lupus, rheumatoid arthritis and multiple sclerosis. Centenarians living in Okinawa, for example, have variants of HLA that tend to protect against those diseases. Perls has found a region on chromosome 4 that centenarians and their siblings and children in the U.S. seem to have in common and that sets them apart from shorter-lived individuals. The finding has not yet been replicated by other groups, but Perls expects to publish a paper in the next month detailing his results.

NATIONALITY: Japanese live longest: 81 years, Zambians shortest: 33 years; immigrants to the U.S. outlive natives by three years

What exactly that stretch of DNA does remains to be discovered, but it may be a key not just to long life but also to the resilience found among U.S. centenarian-study participants, with their 20% smoking rate and imperfect eating habits. That group may be especially genetically blessed, and researchers are eager to tap its secrets.

We certainly need them. For as medical science adds years to our collective lives, we chip away at them by doing things—stewing at our desk jobs, eating fatty processed foods, blowing a gasket in a freeway traffic jam, exercising no more than our fingers at the computer—that centenarians can't imagine. Most of them were born into an America as remote from today's metaphorically as the craggy villages of Sardinia, Okinawa and Nova Scotia are geographically. In the early 1900s people walked miles to work not by choice but out of necessity; cars were still a luxury. People tilled the fields because their farmer parents needed cheap help. People ate what they grew because it was there. Most labor was manual then, and most nutrients were natural. Preserved food was what Aunt

Maud sealed in a jar. Tobacco and alcohol were available, but most of today's centenarians didn't indulge to excess.

They trigger our awe and our nostalgia as representatives of a flinty, hardscrabble culture that hardly exists today. They lived out a parable of man at one with nature. They used their bodies as they were designed and programmed over the millennia: for walking, for working, for being fed from the earth's natural bounty. It makes one wonder whether the next generation of oldsters will last quite as long. They will need not just the luck of the genetic draw but also the strength to renounce the lure of fast-food days and couch-potato nights that add yards of butt lard and shorten lifespans by years.

Will Americans in the supersize age resolve to go medieval on their own bodies? It would help, if they want to live to 100. As Poon says of his research pools, "I don't have any fat centenarians." And if research really does extend life by a vigorous couple of decades, the new millions of centenarians will need a support system that spreads beyond family and friends to include a hugely expensive Social Security and Medicare apparatus. The coming gerontocracy won't come cheap.

But that's for the future. Any child of today who hopes to live into the 22nd century without the aid of medical miracles should look to the past, and consider the lessons today's centenarians took from the 19th century. There's a poetry of common sense in their scheme for immortality. Eat sensibly. Keep walking. Keep knitting. If you can't keep friends, make new ones. Plan so much invigorating work that there's just no time to die. And no regret when you do. —*Reported by Alice Park, New York; Melissa August, Washington; Anne Berryman, Athens, Georgia; Hanna Kite, Okinawa; Chris Lambie, Halifax; Jeff Israely, Sardinia; and Francis X. Rocca, Rome*

PUTTING A PREMIUM ON
HEALTH

Employers are looking to cut healthcare costs by charging less for
those who maintain a healthy lifestyle—and charge more for those who don't

John Dorschner

As healthcare costs soar, some experts are now asking tough questions: Should fat people pay more for health insurance? What about smokers? Should healthy people who go regularly to the gym pay less?

"We believe people should be given the tools to improve their health," says Howard Gruverman, a Fort Lauderdale consultant with Chapman Schewe who advises companies on their health plans. "To the extent they follow the tools, they shouldn't pay more. But if they don't take advantage of [the tools], then they *should* pay more."

Some major South Florida employers—Baptist Health, Ryder System, the University of Miami— already require smokers to pay more for health coverage. But that may be just the beginning.

"The relationship between employer and employee is going to change in the next five years," says Bruce Shanefield, a Miami healthcare specialist with Aon Consulting.

Some consumer advocates are wary.

"This is an area worthy of exploration, but it has to be done with great care," says Ron Pollack of Families USA. Charging smokers more "makes

eminent sense, but there are other areas that could be questionable."

A few companies nationally, like Weyco in Michigan, have fired smokers and warned they will do random tests for nicotine, but large employers here are taking a more complex approach which, at least to begin with, involves more carrot than stick.

Would smokers pay more?

"The main point is to get people healthy," says Maribeth Rouseff, who handles Baptist Health's wellness program. "We have to get away from the notion of a pill to fix everything."

"Our system is based on illness, not wellness, and frankly we need to change that paradigm," says Andy Scibelli of Florida Power & Light. "There is no other place to go with shifting healthcare costs."

Surveys

What's happening is a multistep process. Many employers start with health-assessment surveys—a basic

measure of an employee's health, including weight, blood pressure, and chronic conditions, such as diabetes.

Many consultants would like to see all employees who want health insurance be forced to complete the surveys, but those employers using the survey locally have made them voluntary. "We believe the carrot is stronger than the stick right now," says Pam Rothstein at Ryder.

Employees at the transportation company are invited to fill out a survey on the Internet about health status and "lifestyle choices" that is then analyzed by an independent third party that will not show the data to Ryder, says Pam Rothstein, who handles health benefits. About 20 percent of employees have done the survey in the several months that the program has been available.

As a reward, the employees who complete the survey get their names entered in a drawing, and 10 end up with six months of free health insurance.

Baptist Health offers free health screenings twice a year that include tests to measure for cholesterol, blood sugar, body fat and osteoporosis. About a third of Baptist employees have participated, says Rouseff, and 20 percent go on to complete the

8

health assessment survey. Their reward: A $10,000 death benefit paid to the survivor.

At Florida Power & Light, about 30 percent fill out the survey. They're rewarded by getting their names entered in raffles for items like digital cameras and iPods.

Employers say that answers on the surveys will have no repercussions in the workplace, and they're assuming employee honesty in filling them out. But how many employees want to be honest about their penchant for Big Macs or Pinot Noir?

"A big question is how far you go before it's an invasion of privacy," says Pollack, the consumer advocate. "And how does it get monitored."

Step two: Giving employees advice based on the surveys. Those overweight may get pamphlets on diet and exercise. Diabetics can be instructed on the importance of having blood sugar levels measured regularly. Smokers can be told about a variety of programs to help them stop.

This advice is naturally linked to employers' growing use of wellness programs. Baptist Health and Ryder, for example, have free on-site gyms.

Florida Power & Light offers gyms at small monthly fees, and it gives extra raffle entries for those who make such health-driven steps.

Wellness Coaches

Baptist also has "wellness coaches" who are sometimes stationed outside employee parking garages during shift changes, to chat with employees and pass out brochures on healthy lifestyles. "The coach hopes to look hundreds of employees in the eyes," says Rouseff.

Baptist Health started the emphasis on this wellness program in 2001, after the 10,500-employee organization went mostly to self-insurance. Rouseff says the program has paid off. Instead of annual increases "in the mid-double digits" for healthcare expense, the five-hospital organization now sees changes of 6.5-8 percent annually—a noteworthy achievement.

FPL reports it has averaged 5 percent annual increases the past two years, but attributes that to a wide range of factors designed to make employees more careful consumers of healthcare. Hewitt Associates says the average increase in Florida runs about 12 percent.

Eventually, consultants believe employers need to use the stick: If your cholesterol is too high, start lowering it with statins or diets. If you're too overweight, sign in at the gym three times a week.

And if you don't take those steps, says Gruverman, then employers should have a right to raise your insurance rates, because the history of healthcare indicates you're likely to be costing your employer more.

Right now, the stick is seen only with smokers, and it's a minimal one. The University of Miami and Ryder charge smokers $10 a month more.

Baptist Health charges $10 per biweekly pay period, though Rouseff says studies show smokers really cost an employer an average of $1,200 to $1,500 a year more in health expenses.

UM was an early starter in the smoking field, beginning its surcharge more than a decade ago. "We had about 1,800 acknowledged smokers in 1992," of its 9,000 employees, says benefits manager Bill Walsh, "and now we're down to 600 or 700."

He says that "every dollar" of the extra money from smokers "is dedicated to assist employees who want to break the habit." That includes paying for stop-smoking classes and nicotine patches.

The issue of overweight persons paying extra is more problematic. Tommy Thompson, secretary of Health and Human Services in the first George W. Bush administration, suggested in 2003 that group health plans should be rewarded if they maintained a healthy weight.

Local employers, however, are concerned that weight issues could be what Walsh calls "a black hole."

He and other benefits managers point to complex issues: Is obesity a disease or a lifestyle choice?

What's the right borderline for obesity? What happens if a person slips from normal to obese during the year, or goes from obese to normal?

Exercise

"I'm all for promoting a healthier lifestyle," says Pollack, the consumer advocate. "Promoting more exercise, free membership in gyms. But when you start penalizing people and possibly invading their privacy, that could be a very questionable practice."

Walsh at UM doubts obesity will ever become an issue in premium payments. "I don't see this coming down the pike."

But many other things may be. Scibelli says FPL is considering contributing dollars to employees tax-free health accounts depending on how many steps employees take toward a health lifestyle.

As Shanefield of Aon Consulting says, "You're just seeing the beginning."

Why the Rich Live Longer

There's a stunning new explanation for upscale longevity, and it's quite contrary to what the world's health bureaucrats have been telling us.

By Dan Seligman

ONE OF THE GREAT MYSTERIES OF MODERN MEDICINE: Why do rich people live longer than poor people? Why is it that, all around the world, those with more income, education and high-status jobs score higher on various measures of health? As stated in a World Health Organization pamphlet: "People further down the social ladder usually run at least twice the risk of serious illness and premature death of those near the top."

The traditional answer to these questions has been that greater wealth and social status mean greater access to medical care. But even ten years ago, when this magazine last delved into the topic (FORBES, *Jan. 31, 1994*), the available answers seemed inadequate. If access was the key, then one would have expected the health gap between upper and lower classes to shrink or disappear with the advent of programs like Britain's National Health Service and America's Medicare and Medicaid, not to mention employer-sponsored health insurance. In fact, the gap widened in both Britain and America as these programs took effect. The 1994 article cited a study of British civil servants—all with equal access to medical care and other social services, and all working in similar physical environments—showing that even within this homogeneous group the higher-status employees were healthier: "Each civil service rank outlived the one immediately below." How could this be?

Today the standard answer—or, at least, the answer you are guaranteed to get from the WHO and other large health bureaucracies—is that inequality itself is the killer. The argument is that low status translates into insecurity, stress and anxiety, all of which increases susceptibility to disease. This psychosocial case is lengthily elaborated in *Social Determinants of Health,* a 1999 publication collectively created by 22 medical specialists and endorsed by the WHO. "Is it plausible," the book asks at one point, "that the organization of work, degree of social isolation and sense of control over life could affect the likelihood of developing and dying from chronic diseases such as diabetes and cardiovascular disease?" The authors' answer is a resounding yes. Pushing their case to the outer limits, the authors supply data indicating that in the world of African wild baboons, those who are socially dominant tend to be most healthy (as mainly evidenced in their higher levels of good cholesterol).

This revised standard answer has some plausibility, but also some serious weaknesses. One of its problems is that we lack serious comparative data on tension and anxiety levels in low- and high-status jobs. It is far from clear that barbers, elevator operators and lower-level civil servants suffer more tension than do surgeons, executive vice presidents and higher-level civil servants. Another problem is that psychosocial explanations don't tell us why the health gap would widen when employers and governments provide more health care. Nor do they explain one well-known source of the health gap: the notoriously high rate of smoking in the low-status population.

An explanation not presenting these problems has recently been proposed in several papers by two scholars long associated with IQ studies: Linda Gottfredson, a sociologist based at the University of Delaware, and psychologist Ian Deary of the University of Edinburgh. Their solution to the age-old mystery of health and status is at once utterly original and supremely obvious. The rich live longer, they write, mainly because the rich are smarter. The argument rests on several different propositions, all well documented. The crucial points are that (a) social status correlates strongly and positively with IQ and other measures of intelligence;(b) intelligence correlates strongly with "health literacy," the ability to understand and follow a prescription for disease prevention and treatment; and intelligence is also correlated with forward planning—which means avoidance of health risks (including smoking) as they are identified.

The first leg of that argument has been established for many decades. In modern developed countries IQ correlates about 0.5 with measures of income and social status—a figure telling us that IQ is not everything but also making plain that it powerfully influences where people end up in life. The mean IQ of Americans in the Census Bureau's "professional and technical" category is 111. The mean for unskilled laborers is 89. An American whose IQ is in the range between 76 and 90 (i.e., well below average) is eight times as likely to be living in poverty as someone whose IQ is over 125.

Second leg: Intelligent people tend to be the most knowledgeable about health-related issues. Health literacy matters more than it used to. In the past big gains in health and longevity were associated with improvements in public sanitation, immu-

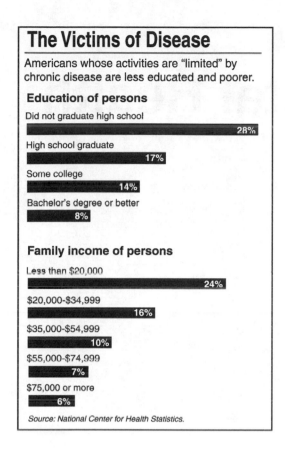

The Victims of Disease

Americans whose activities are "limited" by chronic disease are less educated and poorer.

Education of persons

Did not graduate high school
28%

High school graduate
17%

Some college
14%

Bachelor's degree or better
8%

Family income of persons

Less than $20,000
24%

$20,000-$34,999
16%

$35,000-$54,999
10%

$55,000-$74,999
7%

$75,000 or more
6%

Source: National Center for Health Statistics.

nization and other initiatives not requiring decisions by ordinary citizens. But today the major threats to health are chronic diseases—which, inescapably, require patients to participate in the treatment, which means in turn that they need to understand what's going on. Memorable sentence in the Gottfredson-Deary paper in the February 2004 issue of *Current Directions in Psychological Science:* "For better or worse, people are substantially their own primary health care providers." The authors invite you to conceptualize the role of "patient" as having a job, and argue that, as with real jobs in the workplace, intelligent people will learn what's needed more rapidly, will understand what's important and what isn't and will do best at coping with unforeseen emergencies.

More than half of doctors' prescriptions are taken incorrectly.

It is clear that a lot of patients out there are doing their jobs very badly. Deary was coauthor of a 2003 study in which childhood IQs in Scotland were related to adult health outcomes. A

central finding: Mortality rates were 17% higher for each 15-point falloff in IQ. One reason for the failure of broad-based access to reduce the health gap is that low-IQ patients use their access inefficiently. A Gottfredson paper in the January 2004 issue of the *Journal of Personality & Social Psychology* cites a 1993 study indicating that more than half of the 1.8 billion prescriptions issued annually in the U.S. are taken incorrectly. The same study reported that 10% of all hospitalizations resulted from patients' inability to manage their drug therapy. A 1998 study reported that almost 30% of patients were taking medications in ways that seriously threatened their health. Noncompliance with doctors' orders is demonstrably rampant in low-income clinics, reaching 60% in one cited study. Noncompliance is often taken to signify a lack of patient motivation, but it often clearly reflects a simple failure to understand directions.

A new Test of Functional Health Literacy of Adults can evaluate the problem in a mere 22 minutes. It measures comprehension of the labels on prescription vials, of appointment slips, of what the patient is expected to do before diagnostic tests, etc. The results turn out to be somewhat horrifying. In a sample of 2,659 clinic patients in two urban hospitals, 42% did not understand the instructions for taking medicine on an empty stomach, and 26% did not understand when the next appointment was scheduled. The problem is maximized for patients with chronic illnesses. Asthma, diabetes and hypertension all require patients to make a lot of decisions daily as well as in emergencies, but many patients are simply not up to it. A study cited in the Gottfredson-Deary paper mentions that a high proportion of insulin-dependent diabetics did not know how to tell when their blood sugar was too high or too low or how to get it back to normal.

And then there is the third leg of the IQ argument: the lifestyle question. Smoking, obesity and sedentary living are more prevalent among low-status citizens. A 2001 study by the Centers for Disease Control & Prevention found that college graduates are three times as likely to live healthily as those who never got beyond high school. Not clear is what the government can do about this.

The data on IQ, social status and health present some huge conundrums for policymakers. For years Americans debated what to do for, and about, poor people unable to pay for health care. Ultimately they decided it simply had to be paid for. But now, with money ordinarily not a barrier to medical care, we are discovering another obstacle: "regimen complexity." As this fact of life sinks in, the system will be under pressure to find ways to deliver high-quality care to the low-status population much more simply, understandably—and economically. Not an easy task.

UNIT 2
Stress and Mental Health

Unit Selections

Key Points to Consider

- How have humankind's stressors changed over the last 5,000 years?

- What are the major stressors in your life? How do you manage your stress?

- How can living in a poor, urban environment contribute to stress and illness?

- Give examples that demonstrate the interaction between mental health and physical health.

- Explain how worry can be both a positive and a negative force in shaping one's life.

- Why should suicide be considered a preventable illness?

Student Website

www.mhcls.com/online

Internet References

Further information regarding these websites may be found in this book's preface or online.

The American Institute of Stress
http://www.stress.org

National Mental Health Association (NMHA)
http://www.nmha.org/index.html

Self-Help Magazine
http://www.selfhelpmagazine.com/index.html

The brain is the one organ that still mystifies and baffles the scientific community. While more has been learned about this organ in the last decade than in all the rest of recorded history, our understanding of the brain is still in its infancy. What has been learned, however, has spawned exciting new research and has contributed to the establishment of new disciplines such as psychophysiology and psychoneuroimmunology (PNI).

Traditionally, the medical community has viewed health problems as either physical or mental, treating each type separately. This dichotomy between the psyche (mind) and soma (body) is fading in light of scientific data that reveal profound physiological changes associated with mood shifts. Just what are the physiological changes associated with stress? Hans Selye, the father of stress research, described stress as a nonspecific physiological response to anything that challenges the body. He demonstrated that this response could be elicited by both mental and physical stimuli. Stress researchers have come to regard this response pattern as the "flight or fight" response, perhaps an adaptive throwback to our primitive ancestors. Researchers now believe that repeated and prolonged activation of this response can trigger destructive changes in our bodies and contribute to the development of several chronic diseases. So profound is the impact of emotional stress on the body that current estimates suggest that approximately 90 percent of all doctor visits are for stress-related disorders. If emotional stress elicits a generalized physiological response, why are there so many different diseases associated with it? Many experts believe that the answer may best be explained by what has been termed "the weak-organ theory." According to this theory, every individual has one organ system that is most susceptible to the damaging effects of prolonged stress.

Mental illness, which is generally regarded as a major dysfunction of normal thought processes, has no single identifiable etiology. One may speculate that this is due to the complex nature of the organ system involved. There is also mounting evidence to suggest an organic component to traditional forms of mental illness such as schizophrenia, chronic depression, and manic depression. The fact that certain mental illnesses tend to occur within families has divided the mental health community into two camps: those who believe there is a genetic factor operating and those who see the family tendency as more of a learned behavior. In either case, the evidence supports mental illness as another example of the weak-organ theory. The reason one person is more susceptible to the damaging effects of stress than another may not be altogether clear, but evidence is mounting that one's perception or attitude plays a key role in the stress equation. A prime example demonstrating this relationship comes from research linking cardiovascular disease to stress. "Happier and Healthier" also discusses a mind/body connection and suggests that having a healthy perspective on life can positively impact one's health. The realization that our attitude has such a significant impact on our health has led to a burgeoning new movement in psychology termed "positive psychology." Dr. Martin Segilman, professor of psychology at the University of Pennsylvania and father of the positive psychology movement, believes that optimism is a key factor in maintaining—not only our mental health—but our physi-

cal health as well. Dr. Segilman notes that while some people are naturally more optimistic than others, optimism can be learned.

One area in particular that appears to be influenced by the "positive psychology movement" is the area of stress management. Traditionally stress management programs have focused on the elimination of stress, but that is starting to change as new strategies approach stress as an essential component of life and a potential source of health. It is worth noting that this concept, of stress serving as a positive force in a person's life, was presented by Dr. Hans Selye in 1974 in his book *Stress Without Distress.* Dr. Selye felt that there were three types of stress: negative stress (distress), normal stress, and positive stress (eustress). He maintained that positive stress not only increases a person's self-esteem but also serves to inoculate the person against the damaging effects of distress. Only time will tell if this change of focus in the area of stress management makes any real difference in patient outcome.

While many Americans are benefiting from medical breakthroughs during the last few years, in poor, urban neighborhoods, the stress of living in poverty may be contributing to a variety of illnesses. Many diseases associated with aging are affecting the young in these areas. Stress may be responsible for the higher rates of heart disease, stroke, cancer, asthma, and diabetes. In "Enough to Make You Sick," author Helen Epstein addresses the issues related to living in a poor, urban environment and the increase risk of disease.

Although significant gains have been made in our understanding of the relationship between body and mind, much remains to be learned. What is known points to perception and one's attitude as the key elements in shaping our responses to stressors.

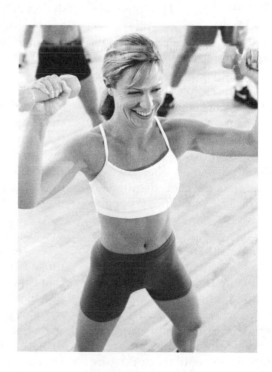

Happier and healthier?

**Your physical well-being may reflect your mental outlook.
And some experts believe you can learn to be happier.**

Happier people are often healthier people, and not just because their good health improves their mood. A growing body of observational research suggests that people who are more optimistic, less hostile, and more satisfied in youth are less likely to develop chronic diseases decades later. Similar studies also suggest that in later stages of adulthood, mental states can influence health events ranging from the minor to the life threatening.

None of this research would be particularly useful if mental outlook were a fixed quality that individuals could not improve or modify. Enter the "positive psychology" movement, which contends that people can learn optimism and happiness at any age. Until fairly recently, psychological study tended to focus solely on mental disorders, such as depression and anxiety, at the expense of inquiry into whether people without disorders could improve the positive mental states, such as happiness, strength, and hope, that make life worth living. Recent work in positive psychology has investigated the factors that distinguish happy from less happy people. Those insights can be helpful for people who want to boost their joy factor, though there isn't much evidence yet about which methods work best long term.

Grounded in scientific research, positive psychology should be distinguished from the kind of mind-over-matter thinking that promised that mental affirmations could cure cancer or warned that people "can't afford the luxury of a negative thought." People with a positive mental outlook are not in a good mood all of the time. But they do have the skills to talk themselves out of a bad mood rather than prolonging it, to take a selfaffirming view of both negative and positive events, and to become absorbed in challenging activities. Clinical experience suggests there are practical methods you can use to brighten your mental outlook.

OPTIMISM PAYS OFF

Dozens of studies have correlated a positive mental outlook with various health outcomes. For example, there's evidence that people who are happier or more optimistic:

• **Have stronger immunity.** Researchers in 2003 assessed the emotional styles of 334 healthy volunteers, then administered a squirt of rhinovirus (a germ that causes colds) in the nose of each participant. Those who scored high on measures of energy, happiness, and relaxation were significantly less likely to develop colds, regardless of their health practices.

• **Are less likely to die of chronic disease.** A decade-long study of some 400 men with HIV found that those who scored highest on a scale that measured positive feelings were less likely to die at any point during the study—regardless of the extent of their illness or use of antiretroviral drugs. A few studies have yielded similar findings for cancer patients.

• **Live longer.** In a landmark study released in 2000, scientists at the Mayo Clinic analyzed the records of 839 patients who had been given psychological tests 30 years earlier. Those who scored highest on a scale of pessimism were roughly 20 percent more likely to die prematurely than were optimists. In a 2001 study, older adults who were hopeful about the future had a significantly lower death rate (11 percent) over the seven-year study period than those who said they weren't hopeful (29 percent), even after researchers adjusted for age, smoking, and health status.

STRESSED AND SICKER

On the flip side, people who are depressed, stressed, angry, or distressed tend to fare poorer. In addition to having an increased risk of heart disease (see next section), they:

• **Get sick—or feel sick—more often.** Data from one long-running, 30-year study show that, compared with optimistic people, pessimists have a higher risk of physical and mental problems.

• **Have more dental problems.** A 2003 Harvard University analysis of more than 42,000 men in the Health Professionals Follow-Up Study found that those who scored highest on an anger questionnaire were 72 percent more likely to develop periodontitis (gum disease) than those who scored lowest.

• **Heal slower from surgery.** A small New Zealand study in the journal Psychosomatic Medicine found that pa-

Pessimistic vs. optimistic interpretations of life events

How you interpret positive and negative life events is the crux of your mental outlook. If you make a mistake, do you call yourself "stupid" or say you're off your game? If you succeed at a project, is it an accident or a reflection of your inner talent? Becoming aware of your "self-talk" tendencies can help ou train yourself to think more optimistically. "People who master this technique are two to eight times less likely to become depressed when they encounter setbacks," says Martin Seligman, Ph.D., professor of psychology at the University of Pennsylvania. The examples below are adapted from Seligman's book "Authentic Happiness."

IS IT TEMPORARY OR PERMANENT? Optimists see negative events as temporary, and positive ones as permanent.

	Pessimistic	Optimistic
Despite trying to stick to a diet, you gain weight over the holidays, and you can't lost it.	Diets don't work	The diet I tried didn't work.
You win a tennis match.	My opponent got tired.	I'm a good player.

IS IT SPECIFIC OR PERVASIVE? Optimists see negative events as specific, and positive ones as pervasive.

	Pessimistic	Optimistic
You miss an important engagement.	Sometimes my memory fails me.	I sometimes forget to check my appointment book.
You run for a community office position and win.	I devoted a lot of time and energy to campaigning.	I work hard at everything I do.

IS IT HOPELESS OR HOPEFUL? Hopeful people view negative events as temporary and specific, positive events as permanent and pervasive.

	Hopeless	Hopeful
You and your spouse get into an argument.	He/she is a tryant.	He/she was in a bad mood.
You get a promotion at work.	I'm lucky.	I'm talented.

tients who were worried before undergoing hernia surgery reported slower, more painful recoveries than those who were less worried. The stressed patients also scored significantly lower on an objective marker of recovery: the levels of the repair protein interleukin-1 in their wound fluid.

• **Are more likely to get Alzheimer's disease.** In a December 2003 study in the journal Neurology, involving nearly 800 older people, those most prone to psychological distress—including anxiety, anger, depression, and feelings of helplessness—were twice as likely to develop Alzheimer's as those who were least prone to such feelings.

HOW FEELINGS AFFECT PHYSIOLOGY

The mechanism through which troubled psychological states can influence health is clearest within the cardiovascular system. Substantial research has tied hostility, anger, impatience, and stress to increased heart risk; somewhat lesser evidence suggests that depression and social isolation may also harm the heart.

High levels of emotional stress, particularly anger, cause a surge in certain hormones, such as adrenaline and cortisol, that prepare your body to face an emergency. That surge causes physiological changes that can, in turn, trigger a heart attack or stroke, especially in people whose arteries are already clogged. Mental duress may also contribute to the development of disease by encouraging unhealthy lifestyle choices that increase heart risk—such as drinking, smoking, overeating, and not exercising.

Negative emotions may begin to affect risk factors as early as one's teens. In a study of more than 3,300 people published in The Journal of the American Medical Association, hostile and impatient young adults were nearly twice as likely as their mellower peers to develop hypertension over a 15-year period.

WHAT CAN YOU FIX?

Thus far there has been little research into whether individuals can change their mental outlook and, if so, whether this improves their health. In the book "Authentic Happiness," University of Pennsylvania psychology professor Martin Seligman, Ph.D., argues that our overall level of happiness depends on three factors: inborn tendencies, circumstances, and factors under our control.

Research suggests that we're born with a hardwired emotional profile, or "happiness thermostat." This is a base state of happiness, a "fixed and largely inherited level to which we invariably revert," writes Seligman. The base state may persist despite strokes of fortune or misfortune. For example, one study shows that over time, winners of large lottery prizes are no happier than nonwinners. And people paralyzed after spinal-cord injuries wind up only slightly less happy, on average, than individuals who aren't so affected, according to Seligman. One's personal happiness range also appears largely independent of material wealth or other "comfortable life" factors. As long as a person's basic economic needs are met, money has surprisingly little effect on happiness.

Life events can trigger or protect against certain inborn tendencies, such as a tendency toward depression or anxiety. And some circumstances—such as extreme poverty, the death of a child, or caring for a relative with Alzheimer's disease—do have a long-range depressing effect on happiness levels.

While it may not be possible to modify your genetic inheritance or control your external circumstances, it may be possible to modify your mental outlook and response to life events. For example, clinical trials have tested the ability of meditation and other behavioral interventions to reduce hostility in heart patients; they've found that these techniques not only reduce measures of hostility but also may lower blood pressure and possibly reduce the risk of heart attack recurrence.

Here are some of the ways psychologists believe that you can increase your happiness quotient, and perhaps simultaneously improve your health.

CULTIVATING POSITIVE EMOTION

Both your thinking and your activities affect your mental state. Thought patterns may be more amenable to change and control than many of us realize. Just as you can interrupt an over talkative friend, you may be able to interrupt your own negative thoughts and interpretations of the world and substitute more positive ones, using what psychologists call "self-talk." Gaining a measure of control may take persistence and perhaps professional

counseling, but the mood improvement may be substantial.

• **Rewrite your past.** Research has shown that our memories seem to be mood related. In other words, when you're in a bad mood, it's easy to remember all your other problems and grievances against the world, while when you're in a good mood, it's easy to recall other good times. So a conscious effort to dwell on good recent and long-term memories may have a powerful effect on your daily mood. Such simple measures as cultivating a sense of gratitude by "counting your blessings" each day may help amplify positive memories. So may efforts to celebrate small victories and achievements—even something as simple as patting yourself on the back. And forgiving and forgetting unpleasant experiences may help mute those memories.

• **Project a brighter future.** What do you say to yourself when you misplace your keys? If what springs to mind is "I'm an idiot," then you're interpreting the bad event as something permanent and universal, a pessimistic view likely to decrease your happiness. The remedy is to argue yourself into a more optimistic explanation: "I'm not stupid. There are many things I do well. I'm just tired and stressed today."

When it comes to responding to positive events, however, the opposite approach is best. If, for example, you've gotten a compliment or a promotion at work, it's OK to generalize. Instead of thinking "I'm just lucky" or "That last report must have impressed the boss," tell yourself, "This is a reward for all my talent, leadership ability, and hard work."

• **Improve the present.** Making room in your day for more genuinely rewarding activities is another important tactic. A lasting source of happiness comes from entering a state of "flow," in which you're so absorbed in an activity that you lose your self-consciousness and even awareness of time. That occurs most readily when you're actively engaged, either mentally or physically,

in activities that use favorite skills and are challenging enough to ward off boredom, but not so difficult that you become anxious.

Research amassed over the past two decades by Mihaly Csikszentmihalyi, Ph.D.—who coined the "flow" concept and currently serves as a professor of psychology at Claremont Graduate University—and his colleagues shows that activities that foster lasting happiness tend to involve creativity, exploration, imagination, strategy, and discovery.

Too often people "get trapped in life doing things that we think we have to do even if we don't like them," says Csikszentmihalyi. "We give up the things we enjoy and end up with a very thin life." To change that, you need to seek out fulfilling activities. Consider one you really enjoyed doing years ago, perhaps painting, reading, gardening, or traveling, but gave up as the pressures of adult life took over. Also think about something you've never had a chance to do, such as learning another language, going on an archaeological dig, or starting an antique-car rehabilitation service in your garage, suggests Csikszentmihalyi. Sample a range of activities you never considered before, consulting the local paper or a nearby community center for ideas. Sign up for a day trip to a nearby ghost town or state park; join a hiking club; tour your city's architectural landmarks.

Or volunteer to teach others something you already know: That, Csik-szentmihalyi says, may bring the best fulfillment there is.

MANAGING NEGATIVE EXPERIENCES

Along with increasing positive thinking and activities, it's important to have tactics for dealing with the stresses of modern life. The way you manage your response to stressful events can either strain or help protect your health.

Anger and hostility are among the most dangerous responses to stress because they strain the cardiovascular system and can prompt reckless and destructive behavior. Taming those emotions involves reasoning with yourself and determining whether your rage is called for and, if so, how to deal with it constructively. Redford Williams, M.D., director of the Behavioral Medicine Research Center at Duke University, recommends asking yourself the following questions when someone does something that makes you angry:

1. Is this important?
2. Is anger appropriate in this situation?
3. Is there anything I can do to modify the situation?
4. Would it be worthwhile to have a confrontation?

If you answered yes to all four questions, you need to practice assertion: Find a constructive way to ask the offending person to change his or her behavior, whether it's a friend who just insulted you, a store clerk who says you can't return an item, or a spouse who tells you to run an errand when you're exhausted. Stay calm and rational as you make a specific request for the outcome you desire.

However, if you answered no to any of the four questions, it may pay to avoid a confrontation and use techniques to quiet your emotions. Talking to yourself ("Hey, this isn't that important!"), exercising, breathing deeply, consciously relaxing your muscles, and seeking support by talking to a friend are some options.

Acting out your feelings for the sake of catharsis is not recommended. "Punching a bag, yelling and screaming, hitting something—these types of things do nothing but make you more likely to behave aggressively afterward," Williams says. In one study, subjects who were verbally insulted and then opted to vent their anger on a punching bag acted more aggressively later than those who declined to punch.

While a variety of techniques have the proven potential to help people cope with stress, more studies are needed to determine which techniques work best, for whom, and for how long. To put together your own portfolio of coping strategies, consider drawing from the following areas:

• **Meditation, relaxation training, yoga, tai-chi.** These all involve "mindfulness," the art of concentrating on the present moment and tuning out external factors.

• **Cognitive training.** A therapist or an adult education course may be able to help you learn to thwart a stress reaction (pounding heart, quick breathing, increased blood pressure) by reasoning with yourself and changing your thought processes. One commonly recommended cognitive tool is "thought stopping," in which you interrupt your worry or anger by literally telling yourself to stop, either aloud or under your breath.

• **Social support.** Club membership, religious or civic activities, volunteer work, or just a few close friends can help protect you from the effects of stress on the body. Animal support counts too: Researchers at the State University of New York at Buffalo found that overall, people with a pet had lower stress levels than those who did not own a pet.

• **Exercise.** People who get regular aerobic exercise have lower levels of stress hormones and smaller increases in heart rate and blood pressure under mental duress. Exercise works as a long-term antidote as well as a quick stress fix.

• **Treatment options.** Chronic anger, hostility, and unhappiness may reflect a serious underlying problem, such as depression or an anxiety disorder. In those cases, individual or group therapy and/or drug therapy may be indicated.

Summing up

There is much observational evidence linking mental outlook to health outcomes. At this point, however, most strategies for improving mental outlook are based only on clinical experience. It's not yet clear whether it's possible for most people to improve their happiness levels, and, more important, if doing so can have a positive impact on their health.

There is, however, fairly good evidence that frequent hostility and anger can stress the cardiovascular system. Learning to cope better with stress has been shown to help lower blood pressure and decrease the risk of heart disease.

People interested in measures to boost their mental outlook should consider the following:

• **Cultivate positive feelings** by focusing on good memories rather than bad, seeking activities that provide engaging experiences, and learning to use an optimistic explanatory style.

• **Create personal strategies** for coping with stress, such as mindfulness practices (e.g. meditation), cognitive techniques, social support, and exercise.

• **Seek professional help** if your negative emotions and outlook seriously interfere with functioning or life satisfaction.

Enough to Make You Sick?

In America's rundown urban neighborhoods, the diseases associated with old age are afflicting the young. Could it be that simply living there is…

By HELEN EPSTEIN

Beverly Blagmon lives in the School Street housing projects in southwest Yonkers, a once-vibrant manufacturing area just north of New York City long mired in unemployment and poverty. Beverly has asthma, diabetes, high blood pressure, rheumatoid arthritis, gout and an enlarged heart, and her blood has a dangerous tendency to clot spontaneously. She is 48, and she had her first heart attack in her late 20's. One of her brothers died of heart failure at 50, and another died of kidney failure at 45, as did a sister who was 35. A young cousin recently died of cancer. In the past three years, at least 11 young people she knows have died, most of them not from gunshot wounds or drug overdoses, but from disease.

Monica, who asked that her last name not be used, moved to the Crown Heights section of Brooklyn from School Street a year ago. She has diabetes, arthritis and asthma. She is overweight, and the pain from a back injury that occurred four years ago makes it hard for her to walk or even bend over a stove. Her elaborately braided hair is tinged with gray. In the past year, six of her friends have died, all of them younger than she is. When asked simple questions about her life—when she was born, where she grew up, when her three children were born—Monica answers in short phrases, wiping tears from her eyes. She is 36.

One researcher calls the grinding everyday stress of living in poverty in America 'weathering,' a condition not unlike the effect of exposure to wind and rain on houses.

Ebony Fasion, 22, and her friend Dominique Faulk, 17, both former residents of School Street, have asthma. Dominique's cousin Jo-Scama Wontong, 19, still lives in the School Street projects. Jo-Scama has lost so many people she loved to disease and accident recently that whenever she thinks about it, she is stricken with panic. "My heart beats so fast, and I can't breathe, and there's just death going through my mind the whole time."

Something is killing America's urban poor, but this is no ordinary epidemic. When diseases like AIDS, measles and polio strike, everyone's symptoms look more or less the same, but not in this case. It is as if the aging process in people like Beverly and Monica were accelerated. Even teenagers are afflicted with numerous health problems, including asthma, diabetes and high blood pressure. Poor urban blacks have the worst health of any ethnic group in America, with the possible exception of Native Americans. Some poor urban Hispanics suffer disproportionately from many health problems, too, although the groups that arrived most recently, like Dominicans, seem to be healthier, on average, than Puerto Ricans who have lived in the United States for many years. It makes you wonder whether there is something deadly in the American experience of urban poverty itself.

The neighborhoods where Beverly, Monica, Ebony, Dominique and Jo-Scama live look like poor urban areas all across the country, with bricked-up abandoned buildings, vacant storefronts, broken sidewalks and empty lots with mangy grass overgrowing the ruins of old cars, machine parts and heaps of garbage. Young men in black nylon skullcaps lurk around the pay-phones on street corners. These neighborhoods are as segregated from the more affluent, white sections of metropolitan New York as any township in South Africa under apartheid. Living in such neighborhoods as southwest Yonkers, central and East Harlem, central Brooklyn and the South Bronx is assumed to predispose the poor to a number of social ills, including drug abuse, truancy and the persistent joblessness that draws young people into a long cycle of crime and incarceration. Now it turns out these neighborhoods could be destroying people's health as well.

There are many different types of disadvantaged neighborhoods in America, but poor urban minority neighborhoods seem to be especially unhealthy. Some of these neighborhoods have the highest mortality rates in the country, but this is not, as many believe, mainly because of drug overdoses and gunshot wounds. It is because of chronic diseases—mainly diseases of adulthood that are probably not caused by viruses, bacteria or other infections and that include stroke, diabetes, kidney disease, high blood pressure and certain types of cancer.

The problems start at birth. The black infant death rate in Westchester County is almost three times as high as the rate for the county as a whole. Black youths in Harlem, central Detroit, the South Side of Chicago and Watts have about the same probability of dying by age 45 as whites nationwide do by age 65, and most of this premature death is due not to violence, but to illness. A third of poor black 16-year-old girls in urban areas will not reach their 65th birthdays. Four times as many people die of diabetes in the largely black area of central Brooklyn as on the predominantly white Upper East Side of Manhattan, and one in three adults in Harlem report having high blood pressure. In 1990, two New York doctors found that so many poor African-Americans in Harlem were dying young from heart disease, cancer and cirrhosis of the liver that men there were less likely to reach age 65 than men in Bangladesh.

Since the time of slavery, physicians have noted that the health of impoverished blacks is, in general, worse than that of whites. Racist doctors proposed that the reasons were genetic, and that blacks were intrinsically inferior and physically weaker than whites. But there is very little evidence that poor blacks or Hispanics are genetically predisposed to the vast majority of the afflictions from which they disproportionately suffer. As the living conditions of blacks have improved over the past century, their health improved in step; when conditions deteriorated, health deteriorated, too. This has helped support the contention among researchers that much chronic disease among minority groups is caused not by genes, but by something else.

That something else may come down to geography. Ana Diez-Roux, an epidemiologist at the University of Michigan, has shown that people who live in disadvantaged neighborhoods are more likely to have heart attacks than people who live in middle-class neighborhoods, even taking income differences into account. Researchers from the Rand Corporation found that neighborhoods where many buildings are boarded up and abandoned have higher rates of early death from cancer and diabetes than neighborhoods with similar poverty rates and similar proportions of uninsured people, but intact housing. Abandoned buildings do not in themselves cause disease, of course, but they are an indicator of neighborhood deprivation and neglect—and this does seem to be associated with poor health, though we don't know why.

In some ways, our public health institutions are in the same position they were in 150 years ago. In the mid-19th century, public health boards were established to fight the great killers of the day—cholera and tuberculosis. The poor were more susceptible to these diseases then, just as they are more susceptible to chronic diseases now. And then, as now, the reasons were unknown. Some believed diseases were acts of God and the poor got what they deserved. If they would only drink less, go to church and stay out of brothels, they wouldn't get sick. Others maintained that the afflictions of poverty were environmental. A stinking mass of invisible vapor, referred to as "miasma," hung in the air over the slums, they claimed, and sickened those who inhaled it.

It was not until the early 1880's, when the German scientist Robert Koch looked down his microscope at swirling cholera and tuberculosis bacteria, that everyone finally agreed about what was going on. The water the poor drank was full of sewage and contained deadly cholera germs; in overcrowded tenements, the poor breathed clouds of tuberculosis bacteria. Malnourished alcoholics tended to be more susceptible to these diseases, but immoral behavior was not their primary cause. Nor was miasma. The primary cause was germs.

We don't have a germ theory for chronic diseases like stroke, heart disease, diabetes and cancer. We know something about what can aggravate these diseases—diet, smoking and so on—but not enough about why they are so much more common among people who live in certain neighborhoods, or what makes, for example, a poor person who smokes the same number of cigarettes a day as a rich person more likely to get lung cancer. Or why several research studies show that smoking, eating, drinking and exercise habits do not fully account for why rich people are healthier than poor people. Even lack of health care cannot entirely explain the afflictions of the poor. Many poor people lack health insurance, and those who have it are often at the mercy of overworked doctors and nurses who provide indifferent care, but inadequate health care cannot explain why so many of them get so sick in the first place.

'You wake up stressed, you go to sleep stressed, you see all the garbage and the dealers ... you say, "What's the use of doing anything?" '

Most poor minority neighborhoods "are less healthy," says Adam M. Karpati, who works in the Brooklyn office of the New York City Department of Health and Mental Hygiene. "You walk down the street and you know it. But what is that thing that you know is going on? What's at play there? That thing you can't name? We don't know that."

Clearly we need to examine this miasma with a different kind of microscope. The best we have at the moment are theories that fall into two main schools of thought. One school holds that the problem has mainly to do with stress; the other holds actual deprivation responsible. These two factors are often intertwined, but the emphasis is important. "There are so many fists in the face of poor African-Americans," says Arline Geronimus, a professor of public health at the University of Michigan who leans toward the stress school, and she proceeded to list them for me. They have enormous family obligations, she explained, and while the middle class are able to purchase child care and care for elderly relatives, the poor cannot. The experience of racism and discrimination in everyday life is also still very real, and very stressful. She says that blacks are faced with a society that institutionalizes the idea "that you are a menace—and that demeans you," she says. Nancy Krieger, a Harvard researcher, found that working-class African-Americans who said they accepted unfair treatment as a fact of life had higher blood pressure than those who challenged it.

Geronimus calls the grinding everyday stress of being poor and marginalized in America "weathering," a condition not unlike the effect of exposure to wind and rain on houses. Listening to Geronimus describe "weathering," I found it hard not to wonder whether anyone really knows what it is. Stress is subjective, a feeling, and it means different things to different people. Philip Alcabes, associate professor of urban public health at Hunter College, says that stress is like the miasma that was once thought to cause cholera in 19th-century slums. "You can't see it, you can't really measure it, but it floats over certain people, especially the poor, and makes them sick."

The people I met who left the troubled neighborhoods of southwest Yonkers felt better, and moving appeared to have made all the difference.

If "weathering" and stress have their modern day Robert Koch, he is probably Bruce McEwen, a neuroendocrinologist at Rockefeller University in New York. McEwen argues that stress hormones threaten the health of poor people, especially blacks and the Hispanic poor. Stress hormones are produced by the adrenal glands in response to signals from the brain. When people feel frustrated, frightened or angry, stress hormones travel through the bloodstream and instruct different parts of the body to prepare for an emergency. They speed up the heart rate and narrow the arteries so that blood gets to the tissues faster; blood sugar rises, so that energy rushes to the muscles and other organs; and some bodily functions, like digestion and the mechanisms that maintain the strength of the bones and other tissues, are inhibited. But not all stress is the same. Occasional periods of intense stress, like what you feel during a near miss in a car, do no harm. However, McEwen's research suggests that constant exposure to stress hormones impairs the immune system and damages the brain and other organs.

Chronic stress also signals the body to accumulate abdominal fat around the waistline, which is more dangerous than fat that lies under the skin, or subcutaneous fat. Abdominal fat worsens many chronic health problems, including diabetes and heart disease, whereas subcutaneous fat does not. It's as if stress hormones were like lye, powerful stuff that in small amounts is useful for cleaning the stove, but that in large amounts will eat right through the floor.

Not everyone believes that stress is a major contributor to the health crisis among the poor. George Davey Smith, a professor of clinical epidemiology at the University of Bristol in England, agrees that the poor live very stressful lives, and that racism is an everyday reality for many people. However, in his view—the second school of thought on the matter—the health crisis among the poor has more to do with living in a deprived environment.

The experience of poverty in America has changed a great deal since the 19th century; the poor now have safe drinking water and live in less crowded dwellings, and many have cars and TV's. However, it's also true that many poor people eat unhealthful food, smoke and abuse drugs. Americans hear a great deal about the importance of making healthy choices in their lives; warnings about cigarettes and high-fat foods issue frequently from the surgeon general's office and fill the pages of magazines and best-selling advice books. There are plenty of people who feel little sympathy for overweight diabetic people, poor or not, who eat regularly at McDonald's. But while there is considerable controversy about the ideal lifestyle regimen, you don't need to know much about impoverished neighborhoods to see the absurdity of choosing to go Atkins or macrobiotic for a person like Beverly Blagmon, who subsists on disability payments. Poor people are more likely to have unhealthy habits because fast food and cigarettes are abundant and cheap in their neighborhoods, and healthy alternatives tend to be limited.

A recent survey conducted in four regions of the United States found that there were three times as many bars in poor neighborhoods as in rich ones, and four times as many supermarkets in white neighborhoods as in black ones. There are fewer parks in poor neighborhoods as well, so it is more difficult to find open spaces in which to exercise, and many of them are dangerous. Forty-one percent of New York's public elementary schools have no consistent physical education program. As Mary T. Bassett, a New York City deputy health commissioner, said to me, public health campaigns that tell people to "just say no" to smoking, or to change their diets and start exercising, can be cruel if they are indifferent to neighborhood circumstances.

Davey Smith also points out that many of the poor black people who are sick today grew up in the 40's, 50's and 60's, when many black people lived in overcrowded dwellings, and were more prone than affluent whites to childhood infections. Some of these infections may have long-term effects on health. Helicobacter pylori, a bacterium that has been associated with both ulcers and stomach cancer in adulthood, is most often acquired in childhood, and this may explain why poor blacks in particular have relatively high rates of both diseases. Adults who were poor as children, even if they are not poor now, are also more prone to stroke, kidney disease and hypertensive heart disease.

I wondered about these alternatives. Presumably both stress and material disadvantage are important causes of ill health among the poor. But which is more important? And what would be the best way to address these problems? If stress is a major cause of ill health, interventions to alleviate it—counseling, antidepressants, even yoga—might be beneficial. A recent article in The British Medical Journal suggested that building self-esteem actually helped a group of Native Americans manage their obesity and diabetes better than did conventional counseling about diet and exercise. On the other hand, if material disadvantage is a major cause of ill health among the poor, then extensive changes in the environment in which the poor live—for example, cleaner buildings and more parks—are needed.

PERHAPS BEVERLY BLAGMON, who lives in the midst of such problems, could help resolve this matter. I asked her what she thought the health crisis in southwest Yonkers was caused by, and she answered without missing a beat. "Racism." We went on to talk about the lack of jobs in the area and the dilapidated state of the housing. I also learned that if stress is a killer, there is plenty of it on School Street, but yoga classes and motivational seminars are not likely to be of much help.

Beverly raised 10 children, eight orphaned nieces and nephews in addition to her own son and daughter. The kids were desperate for attention from the overextended Beverly. "It was hard," she said. "You had to deal with 10 different personalities." All the kids are grown now, and all but two have left home. Now she worries because some of them can't find jobs. When she was young, Yonkers was full of factories that hired many young people. But not anymore.

Then last year, disaster struck. Beverly's 21-year-old daughter was killed in a car accident; shortly thereafter, her nephew was shot and killed right outside her building. "I was totally out of it," she said. "People don't know how much a death can take from you. I went into the hospital right after my daughter's funeral. They didn't know if I'd had a mild stroke or not."

"Life is taken stupidly" all the time around School Street, Beverly said, but this doesn't make it easier to handle. Beverly struggles with these losses, and said her family, friends and even officials from the local Housing Authority have been supportive. But when Beverly talked about life on School Street, what she said is underscored with tension—the constant strain of "us versus them." She sees the police in particular as a constant source of grief. "Some of them are very prejudiced, even now," she told me. She claimed that a few officers harassed children and teenagers, and have even been known to swear at kids and shove them. She recalled, as if it were yesterday, a 1997 fight at School Street. Someone called Beverly to come outside, which she did, along with a visiting friend. Police officers were on the street, some of them shouting, and in the chaos that ensued, she said, a policeman knocked down Beverly's friend, a older woman who is legally blind. "I was freaked out," Beverly said. "The main witnesses were drug dealers, and they couldn't say anything." (The Yonkers police confirmed that the woman later filed a complaint, but said an internal investigation found no wrongdoing.) Beverly said she was infuriated when, shortly after the incident, she saw the mayor of Yonkers praise the police in a televised speech.

People who are not poor often casually ascribe their aches, pains and even more serious afflictions to "stress," but stress, if it is a killer, is a far more serious problem for people like Beverly. When middle-class people feel the police or other authorities treat them unfairly, they often have the resources to hire a lawyer and even effect change. But all too often poor blacks feel ignored when they complain about discrimination and abuse.

How might painful experiences like Beverly's be imprinted on the body? Laboratory animals suffer when stressed with electric shocks or when kept in isolated cages away from their peers, and they sometimes do develop symptoms that resemble human chronic diseases. But how does mouse stress compare to Beverly's stress? Or mine? Or yours? George Davey Smith would argue that it is entirely possible that the afflictions of poor people like Beverly are not due to stress, at all, but to old-fashioned deprivation: crowding, poor nutrition, lack of exercise and exposure to dirty air, germs and vermin. For a while, Beverly's family of 11 crowded into a two-bedroom apartment, until they were eventually moved into a six-room place. Once, money was so short that she begged the welfare office for food stamps. There is nowhere around School Street for kids to run around, Beverly says, except a concrete playground with a set of monkey bars. "Why can't they put up some swings or build a basketball court? You see kids using garbage cans as basketball nets around here." Until two years ago, an incinerator in the building spewed forth horrible fumes that may have contributed to the high rates of asthma on School Street. "When you got ready to polish the furniture, it was black with dust," Beverly recalled. "Every day. Now, how much of that was getting in our lungs? I've been in the hospital every year with acute asthma." The incinerator has been replaced by a compactor, but as a result, life is a constant battle against roaches and mice, whose droppings also worsen asthma. Beverly told me that she recently caught three mice in one day. "I put them on the maintenance people's desk," she said. The elevators are always breaking down, which is hard on the elderly. Once she saw human feces in the hallway.

AFTER TALKING to Beverly, I could only conclude that her life was full of many sorts of trouble, any or all of which might be harmful to health. If only it were possible to devise an experiment that would examine the effects of stress and deprived living conditions on the health of the poor. For nearly 10 years, the U.S. Department of Housing and Urban Development has been conducting an experiment called Moving to Opportunity that seems to be doing just that. HUD researchers wanted to see what happens to poor urban families who move out of neighborhoods like Harlem in New York, Roxbury in Boston or the South Side of Chicago and settle in better neighborhoods. They wanted to know whether moving would help children do better in school, and escape being drawn into crime when they reached adolescence. They also wanted to know whether their parents would climb out of poverty.

HUD did find that people's lives improved in some ways. For example, the children who moved to better neighborhoods in Baltimore did better on standardized tests, and adults there were more likely to get off welfare. But HUD's most remarkable early findings had to do with health. In Boston, poor children who moved to low-poverty neighborhoods were less likely to experience severe asthma attacks. Adults in New York who moved were less likely to suffer from symptoms of depression and anxiety than those who stayed behind, and adults in Boston were more likely to report that they felt "calm and peaceful." The HUD researchers who devised the experiment had not set out to study health, but their findings were so striking that they decided to expand their study to determine whether moving out of poor neighborhoods affected other aspects of health that they did not measure in the first round, including blood pressure, obesity and other factors associated with such chronic afflictions as heart disease, cancer and stroke, like smoking. Those results aren't available yet, but when I heard about the earlier study, I decided to conduct a small experiment of my own.

Staying indoors keeps kids safe from crime but puts them 'at the intersection of the asthma and obesity epidemics,' according to one researcher at Columbia.

I wanted to talk to families, like those who had participated in the HUD program, who had recently moved out of the slums. Did the move affect their health? And if so, why? Did people experience less stress? Did they eat better food? Breathe better air? What might their experiences tell me about the mysterious miasma of contemporary poverty?

My investigation led me to Jerrold M. Levy, the general counsel of the Enhanced Section 8 Outreach Program, or ESOP, which helps low-income families move out of depressed, dangerous inner-city neighborhoods in Yonkers into middle-class areas. ESOP wasn't conducting any studies of these people, of course, but Levy was willing to put me in touch with 10 of the families he'd helped move. He had noticed that the people who moved out of dangerous neighborhoods seemed happier. "A few weeks after they've moved," he says of his clients, who are mostly single mothers, "they come into my office, and it's like one of those programs on late-night TV where they do the makeovers, you know? They have their hair done nicely, they're wearing high heels and makeup, it's like they're transformed. They have a new sense of self-worth and dignity. But will you see changes in their health? I don't think so." Depression and anxiety are major health problems that affect large numbers of poor people, so I thought I would be satisfied just to find people whose mental health improved. And I did find such people. But I also found that most people who moved gained far more than high spirits.

Of the 10 families I met, 9 had at least one member who suffered from a serious health problem before the move that required either medication or hospitalization. Of the 16 people in these families who had health problems, 12 told me that they felt better in significant ways—either their symptoms were less severe so that they no longer required hospitalization, or they were taking less medication. Their health problems included severe asthma, diabetes, high blood pressure, liver cirrhosis and eczema. Emergency-room visits for the asthmatic kids virtually stopped, and some adults with high blood pressure or diabetes reduced the doses of their medications. This was hardly a rigorous scientific experiment. There was no control group, and I was not able to check medical records. Nevertheless, I was stunned by what people told me. These people felt better, and moving appeared to have made all the difference. If moving out of southwest Yonkers were a drug, I would bottle it, patent it and go on cable TV and sell it.

Juanita Moody is now 52. In the summer of 2001, she and her husband, William, moved to a middle-class section of Yonkers from a low-income housing complex on Nepperhan Avenue, where they lived for nearly 30 years. Juanita was crippled by polio when she was a teenager, and during an operation to adjust her spine, she was given a blood transfusion that contained hepatitis C. The virus lay dormant for many years. But two and a half years ago, Juanita's doctor told her that her liver was showing signs of damage and advised her to take interferon, a prescription drug for viral infections. When Juanita found out about the possible side effects, however, she refused. Today Juanita's liver tests are almost normal, suggesting that her hepatitis is not progressing rapidly. "The doctor said I was fantastic, in terms of enzymes," Juanita told me. I did not speak to Juanita's doctor myself, so I could not confirm her diagnosis, but Juanita seemed energetic, and other doctors confirmed that it is possible for hepatitis to slow its progression. In addition, Juanita says that since she moved, her blood pressure has fallen from 140/90, which is considered high, to 130/78, which is almost normal, and the dose of blood-pressure pills she takes has been reduced by half.

Juanita, a born-again Christian, attributes her improved health to prayer and to the new regimen she has maintained since she moved. She has become a health-food nut. Before she moved, her daughter told me, "everything was fried, fried, fried. Before she'd eat at McDonald's and stuff, but not now." Now she drinks fruit and vegetable juices, and her kitchen cabinets are full of natural remedies: vitamins C and E, zinc, magnesium, calcium, alpha lipoic acid and milk thistle, which she says is excellent for the liver.

Juanita says she began focusing more on her health after she moved. When she lived on Nepperhan, there were too many other things to worry about, including frequent robberies and killings in and around the complex itself. The building managers put up a fence to keep drug dealers out, "but the crackheads living inside the building gave the dealers the keys." The elevators were often broken, which meant that someone would have to carry Juanita and her wheelchair up and down three flights of stairs.

Juanita's new apartment is not in a luxury building. It's on a busy road, near two gas stations and a shopping mall, and has few amenities. But it is safe and has nice, leafy views. On Nepperhan, "it was stressful just to walk out of that place. You were always scared for the kids....You wake up stressed, go to sleep stressed, you see all the garbage and the dealers. That is depressing. In a bad environment like that you say, 'What's the use of doing anything?'" Living in her new apartment building gives her a very different feeling. "It inspires you to do all you can—spiritually, healthwise, any kind of way."

It is well known that junk food can make anxious people feel better. Researchers from the University of California recently discovered one possible reason. In response to constant stress, the brain makes a hormone called corticotropin-releasing factor, which instructs the adrenal glands to manufacture stress hormones, including adrenaline and cortisol. These hormones cause a range of physiological changes that over long periods can be harmful. When people with high levels of cortisol eat sugary, fatty foods, fat is deposited in the abdomen. The researchers theorize that these abdominal fat cells can temporarily inhibit the brain from making corticotropin-releasing factor, reducing feelings of stress and anxiety. If this theory is correct, it could explain how the stress of poverty creates a biological urge to overeat, thus putting poor people at greater risk of obesity and its consequences—diabetes, heart disease, stroke and certain types of cancer. Perhaps this explained why Juanita found it easier to change her diet once she moved out of the stressful atmosphere of Nepperhan Avenue. She admitted that doctors had been telling her over the years that she should consume less fattening food. "But they can tell you, and you don't do it," Juanita said.

Noemi, 31, moved with her two teenage children and her 76-year-old aunt, Raimunda, from Burnham Street in Yonkers to a better neighborhood in northwest Yonkers only three months before I met her in August. Noemi, who asked that her last name not be used, has had diabetes since childhood. Shortly after she moved, her doctor reduced her dose of insulin by three units. Noemi thinks it's because she feels less stressed in the new neighborhood. "Stress affects your blood sugar," she explained. "It makes your sugar go up so you need more insulin." She drove me from her new neighborhood of neatly mowed lawns, bushy trees and two-car garages to the place she used to live. "Look at the neighborhood here," she said, as we drove by industrial garages, boarded-up buildings and vacant lots. An enormous, dented, wheezing Lincoln car screeched by. "I had to be worried all the time, you know. Are the children gonna get hit by a car? Is something gonna happen? We've lived in neighborhoods with a lot of drugs, a lot of people getting killed. You'd read about it in the paper the next day and think: Oh, God! That's only two blocks from here."

Noemi's aunt Raimunda speaks no English, although she has lived in the United States for more than 15 years. She has high blood pressure and heart disease. I asked Noemi to ask Raimunda how she was feeling these days. "She says her thing with the head is gone," Noemi translated. "Before she used to get dizzy, but not anymore. Not for the past couple of months." When I asked Raimunda why she thought the dizzy spells went away, she, unlike Noemi and Juanita, did not mention stress. Instead, she said she thought the improvement had something to do with diet. "She thinks the chicken is better here—easier to digest," Noemi said. "But what she doesn't know is that since we moved, I still buy the chicken in the same place."

After meeting Noemi, Raimunda and Juanita, I began to see more clearly what Arline Geronimus, the University of Michigan researcher, was talking about. Perhaps the miasma that is killing the poor really is stress after all. Then I spoke to the mothers of six children who had severe asthma. Every one of them had significantly fewer and less severe attacks after the families moved out of southwest Yonkers. Reduced stress could be partly responsible—stress can worsen asthma—but it seemed clear to me a cleaner environment was also responsible. The children ranged in age from 3 to 16; they all moved out of

southwest Yonkers and settled in different parts of Westchester. The mothers, who asked that their last names not be used, saw astonishing changes, and hearing their stories convinced me that the only way to deal with the staggering epidemic of asthma that afflicts 30 percent of children in some New York City neighborhoods is to clean up the rundown, roach-infested buildings where so many of these children live.

Carmen and her 4-year-old son moved to a middle class section of Westchester in the spring of 2002. In Yonkers, her son would have severe asthma attacks every month and would have to sit for hours every day breathing through a nebulizer. Since they moved, she says he has needed the nebulizer only twice. Two years ago, Monique, her 3-year-old son and 8-year-old daughter moved from Cedar Street in Yonkers to Peekskill. When they lived on Cedar Street, her son's severe asthma came complete with projectile vomiting. The attacks started just a few months after he was born, and they terrified Monique. She blames her former landlord. "There was no hot water for two weeks once, there were leaks in the roof, so it was damp all the time. Sometimes there was water coming through the roof, and mice playing in the living room," she says. "There were cockroaches everywhere, even in the refrigerator. The landlord did nothing until I called the health department. It was stressful having all those roaches around. You didn't know if they were crawling all over you at night." As soon as the family moved up to Peekskill, the boy's attacks became less severe. Although he is still on medication, the violent attacks and the vomiting have stopped.

Cockroaches and vermin do worsen asthma, and this might explain why Monique's son was so sick. But there could be another reason that so many children in poor neighborhoods have asthma, and why they get better when they move. In the past decade, rates of childhood asthma, as well as obesity and diabetes, have soared in the very neighborhoods that were worst affected by the crime waves of the 70's, 80's and 90's. One possible explanation, says Daniel Kass, a research scientist for the New York City health department, "is that asthma follows the crime epidemic, because it goes wherever people spend a lot of time indoors."

Poor parents, terrified that their kids will be killed on the street, tend to keep them inside, with the windows shut and the TV on, where they are constantly exposed to contaminants in indoor air, which some researchers believe can be as damaging as industrial pollution. Not only are sedentary, overweight kids more at risk for asthma, but kids with severe asthma tend to exercise less and are thus prone to obesity. Mothers trying to protect their kids from crime may not realize they are putting their future health at risk. As Mindy Fullilove, professor of clinical psychiatry and public health at Columbia University explained, "The best parents—the people who are the most upright, the churchgoers, the most protective mothers—keep their kids inside, and they are at the intersection of the asthma and obesity epidemics."

I thought of Trevor Jackson Jr., a 14-year-old boy with serious eczema who moved from southwest Yonkers up to Cortland Manor in northern Westchester two years ago. "This is a much better atmosphere," his mother, Dawn, told me. Their new apartment is in a large house with a wide sloping lawn surrounded by trees. "The kids can just go outside anytime. The little one wouldn't go to sleep when we first got here." He wanted to be outside all the time. In Cortland Manor, "kids have a better chance to grow," Trevor's father, Trevor Sr., says. "We see deer in the yard, woodchucks, otters, frogs. There's just life up here."

I WAS BEGINNING to see that the problems of stress and material deprivation were inseparable parts of the contemporary miasma of poverty. But how did these neighborhoods become so unhealthy? New York City is one of the most segregated metropolitan areas in the country. Blacks, whites and other ethnic groups interact every day, but to a large extent they live separately. At the same time, the city has also become more segregated by wealth, so that many black and Hispanic neighborhoods are also the poorest.

The Harvard sociologist William Julius Wilson has described how, thanks to the civil rights movement of the 60's, many middle-class blacks have been able to find jobs and housing outside traditional black areas, leaving behind the most impoverished, poorly educated people. This concentration of disadvantage—racial, social and economic—combined with the loss of many unskilled manufacturing jobs, is what Wilson says contributed to the many social problems associated with poverty today, including drug abuse, crime and single motherhood. Mindy Fullilove says that these trends contributed to widening health inequalities as well. As racial and economic segregation increased, health problems became concentrated in the most deprived areas, as if the miasma were condensing over them. Indeed, I wondered if the miasma might not turn out to be segregation itself.

In order to understand the health crisis among America's urban poor, Fullilove explains, you can't just consider what's going on now. "You have to look at the history of these neighborhoods" and think about the people who live there and what has happened to them in the past. "The history of each neighborhood will determine its pattern of disease. A city like New York suffers from an overlay of epidemics."

In the 70's, 80's and 90's, poor minority neighborhoods throughout the country experienced a protean health crisis. Rates of some chronic and infectious diseases began increasing for the first time since World War II. Even older blacks who made it into their 60's, and who once had as good a chance of reaching their 75th birthdays as 60-year-old whites, began dying at higher rates.

Fullilove says that urban-renewal projects that helped create concentrated poverty, along with redlining—discrimination by banks and insurance companies—and public-service cuts in poor neighborhoods led to catastrophic changes in the way the poor lived, and destroyed the foundation that made poverty endurable. The migrancy of poor people, displaced by fires, evictions and other calamities, destroyed informal community mechanisms for caring for children and controlling the behavior of adolescents and young adults, and this made it harder than ever for the poor to cope. "It was like a massive refugee situation," Fullilove says.

At the same time, as the middle class increasingly campaigned for restrictions on cigarette and alcohol advertising, those companies spent more of their marketing dollars in poor neighborhoods. As Rodrick and Deborah Wallace wrote in their book "A Plague on Your Houses," politicians looked the other way when companies posted huge, colorful billboards—depicting exuberant black people smoking cigarettes and drinking beer—outside schools and churches in Harlem, Brooklyn and the South Bronx. Construction on central Harlem's first full-size supermarket did not begin until 2002, but in the 90's there were more than a hundred places where a child under 18 could buy cigarettes, including individual "loosies," which are cheap but illegal.

The wave of crime and drugs of the 80's and 90's has subsided considerably, and some once-grim urban neighborhoods are even prospering. But poverty has risen in many suburban minority enclaves, and the health problems of the poor have not gone away.

Much has been written about how such social problems as joblessness and drug abuse worsen health problems, but it is also possible that the converse is true. Both Beverly and Monica have lost jobs as a result of illness, and many sick people fall into poverty. Anne Case, a Princeton University economist, has shown that unhealthy young people are far less likely to succeed in school and find good jobs later on. Thus, illness can trap poor families in cycles of disease, death and poverty for generations.

Adam Karpati of the New York City health department says that even though we don't know what the miasma is, there is still a great deal we can do to improve the well-being of the poor. In the 19th century, it was not the discovery of germs that led to the greatest advances in public health, but a series of profound changes in the way the poor lived—a virtual social revolution. Then, as now, health and poverty were inseparable from each other, and better housing, sewers, decent wages, better working conditions and improved nutrition saved millions of lives. Today much could be done to improve the environment and make life less stressful for the poor. The health department is working to reduce mold and roach infestation in public housing, as well as encouraging doctors and community organizations to address such problems as obesity, asthma and diabetes. These admirable programs, however, are modest in scale, and in the current fiscal climate, their financing is far from secure.

More ambitious changes are needed, but at present, our government is permitting matters to get even worse. Since 2000, millions of jobs have been lost, and nearly three million people have joined the ranks of the poor, who now account for more than 12 percent of the U.S. population and 24 percent of African-Americans. This means fewer families will be able to move out of poor neighborhoods on their own. For now, the federal Section 8 program—which provides subsidies for people to pay for private housing—is the only hope most people have of getting out of these neighborhoods, but even its future is in doubt. Possible budget cuts could mean thousands of Section 8 recipients will lose their vouchers next year, and in the longer term, Republicans in Congress hope to devolve the program to the states. This will almost certainly mean the program will shrink. Last month, moreover, HUD also suspended rental supplements that Jerrold Levy says have made programs like ESOP possible. "This will reinforce the ghettoization of poor people," Levy says.

Rising unemployment and budget cuts will not only harm people's health. They will also cost Americans money. Take diabetes and asthma as examples. Around one million people succumb to Type 2 diabetes each year, with African Americans, Hispanics and Native Americans most at risk. The bill for treating the nation's 11 million known diabetics comes to $92 billion for medications and doctors' visits plus $40 billion in lost productivity due to absences from work and premature death. The yearly bill for the nation's asthma epidemic is $14 billion. As Beverly pointed out to me, shortsighted cuts, amounting to a few hundred million dollars, from the HUD budget mean programs to refurbish public housing, organize recreation for children and build playgrounds have been halted. The exterminator teams that used to come every month now come once every two months, and the roaches are flourishing as never before.

Whatever the miasma is that afflicts America's minority poor, it is at least partly a legacy of the segregation of America's cities. These neighborhoods, by concentrating the poor, also concentrate the mysterious, as yet poorly understood, factors that make them sick. You'd almost think this new miasma was caused by some sort of infection, because of the way it seems to strike certain neighborhoods and certain types of people. I recently came across a research article by Angus Deaton of Princeton University, reporting that white people who live in cities with large black populations have higher death rates than whites with the same income who live in cities with smaller black populations. It made me wonder whether the deprived, polluted, roach-infested, stressful conditions in which poor blacks live aren't affecting all of us, to some degree. And even if we never find out what the miasma is, this possibility should scare us into treating this as the health emergency it is—if nothing else will.

Helen Epstein writes frequently about public health for The New York Review of Books. This is her first article for the magazine.

Are you OK?

It's easy to minimize the emotional symptoms that can interfere with your health and well-being. Here's how to check yourself and where to seek help.

If you have a persistent cough or a sore that won't heal, you're likely to seek prompt medical attention. But when it comes to persistent emotional symptoms, such as tension, worry, gloom, and discouragement, Americans are notoriously reluctant to seek help. That's unfortunate, because treatment can often make a profound difference in your level of happiness and, indeed, your overall health. Emotional problems cannot only interfere with recovery from disease, but new research also shows they can increase your risk of heart disease, diabetes, dementia, and other disorders.

Negative emotions are, of course, a normal part of life for most people, especially those coping with illnesses or recovering from accidents or other trauma. Most of the time bad moods are fleeting, even if the underlying situations that cause them are not. Sometimes, however, bad moods become continuous and disabling, and it's not always obvious when to seek help. The percentage of U.S. adults reporting "frequent mental distress" is on the rise, from 8.4 percent in 1993 to 10.1 percent in 2001, according to an October 2004 report by the federal Centers for Disease Control and Prevention. Unfortunately, only a third of the 44 million Americans a year who are beset by anxiety, depression, or other psychological disorders get the help they need.

That is particularly unfortunate for those whose emotional symptoms are related to a physical disease. Certain medications, including beta-blockers and corticosteroids, and illnesses, such as thyroid disease, diabetes, and cancer, can also cause depressive symptoms. And it's now well established that emotional problems can complicate the treatment of and delay recovery from many diseases, including some that are life-threatening. Individuals who become depressed in the wake of a heart attack, for example, typically take longer to recover. Arthritis sufferers who become depressed tend to experience greater disability than do similar patients who stay upbeat. Depression also seems to delay the knitting of broken bones and to speed the progression from HIV to AIDS.

Evidence is mounting that emotional problems can cause as well as exacerbate physical illness. A 2003 report

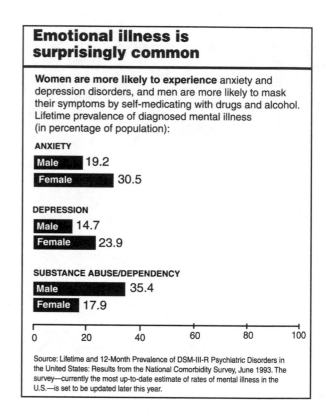

Emotional illness is surprisingly common

Women are more likely to experience anxiety and depression disorders, and men are more likely to mask their symptoms by self-medicating with drugs and alcohol. Lifetime prevalence of diagnosed mental illness (in percentage of population):

ANXIETY
Male 19.2
Female 30.5

DEPRESSION
Male 14.7
Female 23.9

SUBSTANCE ABUSE/DEPENDENCY
Male 35.4
Female 17.9

0   20   40   60   80   100

Source: Lifetime and 12-Month Prevalence of DSM-III-R Psychiatric Disorders in the United States: Results from the National Comorbidity Survey, June 1993. The survey—currently the most up-to-date estimate of rates of mental illness in the U.S.—is set to be updated later this year.

from the National Institute of Mental Health found depression to be just as significant a risk factor for cardiovascular disease as high blood pressure and elevated cholesterol. And research suggests that depression and possibly anxiety as well may raise the risk of developing osteoporosis and even Alzheimer's disease. A study of almost 2,000 people has also found that depression doubles the likelihood of developing diabetes.

"Antidepressants work for a large majority of people, but they're not wonder drugs. Side effects include loss of libido."

"Depression is an illness that has profound physiological effects all over the body," says Steven P. Roose, M.D., professor of clinical psychiatry at Columbia University's College of Physicians and Surgeons in New York City. For example, depression impairs circulation by making platelets "stickier." And in people with anxiety or depression, the body secretes extra cortisol, a stress hormone that can damage the blood vessels. Ominously, these physiological changes can occur even in the absence of full-blown mental illness. Says Roose, "Risk increases proportionally to the severity of your symptoms."

PROTECTING EMOTIONAL HEALTH

One strategy for keeping emotional distress in check is to be reflective about your moods and relationships. "That means observing negative patterns in your life and understanding the things that control you and hold you back," says Gail Saltz, M.D., associate professor of psychiatry at Weill-Cornell School of Medical Sciences in New York City. "If you can become aware of the patterns, you can direct them so that you can be your own pilot and not be driven by them."

The self-check questions for emotional symptoms is designed to alert you to symptoms that need evaluation. And the table treatment strategies for emotional disorders summarizes symptoms and treatments for the most common forms of emotional disorders. Here are some ways to find the right treatment.

OVERCOMING BARRIERS TO TREATMENT

Many Americans view an emotional problem as a personal weakness rather than a medical problem, Saltz says. "We'll spend tons of money on a great haircut but won't do what's needed to evolve into someone who is more aware of emotional issues and therefore better able to get what we really want out of life," she adds.

Some people are so fearful of being labeled mentally ill that they deny the problem exists. Others deny that the problem is severe enough to warrant treatment. Financial barriers to treatment can also be significant. A single session with a psychiatrist can easily cost $100, and the cost of many antidepressants can run several dollars a pill. So those without insurance may find it difficult to afford help.

Another force that discourages treatment is the fear that unauthorized release of a person's medical records might jeopardize his or her employment or insurability. Despite prohibitions against this practice, violations continue. "Unauthorized disclosure of sensitive mental-health information can be devastating," says Ron Honberg, legal director of the National Alliance for the Mentally Ill. "It's a major concern."

Physicians who are too quick to offer drug treatment as the only option may be another barrier. Those who wish to avoid drug treatment should know that many studies have shown that various types of counseling and talk therapy can effectively relieve a range of emotional disorders. Talk therapy may take longer to have an impact than prescription drugs, but it also causes fewer side effects and can be a reasonable alternative when symptoms are not severe.

BEST THERAPY OPTIONS

Modern antidepressants, including selective serotonin reuptake inhibitors (SSRIs) like fluoxetine (*Prozac*) and sertraline (*Zoloft*), are often prescribed for depression and anxiety disorders. "They do work for a large majority of people," says Eric J. Nestler, M.D., Ph.D., chairman of the department of psychiatry at the University of Texas Southwestern Medical Center in Dallas, though they're not "wonder drugs." Side effects include weight gain and loss of libido, and recent evidence suggests that they may raise the risk of suicidal behavior in the first few weeks of treatment. A change in prescription can sometimes diminish side effects, and Nestler encourages people who could benefit from antidepressants not to be afraid of them.

A Consumer Reports survey of 3,079 readers with depression or anxiety found that **drug therapy** relieved symptoms faster than talk therapy. The majority of peo-

Treatment strategies for emotional disorders

Disorder, symptoms	Drug treatment	Best talk therapy
Alcohol dependency: Inability to cut back on drinking, strain on work or home life, resulting medical problems.	Acamprosate (*Campral*), disulfiram (*Antabuse*), or naltrexone (*ReVia*).	Counseling by physician, Alcoholics Anonymous or similar program.
Anxiety disorder (generalized): Persistent and uncontrollable worrying, trembling, headaches, insomnia, stomach trouble.	SSRI antidepressant, such as escitalopram (*Lexapro*) or paroxetine (*Paxil*) benzodiazepine sedatives, such as alprazolam (*Xanax*) or lorazepam (*Ativan*).	Cognitive-behavioral therapy, relaxation therapy.
Bipolar disorder: Boundless energy, sleeplessness, impulsive or reckless behavior regarding money, sexuality, and other areas.	Lithium (*Eskalith*), lamotrigine (*Lamicta*l), or valproic acid (*Depakene*).	Psychotherapy, support groups.
Depression: Sadness, hopelessness, changes in appetite, weight, or sleep patterns.	SSRI antidepressant, such as citalopram (*Celexa*) or fluoxetine (*Prozac*), bupropion (*Wellbutrin*); possibly dietary supplement St. John's wort or SAM-e for mild-to-moderate symptoms.	Cognitive-behavioral therapy, interpersonal therapy.
Obsessive-compulsive disorder: Recurrent thoughts, repetitive and irrational behaviors.	SSRI antidepressant, such as fluoxetine (*Prozac*) or sertraline (*Zoloft*).	Cognitive-behavioral therapy
Panic disorder: Heart palpitations, profuse sweating, shortness of breath, avoidance of situations that induce panic.	SSRI antidepressant, such as fluoxetine (*Prozac*) or sertraline (*Zoloft*); tricyclic antidepressant, such as desipramine (*Norpramin*); MAOIs, such as pheneizine (*Nardil*) or tranylcpromine (*Parnate*).	Cognitive-behavioral therapy
Post-tramatic stress disorder: Reliving a trauma through flashbacks or nightmares, avoiding things pertaining to the trauma, feeling emotionally numb, feeling irritable, trouble sleeping or concentrating.	SSRI antidepressant, such as paroxetine (*Paxil*) or sertraline (*Zoloft*), tricyclic antidepressant, such as imipramine (*Tofranil*); MAOIs, such as pheneizine (*Nardil*) or tranylcpromine (*Parnate*).	Cognitive-behavioral therapy, interpersonal therapy; possibly "critical incident debriefing."
Social phobia: Avoidance of social gaterings because of heart palpitations, trembling, sweating, or blushing.	SSRI antidepressant, such as paroxetine (*Paxil*) or sertraline (*Zoloft*); beta-blocker, such as propranoiol (*Inderal*).	Cognitive-behavioral therapy

ple who described their therapy as "mostly medication" had good outcomes. But it took trial and error to find the right medication. And the rates of adverse drug effects were much higher than those noted on the medications' package inserts.

Talk therapy rivaled drug therapy in effectiveness. Respondents who said their therapy was "mostly talk" and lasted at least 13 sessions had better outcomes than those whose therapy was "mostly medication." Therapy delivered by psychologists and clinical social workers was perceived as being just as effective as that given by psychiatrists. Other professionals who offer therapy include psychoanalysts, psychiatric nurses, and marriage and family counselors.

If you need therapy, don't just pick a name from an ad or the Yellow Pages. Difficult as it may be when you're in distress, try to approach therapy as an active consumer. Ask your doctor and friends for referrals, and speak to potential therapists over the phone or in the office. (Many will meet with you briefly without charge.) Even a brief

interview should tell you if you'd be comfortable sharing your most intimate thoughts and feelings.

No one type of therapy is best for all people. Many therapists favor a particular theoretical approach, although they often use a combination. Clinical trials have proved that two types of therapy are most consistently effective: cognitive behavioral therapy and interpersonal therapy. Both are designed to produce a meaningful improvement within 15 to 20 sessions. Both teach people to manage their moods—to think and behave their way to better mental health.

Cognitive behavioral therapy focuses on training patients to identify and consciously correct the distorted thought patterns associated with anxiety or depression. Anxious people tend to overestimate the likelihood of a catastrophe, while depressed people tend to react to setbacks or disappointments with extreme self-criticism and a feeling of hopelessness out of proportion to the situation. The therapy typically involves specific "homework" assignments. For instance, a depressed person might be assigned to arrange an enjoyable social activity or become more assertive on the job. Or an anxious person might be assigned to take steps to confront a feared situation.

Interpersonal therapy, used primarily for depression, focuses more on the patient's relationship problems with others, such as spouses, children, or co-workers. It can be especially effective when depression results from a major life transition, such as the birth of a child, divorce, loss of a job, or bereavement. Therapy typically involves learning to change one's manner of dealing with family and friends, adapting to changed life circumstances, or building up one's social skills.

WHAT YOU CAN DO

• Avoid unhealthy situations that can trigger negative emotions. These include chronic stress, unacknowledged anger, poor sleep habits, and lack of exercise.

• Monitor moods. As a general rule, it's time to consult your doctor if emotional problems persist beyond two weeks or interfere significantly with everyday life. In cases of bereavement and other severe loss, however, several months of depressed feelings are not unusual.

• Listen to a friend. Emotional problems can blunt your powers of observation and judgment, so you may not recognize symptoms that are obvious to others. If someone you trust voices concern or observes that you seem unusually sad or tired, don't be quick to dismiss his or her viewpoint.

• Comparison shop for a therapist. Referrals from health professionals and friends are a good starting point. Consider whether you have preferences regarding your therapist's gender, academic background, therapeutic approach, or other characteristics. Interview prospective therapists until you find someone you feel is a good fit.

DEALING with DEMONS

Seen as a public health problem, suicide is preventable—at least that's an approach several states are starting to take.

Christopher Conte

In the mid-1990s, the United States Air Force was hit by a deadly epidemic: Every year between 1991 and 1996, about 60 airmen took their own lives, making suicide the second leading cause of death among the service's 350,000 members.

Eager to reduce the terrible toll, the service conducted "psychological autopsies" of the victims. These linked most of the suicides to problems airmen were having with the law, finances, intimate relationships, mental health, job performance and alcohol and drugs. The study also found most of the airmen were socially isolated and lacked the skills needed to cope with stress.

With these findings in hand, the service launched a counterattack. Top Air Force officials began urging airmen to seek assistance when they encountered personal difficulties, assuring them that doing so would not hurt their chances of promotion. The service also started training all its members in suicide risk-awareness and prevention, and it established "stress management" teams to help airmen and their families deal with potentially traumatic events.

These and other efforts worked. The suicide rate, which had been 14.1 per 100,000 active-duty service members from 1991 to 1996, fell to 9.1 per 100,000 from 1997 to 2002. Air Force

officials attribute the improvement to the breadth of the program. "Suicide prevention," says one service manual, "is everyone's business."

The Air Force experience is getting a lot of attention these days in state capitols. At least 20 states have adopted suicide-prevention plans, most of them in the past few years, and many other states are working on the issue, too. Their efforts are driven by the belief that public health strategies, which involve looking for patterns that may point to the sources of disease and launching broad-based public information campaigns to encourage healthier living among the population at large, may hold the key to reducing suicide—just as they have been used to reduce heart attacks, strokes and lung cancer.

Public health campaigns to discourage smoking, bad diet or unsafe sexual practices have become a familiar and remarkably successful part of American life, but the use of such strategies against a psychological disorder represents a significant new departure. If successful, it could usher in one of the most fundamental shifts in thinking about the role of state mental health programs in decades—one in which mental health agencies increasingly offer their services to the entire population rather than to the

small group of people diagnosed as having severe mental illness.

"We have been missing opportunities to use public health promotion and prevention in the mental health sector," notes Alan Radke, who, as medical director for the adult mental health division of Hawaii's Department of Health, has been spearheading a broad review of prevention strategies for the National Association of State Mental Health Program Directors. "If we can demonstrate that the use of health promotion and prevention strategies works with suicide, from those learnings we can address any number of other conditions."

AN OUNCE OF PREVENTION

That's a big "if." The overall suicide rate has been stuck between 10 and 13 per 100,000 people annually for the past 50 years, and despite a handful of promising signs such as the Air Force program, there is no conclusive evidence that any strategy to reduce it will work. Indeed, suicide-prevention advocates sometimes seem to be acting more on faith than scientific proof. "When I started, I worried that this is too hard to fix and too big to understand," concedes Jerry Reed, executive director of the Suicide Prevention Action Network—USA, a lobby group that represents "suicide survivors," as family

TRAIL OF ANGUISH

State-by-state suicide death rates, 2001

BETWEEN 14 AND 23 DEATHS PER 100,000 PEOPLE
- Alaska
- Arizona
- Arkansas
- Colorado
- Florida
- Idaho
- Montana
- Nevada
- New Mexico
- Oklahoma
- Oregon
- West Virginia
- Wyoming

BETWEEN 12 AND 14 DEATHS PER 100,000 PEOPLE
- Delaware
- Kentucky
- Maine
- Missouri
- New Hampshire
- North Carolina
- North Dakota
- South Dakota
- Tennessee
- Utah

BETWEEN 11 AND 12 DEATHS PER 100,000 PEOPLE
- Alabama
- Georgia
- Hawaii
- Indiana
- Mississippi
- South Carolina
- Vermont
- Virginia
- Washington
- Wisconsin

BETWEEN 6 AND 11 DEATHS PER 100,000 PEOPLE
- California
- Connecticut
- Illinois
- Iowa
- Kansas
- Louisiana
- Maryland
- Massachusetts
- Michigan
- Minnesota
- Nebraska
- New Jersey
- New York
- Ohio
- Pennsylvania
- Rhode Island
- Texas

Source: Suicide Prevention Action Network Inc.

members of suicide victims call themselves. "But sometimes you have to act like a little bird, and hope when you leave the nest that you'll sprout wings before you hit the ground."

Although the prospects for success seem uncertain, advocates can offer some compelling reasons to tackle the problem. Suicide is the 11th leading cause of death in the United States, accounting for about 30,000 deaths a year. That's more than die from homicide (about 20,000 annually) or AIDS (14,000 a year). Moreover, researchers estimate that as many as 25 people attempt suicide for every one who actually kills himself. In 2002, some 250,000 people required medical treatment following suicide attempts, according to the Centers for Disease Control and Prevention.

And surveys by the CDC show that 20 percent of teenagers have seriously considered killing themselves. (Much of the current push to combat suicide stems from a tripling of the rate among people aged 15 to 24 between 1950 and 1993, even though it has since leveled off.)

Suicide survivors have played a central role in planting the idea that suicide is a community problem, rather than a private, individual matter. That is no small step, because suicide has long carried a stigma. "It took me a couple of years before I could even talk about it," says Massachusetts state Senator Robert Antonioni, who lost a brother to suicide and has since persuaded the Massachusetts legislature to spend close to $1 million on suicide-prevention efforts over the past several years.

The important point, adds Kentucky state Senator Tom Buford, who steered a suicide-prevention bill through his state legislature this year partly in honor of his father who killed himself years ago, is that although "you feel you're living in sinful territory because somebody in your family committed suicide, after a while you see it's just an illness that needs to be treated."

Because the majority of people who are suicidal go undiagnosed until it's too late to treat the illness, researchers say the only effective strategy may be to stress prevention in messages aimed at the entire population. "By reducing the risk for a lot of people, you get more bang for your buck than concentrating on the few who are at high risk," explains Kerry Knox, an assistant professor of preventive medicine at the University of Rochester.

The idea that broad strategies work more effectively than narrow ones against a hidden enemy is a fundamental tenet of public health. Epidemiologists liken society's approach to suicide today to its understanding of cardiovascular disease 30 years ago. Then, strokes, heart attacks and high blood pressure were treated largely on a case-by-case basis. The results were far from satisfactory because, as with suicide, these afflictions often went undetected until victims suffered crippling or fatal symptoms. But research in the 1970s and '80s showed that public information campaigns designed to promote low-cholesterol diets, exercise and screening for high blood pressure among the population at large were an effective way to prevent cardiovascular disease—even though many of the people who hear such warnings probably face little risk.

At first blush, suicide seems different because it isn't a medical disease. But the latest research suggests that it may not be so different. Like cardiovascular disease, it apparently results from both biological and environmental causes. People who commit suicide or attempt it have abnormalities in the prefrontal cortex area of their brains, which controls "inhibitory" functioning. Because of this biological condition, "they are less able to restrain themselves and more likely to have strong feelings," observes J. John Mann, chief of neuroscience at the New York State Psychiatric Institute. "When they get depressed, they get more depressed than most people." He concludes that suicide may be the product of "stress-diathesis"—that is, a confluence of "stressors" arising from the environment and a "diathesis," or predisposition for suicidal behavior.

Knox and Mann both serve on a suicide-prevention working group convened by the New York State Office of Mental Health (the Psychiatric Institute, considered one of the foremost research institutions in its field, is part of the state

agency). Although they come from a public health and a neurobiological background, respectively, they agree that, as Mann puts it, "You need a combination of strategies to have an impact on the suicide rate." While he believes the day isn't far off when doctors will be able to detect people who have suicidal proclivities by reading their brain scans, the technology will be of little value unless people are willing to seek help for themselves or recognize when people they know need it. "You need to educate the public to understand there are such things as psychiatric illnesses, and that they can lead to suicide," he says. "That requires the involvement of government."

THE CPR METHOD

Most states have started their suicide-prevention efforts with broad-based educational campaigns. This spring, for instance, New York State issued "SPEAK," which stands for Suicide Prevention Education Awareness Kits—packets of materials that explain the connections between depression and suicide and encourage help-seeking among teens, men, women and older people. Some states also offer advice to the news media on how to report on suicide. Guidelines adopted by Maine, for instance, seek to minimize the danger of "suicide contagion" by encouraging the press to refrain from describing how a person killed himself, glorifying a suicide and using such phrases as "successful suicide."

Some states have gone beyond educational programs to concentrate on strengthening the bonds that make for more supportive communities. In Alaska, where religious disillusionment and social breakdown are believed to lie behind high suicide rates among some native peoples, the state provides funds for village elders to teach children about their heritage. "This builds pride and relationships, so that if a kid gets in trouble later, he'll have somebody to turn to," explains Susan Soule,

Alaska's program coordinator for suicide prevention and rural human services.

In the lower 48, suicide-prevention programs seek to accomplish the same objective by training "gatekeepers"—clergy, doctors, teachers, social workers and others—who might come into contact with people who are suicidal. Paul Quinnett, president and chief executive of the QPR Institute in Spokane, Washington, believes that doctors, psychologists and social workers should be required to receive suicide-prevention training as a condition of being licensed. QPR, a deliberate take-off on the familiar emergency treatment CPR, stands for "Question, Persuade and Refer," a simple methodology for detecting people at risk of suicide and helping them get professional assistance.

North Dakota has provided its own version of suicide-prevention training to 28,000 people since 2000 on a budget of just $75,000 a year. The program seeks official gatekeepers as well as informal leaders—people who tend to pull communities together by force of personality rather than official position. "We go into schools and ask, 'Who is the person who makes things happen?'" says Mark Lomurray, the state's suicide-prevention project leader. "That's who we train." While Lomurray can't prove a causal connection, he notes that the number of suicide deaths in North Dakota has fallen by almost half since the program began.

A BROAD REACH

It is too early to say if all the efforts surrounding suicide prevention will pay off, but if they do, state mental health programs may well need more money. "Right now, we do a good job identifying people who are suicidal, and we can refer them for services if there's a crisis," notes Cheryl DiCara, director of Maine's Youth Suicide Prevention Program. But for people who are troubled and haven't reached the crisis point, she says, "there's not a lot we can do."

Prevention advocates say that public health strategies may save money in the long run by reducing the need for acute care. But that implies new methods of serving people who don't need institutionalization. New York State offers some clues about where this more expansive orientation might lead. Traditionally, the Office of Mental Health has focused exclusively on helping people with severe mental disorders. After the September 2001 terrorist attacks, however, the department, with funding from the Federal Emergency Management Agency, began offering post-trauma counseling to the entire population of New York City and 10 surrounding counties. In two years, more than a million people availed themselves of these free counseling and educational services.

"We're reaching out to a much broader constituency than we ever did previously," notes Sharon Carpinello, New York's mental health commissioner. She expects the agency to become involved in a variety of new public health endeavors. In addition to suicide prevention, the agency is developing a disaster preparedness and "resiliency" campaign for the entire state and a separate campaign aimed at combating eating disorders in young women.

John Allen, who serves as the office's liaison with outside groups, says the new public health focus has brought enormous changes to his job. In the past, he mainly worked with a few small groups that represented patients in mental hospitals. But the post-9/11 project took him into the mainstream. One of his most important partnerships was with the New York State Thruway Authority, which helped the office distribute brochures to commuters. And the suicide-prevention program is bringing him into contact with major employers, local civic organizations and chambers of commerce.

As the department increasingly operates in a bigger arena, some prevention advocates hope it will start asserting itself on matters that previously have been beyond its ability to influence—including proposals to require insurance companies to offer the same coverage for mental illness treatments as they provide for medical care. The idea, of course, is very controversial because of the possible costs, but it's nothing compared with another issue that some prevention advocates have in their sights: gun control.

At the moment, there is no consensus even among suicide experts that stricter gun control would reduce the suicide rate over the long run. The best evidence is that making the leading instrument of suicide less available might have an impact for a while but that the improvement might dissipate over time as people switch to alternative methods to kill themselves. But the simple fact that the idea is even being discussed is a measure of how optimistic the mental health community is about the potential of public health strategies.

"I think we have to stay away from the more controversial strategies until society changes a little bit, but I don't feel totally hopeless," says Madelyn Gould, a research scientist at the New York State Psychiatric Institute who has participated in the state's suicide-prevention working group. "After all, who would have thought a couple of decades ago that anti-smoking campaigns would be so successful that today you can't even smoke anymore in bars in New York City?"

Christopher Conte can be reached at crconte@earthlink.net

Too Young To Be Stressed

by Aparna Bagdi

"For children, the pressures are beginning to tell." "Required: Stress busters for smart kids." "Shrinks called in as exam fever turns into epidemic."

The above headlines are not a sampling from sensationalized items on a television news show; instead, they led off articles that appeared in a mainstream national newspaper from India. Over the past few years, the *Times of India* has published many articles and editorials on the topic of childhood stress. According to Ramanathan (2002), a recent study conducted by the All India Institute of Medical Sciences reveals that nearly 35 percent of children ages 8-14, especially in urban areas, are stressed enough to need clinical attention. What is startling about such findings are the sheer numbers of children under stress, the early onset of their symptoms, and the extreme measures to which some children will go to cope (negatively) with their stress. This article explores some of the circumstances affecting the lives of children in India and some of the possible reasons for heightened childhood stress levels in a culture where, traditionally, the young are adored and indulged.

A recent study conducted by the All India Institute of Medical Sciences reveals that nearly 35 percent of children ages 8-14, especially in urban areas, are stressed enough to need clinical attention.

Cultural Context

Culture is a way of life shared by members of a certain population. The definition of culture encompasses the thoughts, emotions, behaviors, and customs shared by the people, as well as their social, economic, political, and religious institutions. As children grow and mature, they absorb the mindset, behaviors, and customs of the society in which they develop, and they begin to gain an understanding of their culture. Parents and other child-rearing agents consciously, or unconsciously, promote the competencies required to absorb cultural values and perform cultural tasks through culturally standardized techniques for raising children that have been developed over time and passed down from generation to generation. Children learn the ways of people in their culture by participating in cultural tasks and activities (Ogbu, 1988). The family is the primary unit through which customs, beliefs, habits, values, and modes of behavior are transmitted from one generation to the next through the process of socialization (Saraswathi & Dutta, 1988; Tandon, 1981). Therefore, while studying any aspect of child development, it is essential to examine it from within the child's cultural context (Ogbu, 1988).

Bronfenbrenner's (1979) social ecological theory has significance for studying how children cope with stress. According to this theory, children grow up in a dynamic world wherein they influence the environment around them and, in turn, are influenced by the environment. This reciprocity involves a process of mutual accommodation between children and their environment. The immediate setting, as well as the larger context of the setting, influences a child's development. Consequently, children's reactions to stress can be influenced by their immediate family and friends, and by the community in which they live. Several global considerations also may affect family functioning and child development. Examples of influential factors range from the home and school to the political climate of the country, international laws, and different social systems.

For an Indian child, the family's subculture (i.e., the community and society in which the child is born and brought up) determines the family's status in society, which acts as a filter in providing the child with his/her first role models, informal and formal education, and experiences within the culture. Traditionally, families in India have been classified as extended or joint in nature. Joint families consist of one or more married couples residing with their children and other close relatives, such as grandparents, aunts, and uncles, all in one home. A nuclear family structure, which is becoming increasingly common, constitutes a single married couple and their children (Ahuja, 1993; Bisht & Sinha, 1981; Muttalib, 1990). The structural differences between the joint family and the nuclear family lead to different interaction patterns among members of the two family types. Children in joint families are often indulged and overprotected, which encourages the child's dependence on the mother and other family members. In nuclear families, the child is in more direct contact with his or her parents, and the number of adult role models decreases. As compared to children from joint families, children from nuclear families are encouraged to function in an individualized manner, take initiative, and act independently. Fathers play an important role in nuclear families since they are often more approachable and psychologically available to their children (Bisht & Sinha, 1981). Thus, children's experiences growing up in such a complex society can be unique.

Stress in the Indian Context

While it is true that most parents in India look forward eagerly to the birth to their child, many start worrying about the child's future and the pressures of caring for him/her even before the child is born. The joy in anticipating the arrival of the child is often replaced with perturbation and anxiety (Sethi, 1996). Many factors contribute to augmented parental anxiety, including, but not limited to, the pressures of providing a good family and school life for the child, ensuring the child's academic success (and later in life as well), and trying to find a balance between a busy family life and a demanding work routine. In general, parents in India set very high expectations for their children to do well in school, in extracurricular activities as well as in studies, and these high expectations often lead to worried children and anxious parents (Adhyaru & Nandakumar, 2003).

For most Indian children, formal education starts at the preschool level. Literacy data from the 1991 census reveal that the literacy rate for girls is lower by nearly 20 points as compared to that of boys. The rate of increase in literacy during the last decade also has been slower for females (Guha, 1996). Government and nongovernment agencies are attempting to provide education incentives for children, in the form of free textbooks, uniforms, and meals. However, children face tremendous pressure and competition to gain admission into preschools. Each successive academic year adds to children's emotional strain. The stress reaches monumental proportions by the time students reach grades 10 through 12, performance in which determines the student's career and future success (Saraswathi & Pai, 1997).

Children as young as 3 are faced with pressure at home and in school. The rising number of applicants and the limited number of available seats in nursery schools have resulted in cramped, overcrowded classrooms. An even more difficult issue concerns admission to primary schools, which is based on child interviews. Consequently, good nursery schools are now expected to train young children for primary school admission interviews. During these interviews, children are forced to sit still and answer questions regarding colors, pictures, and fruits, and to recognize and write the alphabet. Many children are rejected because they are too young and therefore unprepared for these tasks. However, getting admission into good schools is considered crucial in order to ensure exposure to a scholarly environment and a good academic career. Parents therefore feel compelled to force their children to perform, even if a child is not developmentally ready. The demands on parents to prepare their children for rigorous entrance interviews have resulted in increased stress levels for both parents and children (Sharan, 1991; Times News Network, 2002). Even kindergartners have demonstrated feelings of inadequacy after being rejected during the interview process (Matthews, 1991).

Once in school, young children face enormous pressure from parents and teachers to work hard and do well. The child's worth is measured in terms of school grades. Children as young as 4 are overburdened with homework, tuition (coaching) classes, and scholarship exams. Although the government has banned classes meeting after 7:00 p.m., some schools begin the school day as early as 6:30 a.m. and operate well into the night (Ramanathan, 2002). A factorial study about the sources of academic stress among high school boys, conducted by Rajendran and Kaliappan (1991), revealed four major factors that contributed to high stress levels: personal inadequacy (e.g., difficulty in keeping up with class work); fear of failure (e.g., fear of failing class tests or exams); interpersonal difficulties (e.g., receiving criticism from teachers); and inadequate study facilities (e.g., time taken to travel to school).

Consequently, school is no longer merely challenging, but distressing, competitive, and anxiety-provoking. For many children, examinations symbolize emotional trauma and anxiety. The stringent ranking system used by several schools also influences children negatively. For older children, every point they receive can influence their chance of getting into a good school and ensuring their place in a shrinking job market. Being labeled as "average" or "below average" may overwhelm the child and cause low self-esteem. At this level, competition becomes unhealthy. Teamwork is considered to be unimportant, so the tendency to become more individualistic increases; moreover, tolerance toward peers decreases. Playing with friends is replaced by watching television, playing computer games, or reading books that are restricted to topics of general knowledge or education. As a result, the positive aspects of play—relaxing, coping with fear, giving vent to aggression, dealing with competition, learning social rules, cooperating, and learning to handle difficult situations—are lost (Jain, 1996; Matthews, 1991).

Extremely high parental expectations can greatly augment children's anxiety levels. According to Saksena (2002), some parents put unrealistic expectations on their child just so they can brag about their child's "smartness." Pushy and overenthusiastic parents may consciously or unconsciously hinder their children's development and make them more prone to early burnout and mental fatigue. Child psychologists warn that tremendously high parental expectations cause children to feel even more pressure than they do from examinations. The Times News Network (February 23, 2003) quotes Sumit Chandra, a child psychologist based in the city of Lucknow, India, as saying, "Parents often tell me that suddenly their child has been acting strange and has not been concentrating on his studies. But none of them understand that this is an obvious fallout of the expectation pressure they put their child through. Every year I see kids buckle under tremendous anxiety to perform well in their exams." Additionally, parents sometimes give their children subtle messages that they have failed them by not doing well in school. Children often react by becoming depressed and uninterested in school activities (Abraham & Neogi, 1997; Jain, 1996; Matthews, 1991; Saksena, 2002).

Some mental health experts believe that parents need to be counseled as much as children do. Many parents respond to high stress situations (such as board examinations) with extreme nervousness, which is then transferred to their child. When all means of recreation are blocked in favor of a constant routine of studying for exams, and children's time to play and talk with friends is minimized, the result is that children's ability to effectively cope with exam stress is compromised (Mukherjee, 2003).

Factors such as competition, changing family patterns, and unhealthful lifestyles (such as a poor diet, excessive exposure to television, and limited exercise) contribute to the physical manifestations of stress (Singh, 2002). Major Indian metropolitan cities, such as Bombay and Calcutta, are plagued by problems of overcrowding and pollution. High incidences of physical and psychological symptoms in response to the crowding and noise have been observed (Lam & Palsane, 1997). In addition, such social problems as parental alcohol abuse, parental depression, and poverty also add to tension at home and the inability of children to keep up with academic activities. And then there is the ongoing problem of homeless children. For children living on street corners, education is not a part of their everyday lives. Instead, miserable working and living conditions, violence, crime, and drugs are a reality. Along with having few resources, poor children are also faced with lack of a support system and good role models (Abraham & Neogi, 1997; Sethi, 1996).

The age of clients visiting psychiatrists in cities such as Bombay is falling steadily. The number of children requiring treatment in the form of medications and/or counseling is increasing (Abraham & Neogi, 1997). Mental turmoil and resulting stress on children leads to physical manifestations, including stuttering, giddiness, fainting, palpitations, migraines, gastro-intestinal complaints, and bed-wetting. Stress-related maladies such as depression, hysterical behavior, abdominal pains, peptic ulcers, hypertension, and asthma have begun to affect children as young as 7. Children unable to cope with psychological tensions may suffer from severe headaches, insomnia, recurring nightmares, and moodiness; often, they do not want to go to school. Adolescent girls who are unable to cope with academic pressures may compensate by trying to be trendy, and trying to imitate fashion models and actresses. As a result, the rate of anorexia nervosa in girls older than 12 is rising. Higher incidences of dropping out of school, running away from home, and suicide attempts can also be the unfortunate result of extreme stress and inability to cope with it (Abraham & Neogi, 1997; Jain, 1996; Matthews, 1991; Sharan, 1991, Singh, 2002).

Despite the abundant newspaper coverage of these behaviors, little research-based literature regarding childhood stress and coping in the Indian cultural context can be found. One recent multi-method study was conducted with 8- to 11-year-olds in Bombay. Information for this childhood stress-coping study was gathered through questionnaires and small focus group sessions. Children were asked to talk about situations that make them feel sad, bad, upset, nervous, or anxious. Children also were asked to talk about what they did in order to help themselves feel better. The results of the study indicated that children are very willing and, indeed, capable of discussing their feelings and talking about things that upset them. The findings reveal that both girls and boys reported feeling stressed in several different aspects of their lives. The results also clearly indicate the need for significant adults, such as parents and teachers, to assist children in learning effective ways of coping with stress (Bagdi, 1998).

Credible efforts to address these important issues are being pursued. The South Point School in Calcutta has organized a six-day-long Art of Living workshop called Art Excel (or All-Round Training in Excellence) (Roy, 2003). The workshop is customized for children ages 9-15 and focuses on such coping mechanisms as breathing techniques and asanas (yoga exercises), as well as simple interactive games to improve physical agility, memory, and concentration. Programs such as Art Excel instill positive coping mechanisms and help children deal effectively with everyday stressors.

Conclusion

It is paradoxical that a culture that believes in adoring and indulging their young ones (Kakar, 1979) should also have inherent social mechanisms that create high levels of stress and anxiety in children. Although the social and educational systems of Indian society try to support and nurture the growth and development of children, it is evident that academic and career success comes at a high price for many children in India.

The goals of high academic achievement and a successful career are laudable. After all, many Indian children do grow up to be successful scientists, researchers, doctors, and educators. To ensure that success, however, it is critical that children and parents receive appropriate supportive structures and learn the crucial life skills of positive coping. Children in India appear to be growing up much too stressed, much too soon. We, as responsible adults, need to figure out a way to give their childhood back to them.

References

Abraham, M., & Neogi, S. (1997). The tension is killing. *The Week, 15*(7), 16-20.

Adhyaru, P., & Nandakumar, P. (2003, February 27). *Shrinks called in as exam fever turns to epidemic. The Times of India.* Retrieved July 18, 2003, from http://timesofindia.india times.com/cms.dll/html/uncomp/articleshow?msid=38703643

Ahuja, R. (1993). *Indian social system.* New Delhi: Rajwat Publications.

Bagdi, A. (1998). *Children's perceptions of stressful events and how they cope with them: An Indian experience.* Unpublished doctoral dissertation, Syracuse University.

Bisht, S., & Sinha, D. (1981). Socialization, family, and psychological differentiation. In D. Sinha (Ed.), *Socialization of the Indian child* (pp. 41-54). New Delhi, India: Concept Publishing.

Bronfenbrenner, U. (1979). *The ecology of human development: Experiments by nature and design.* Cambridge, MA: Harvard University Press.

Guha, S. (1996). The girl child is not a lesser child. In J. P. Singh (Ed.), *The Indian woman: Myth and reality* (pp. 88-109). New Delhi, India: Gyan Publishing House.

Jain, M. (1996). The adult child. *India Today, 21*(7), 92-97.

Kakar, S. (1979). Childhood in India: Traditional ideals and contemporary reality. *International Social Science Journal, 31,* 444-456.

Lam, D. J., & Palsane, M. N. (1997). Research on stress and coping: Contemporary Asian approaches. In H. S. R. Rao & D. Sinha (Eds.), *Asian perspectives on psychology* (pp. 74-92). New Delhi, India: Sage.

Matthews, V. (1991, April 14). Do exams pass the test? *The Sunday Times of India.*

Mukherjee, A. (2003, March 02). Parents don't fret, have faith. *The Times of India.* Retrieved July 18, 2003, from http://timesofindia.indiatimes.com/cms.dll/html/uncomp/articleshow?msid=39001479

Muttalib, M. A. (1990). *Child development: A study of health culture of low income urban settlement.* New Delhi, India: Sterling Publishers.

Ogbu, J. U. (1988). Cultural diversity and human development. *New Directions for Child Development, 42,* 11-28.

Rajendran, R., & Kaliappan, K. V. (1991). A factorial study of sources of student academic stress. *Journal of Psychological Researches, 35,* 53-57.

Ramanathan, G. (2002, December 03). Stress gets the children. *The Times of India.* Retrieved July 18, 2003, from http://timesofindia.indiatimes.com/cms.dll/html/uncomp/articleshow?msid=30113530

Roy, B. (2003, June 3). Stress buster yoga for kids. *The Times of India.* Retrieved July 18, 2003, from http://timesofindia.indiatimes.com/cms.dll/html/uncomp/articleshow?msid=2803

Saksena, I. (2002, August 28). Required: Stress busters for smart kids. *The Times of India.* Retrieved July 18, 2003, from http://timesofindia.indiatimes.com/cms.dll/html/uncomp/articleshow?msid=20495256

Saraswathi, T. S., & Dutta, R. (1988). Invisible boundaries: Grooming for adult roles. *A descriptive study of socialization in a poor rural and urban slum setting in Gujarat.* New Delhi, India: Northern Book Centre.

Saraswathi, T. S., & Pai, S. (1997). Socialization in the Indian context. In H. S. R. Kao & D. Sinha (Eds.), *Asian perspectives on psychology* (pp. 74-92). New Delhi, India: Sage.

Sethi, H. (1996). Comment: Seeking a lost childhood. *Seminar, 443,* 46-47.

Sharan, A. (1991, April 2). The overburdened child. *The Independent Journal of Politics and Business,* p. 17.

Singh, H. (2002, April, 22). For children, the pressures are beginning to tell. *The Times of India.* Retrieved July 18, 2003, from http://timesofindia.indiatimes.com/cms.dll/html/uncomp/articleshow?msid=7697271

Tandon, T. (1981). Process of transmission of values in the Indian child. In D. Sinha (Ed.), *Socialization of the Indian child* (pp. 11-30). New Delhi, India: Concept Publishing.

Times News Network. (2002, August 16). NCERT module for preschool. *The Times of India.* Retrieved July 18, 2003, from http://timesofindia.indiatimes.com/cms.dll/html/uncomp/articleshow?msid=19299179

Times News Network. (2003, February 23). Great expectations. *The Times of India.* Retrieved July 18, 2003, from http://timesofindia.indiatimes.com/cms.dll/html/uncomp/articleshow?msid=38332456

Aparna Bagdi is Assistant Professor, Department of Individual and Family Studies, University of Delaware, Newark.

UNIT 3
Nutritional Health

Unit Selections

Key Points to Consider

- What are trans fats and why are they unhealthy?

- What foods are considered healthy? Unhealthy?

- What dietary changes could you make to improve your diet? What is keeping you from making those changes?

- Do you think that fast food restaurants should be forced to limit the amount of fat and sodium in the food items they sell? Why or why not?

Student Website

www.mhcls.com/online

Internet References

Further information regarding these websites may be found in this book's preface or online.

The American Dietetic Association
    http://www.eatright.org
Center for Science in the Public Interest (CSPI)
    http://www.cspinet.org/
Tufts University Nutrition Navigator
    http://www.navigator.tufts.edu

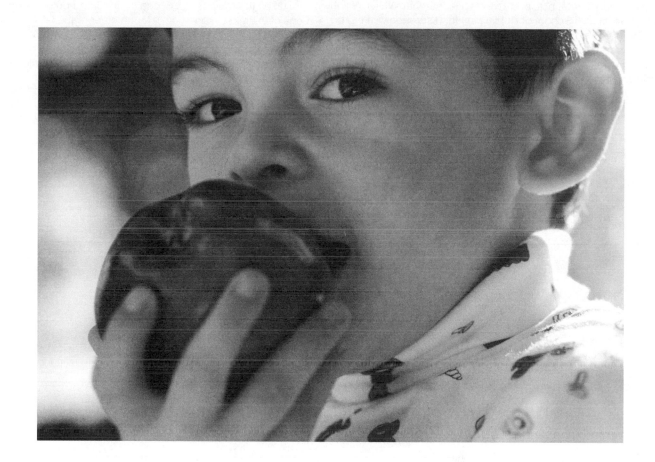

For years, the majority of Americans paid little attention to nutrition, other than to eat three meals a day and, perhaps, take a vitamin supplement. While this dietary style was generally adequate for the prevention of major nutritional deficiencies, medical evidence began to accumulate linking the American diet to a variety of chronic illnesses. In an effort to guide Americans in their dietary choices, the U.S. Dept. of Agriculture and the U.S. Public Health Service review and publish Dietary Guidelines every 5 years. The year 2005 Dietary Guidelines' recommendations are no longer limited to food choices; they include advice on the importance of maintaining a healthy weight and engaging in daily exercise. In addition to the Dietary Guidelines, the Department of Agriculture developed the *Food Guide Pyramid* to show the relative importance of food groups.

Despite an apparent ever-changing array of dietary recommendations from the scientific community, five recommendations remain constant: 1) eat a diet low in saturated fat, 2) eat whole grain foods, 3) drink plenty of fresh water daily, 4) limit your daily intake of sugar and salt, and 5) eat a diet rich in fruits and vegetables. These recommendations, while general in nature, are seldom heeded and in fact many Americans don't eat enough fruits and vegetables and eat too much sugar and fat.

Of all the nutritional findings, the link between dietary fat and coronary heart disease remains the most consistent throughout the literature. The article "The Trouble with Trans Fat," addresses recent research on trans fatty acids, a type of saturated fat. These fats occur naturally in limited amounts in some meats and dairy products. The majority of these fats, however, enter the diet via a process known as hydrogenation. Hydrogenation causes liquid oils to harden into products such as vegetable shortening and margarine. In addition to these products, trans fats are found in many commercially prepared and restaurant foods. Current recommendations suggest that the types of fats consumed may play a much greater role in disease processes than the total amount of fat consumed. As it currently stands, most experts agree that it is prudent to limit our intake of trans fat that appears to raise LDLs, the bad cholesterol, and lower HDLs the good cholesterol and thus increases the risk of heart disease. There's also evidence that trans fats increase the risk of diabetes.

One of the major contributors of trans fat to the American diet is our appetite for fast food, and with the explosive growth of fast-food restaurants serving fried and high fat foods, it is no wonder that fat has gotten a bad name.

While the basic advice on eating healthy remains fairly constant, many Americans are still confused over exactly what to eat. Should their diet be low carbohydrate, high protein, or low fat? When people turn to standards such as the *Food Guide Pyramid*, even here there is some confusion. The *Pyramid,* designed by the Department of Agriculture over 20 years ago, recommends a diet based on grains, fruits, and vegetables with several servings of meats and dairy products. It also restricts the consumption of fats, oils, and sweets. Researcher Walter Willett, from the Harvard School of Public Health, disagrees with the basic tenets of the Pyramid and has actually designed his own version illustrated in "What Does Science Say You Should Eat?" Willett's version draws a distinction between good and bad fats, between whole-grain and refined carbohydrates, and between healthful and less healthful sources of protein. He also moves potatoes into the starch category as opposed to the vegetable category.

Of all the topic areas in health, food and nutrition is certainly one of the most interesting, if for no other reason than for the rate at which dietary recommendations change. Despite all the controversy and conflict, the one message that seems to remain constant is the importance of balance and moderation in everything we eat.

The trouble with trans fat

A new item will soon be appearing on food labels. FDA regulations passed in July 2003 require that food manufacturers begin listing—by no later than January 1, 2006—the trans fat content of their products. Currently, it's included as part of "Total Fat" and is not listed separately. The new requirement has many people wondering, What exactly is trans fat? We've heard it's bad, but what's wrong with it? How much is safe to eat?

What's trans fat?

Trans fat, also known as trans unsaturated fatty acids or trans fatty acids, is naturally found in small amounts in meat and dairy products. But it got its start as a major component of the diet about 100 years ago when food chemists were looking for a cheap alternative to butter. They discovered that by heating vegetable oil and bubbling hydrogen through it, they could create a new type of fat that stayed solid at room temperature and had a longer shelf life. The process, called hydrogenation, converts healthy vegetable oil into unhealthy trans fat.

Today, trans fat is not confined to stick margarines and solid shortenings such as Crisco. Fats found in cooking oils and in commercially prepared foods are often partially hydrogenated to improve flavor and texture and preserve freshness.

Why is trans fat bad for you?

Trans fat packs a one-two punch to the arteries. Saturated fat—the former king of the bad fat hill—does damage by raising LDL (bad) cholesterol, but it redeems itself somewhat by boosting HDL (good) cholesterol. Trans fat both *raises* LDL and lowers HDL— the worst possible combination.

Long-term studies have now shown the resulting impact on health. More than 10 years ago, Harvard researchers with the Nurses' Health Study observed a close correlation between heart disease and a high intake of foods made with partially hydrogenated fats. Analyzing diet and health data from 85,095 women, the investigators found that even after accounting for other risk factors, women who consumed the most trans fatty acids had a 50% greater risk for heart attacks than those who consumed the least. Harvard School of Public Health researchers estimate that hydrogenated fat is responsible for at least 30,000 premature heart disease deaths annually in the United States.

Nutrition Facts
Serving Size 1 cup (228g)
Servings Per Container 2

Amount Per Serving	
Calories 250	Calories from Fat 110

	% Daily Value*
Total Fat 12g	18%
Saturated Fat 3g	15%
Trans Fat 3g	
Cholesterol 30mg	10%
Sodium 470mg	20%
Total Carbohydrate 31g	10%
Dietary Fiber 0g	0%
Sugars 5g	
Protein 5g	

Vitamin A	4%
Vitamin C	2%
Calcium	

Under the new FDA rule, the Nutrition Facts panel will list the amount of trans fat in a serving on a separate line, beneath saturated fat. If trans fat content is less than 0.5 grams per serving, it may be listed at 0 g.

A study published in the October 2003 *American Journal of Clinical Nutrition* linked trans fat to increased waist size in men—another risk factor for heart disease. Dr. Walter Willett, one of the researchers involved in the study and a professor of epidemiology and nutrition at the Harvard School of Public Health, says this effect is probably the same in women. It's not just a matter of taking in more calories. Trans fat appears to affect the body in a specific way that increases abdominal fat.

There's also evidence that trans fat contributes to insulin resistance, raising the risk of type 2 diabetes.

Scientists are beginning to learn more about how trans fat spoils your cholesterol profile. One cause is an increase in the activity of an enzyme called CETP (cholesterol ester transfer protein), which moves cholesterol from HDL to LDL— not a heart healthy move. New research has also linked trans fat to increases in the number of small, dense LDL particles—the kind most likely to contribute to blocked arteries.

How much is too much?

The Institute of Medicine's Food and Nutrition Board says there's no safe level of trans fat intake, and the gov-

Grams of fat per serving of some common foods

Product	Serving size	Total fat	Sat. fat	Trans fat
French fries (fast food	medium	26.9	6.7	7.8
Doughnut	1	18.2	4.7	5.0
Cake, pound	1 slice	16.4	3.4	4.3
Shortening, solid	1tbsp	13.0	3.4	4.2
Wheat crackers	50g	10.0	2.0	4.0
Potato chips	small bag	11.2	1.9	3.2
Margarine, stick	1tbsp	11.0	2.1	2.8
Cookies (cream-filled)	3	6.1	1.2	1.9
Ramen noodle soup	42g	7.2	3.2	0.9
Margarine, tub	1 tbsp	6.7	1.2	0.6
Granola bar, chocolate chip	1 bar (1.5 oz)	7.1	4.4	0.4
Butter	1 tbsp	10.8	7.2	0.3
Milk, whole	1 cup	6.6	4.3	0.2
Mayonnaise (soybean oil)	1 tbsp	10.8	1.6	0

Sources: USDA National Nutritional Database; FDA Center for Food Safety and Applied Nutrition.

ernment sponsored National Cholesterol Education Program urges people to eat as little trans fat as possible. The FDA doesn't recommend eliminating trans fat from the diet because that could result in an inadequate intake of other important nutrients in people who eat a lot of commercially prepared foods. However, the agency doesn't have enough information to establish a "% Daily Value" (recommended daily intake) for trans fat. Therefore the new product label will list only the amount of trans fatty acids in the product. Listing is not required if the total fat content is less than 0.5 grams.

Is there an allowable intake?

What does it mean to know that a serving of chips has 4 grams of trans fat? Many nutrition experts say you should avoid any food with even 1 gram of the stuff. The body doesn't need it, so you should get your consumption as close to zero as possible while maintaining a nutritionally sound diet.

"One of the most important things people can do to improve their health is to avoid trans fat. And that's possible—it just takes awareness," says Willett. He is referring to synthetic trans fat, not to the kind found naturally in beef and dairy products, which may not have the same effects on the body. According to Willett, you should limit your consumption of these foods because of their saturated fat, but they needn't be eliminated.

The good news is that the FDA's announcement has already had an effect. Food makers are scrambling to eliminate trans fat from their products. Many trans fat-free margarines are already available, and some snack and baked goods manufacturers are moving to cut back on their use of trans fat.

How to avoid trans fat

In principle, it should be easy. After all, humans did without synthetic trans fats until 100 years ago. But now it's more complicated because packaged and convenience foods—especially cookies, cakes, crackers, chips, and other snacks—are ubiquitous and usually loaded with trans fat. Trans fat is also found in many restaurant and fast foods, certain cereals, and even some energy and nutrition bars.

Since the new trans fat labeling is strictly voluntary until 2006, how do we know what foods to avoid now? If we stop eating margarine, fried foods such as doughnuts and French fries, and certain prepared foods, we'll cut out at least half the trans fats available in the American diet. (Beef and dairy products generally account for the other half.)

Here are some additional strategies for lowering your intake of trans fat:

- *Be label savvy.* If a product lists shortening or partially hydrogenated or hydrogenated oil as one of its first ingredients, it has a lot of trans fat. Avoid it, or eat it only in very small quantities. If you're eating out, beware of foods fried in partially hydrogenated oils. Some fast food establishments list nutrition information on wall posters or make it available in a handout.

- *Do some math.* Some labels include enough information to allow you to figure out trans fat content, even if it's not listed. If the grams of polyunsaturated fat and monounsaturated fat are given, add them to the grams of saturated fat and subtract the sum from "Total Fat." What's left is trans fat.

- *Choose the better spreader.* Generally, the softer a margarine is at room temperature, the better—that is, the lower in trans fat. One that's labeled trans fat-free is your best bet. Or try using olive oil on your bread or cooked vegetables. If you must choose between butter and a margarine whose trans fat "credentials" are not clearly marked, go with the butter —products that are free of trans fat usually feature that fact prominently on the label, and gram for gram, trans fats are worse than the saturated fats in butter.

- *Fry and saute wisely.* Use canola oil or olive oil. And be on the lookout for true-but-tricky advertising in restaurants and on packages of frozen fried foods. Food that's fried in partially hydrogenated vegetable oils is often labeled "cholesterol free" and "cooked in vegetable oil."

- *Make it yourself.* Trans fat is also found in unexpected places—commercial breads, soups, cereals, bean and other dips, salad dressings, and packaged entrees. Whenever possible, make these foods from scratch, using non-hydrogenated fats.

More questions about trans fat? Visit the FDA's Web page, www.fda.gov/oc/initiatives/transfat

From *Harvard Women's Health Watch*, Volume 11, Number 7, March 2004, pp. 1-3. Copyright © 2004 by Harvard Health Publications Group. Reprinted by permission.

10 MYTHS THAT WON'T QUIT

By Bonnie Liebman

Old myths die hard. And when it comes to diet and health, the misconceptions are endless. Even if you steer clear of claims on herbs and supplements, the "conventional wisdom" isn't always wise.

Some myths have been around for decades ("vitamin C prevents colds"). Others are relatively new ("drink green tea to ward off cancer").

Some of the most persistent myths are generated by the food industry. That's why many people believe that salt doesn't raise blood pressure, chocolate is good for you, eggs are harmless, and pork is "the other white meat."

Here are 10 myths that we can't seem to shake.

1. Soy foods prevent breast cancer.

Most women will do whatever they can to reduce the risk of breast cancer. Maybe that's why they're so willing to believe that the plant estrogens (phytoestrogens) in soy can keep the disease at bay. Yet so far, the evidence is weak.

Researchers in the Netherlands recently reviewed 13 studies—largely from China and Japan—that looked at soy and the risk of breast cancer.[1]

"Overall, results do not show protective effects, with the exception maybe for women who consume phytoestrogens at adolescence or at very high doses," concludes Petra Peeters of the University Medical Center in Utrecht.

What's more, if you exclude studies that asked women who already have breast cancer what they used to eat, that leaves only four studies that asked healthy women about soy and then waited to see who got cancer, she adds. "And none of them found statistically significant breast cancer reductions.'

The bottom line: it's still too early to say whether soy—or other phytoestrogens—might protect the breast.

What else might soy do?

■ **Prostate cancer.** Soy's impact on the risk of prostate cancer is still muddy, in part because most Americans eat too little soy for studies to detect any lower risk. However, researchers have tested soy's impact on PSA (prostate-specific antigen) levels, with mixed results.

In a recent study, soy grits (about two ounces a day) lowered PSA by 13 percent in eight men with prostate cancer.[2] In studies on healthy men, though, PSA didn't budge.[3] And experts are now questioning whether small changes in PSA levels matter.

■ **Hot flashes.** So far, well-designed studies have found that soy (or plant estrogens from supplements like red clover) has little impact on hot flashes and other symptoms of menopause.

Researchers at the University of Minnesota recently examined 20 trials on menopause and soy foods, beverages, powders, or extracts. Nearly all came up empty.[4]

"The available evidence suggests that phytoestrogens available as soy foods, soy extracts, and red clover extracts do not improve hot flushes or other menopausal symptoms," conclude Minnesota's Erin Krebs and colleagues.

The bottom line: soy foods do seem to lower cholesterol, so they may help protect your heart. But whether they do more is a question mark.

2. Olive is the healthiest oil.

Fish oil is probably the healthiest, but you can't pour it on your salad or cook with it. Olive is certainly *one* of the good oils. Whether it's the best is unclear.

"**M**yths" may be the wrong word.

It's not that these beliefs are dead wrong. More often, they're promising theories that are backed by too little evidence. Or they're outdated ideas that have crumpled under the weight of recent research.

In this issue, we clarify the evidence on 10 assumptions that people rarely question.

"The data suggest that any oil that's high in unsaturated fats—whether it's polyunsaturated or monounsaturated—is associated with a decreased risk of cardiovascular disease," says Alice Lichtenstein of the U.S. Department of Agriculture Jean Mayer Human Nutrition Research Center on Aging at Tuffs University in Boston.

"Canola is probably better than olive oil because it's lower in saturated fat," Lichtenstein explains. What's more, canola has more polyunsaturated fat than olive oil, "and polys lower LDL ['bad' cholesterol] more than monos."

So why not stick with soy and canola? Both have more of a polyunsaturated fat called alpha-linolenic acid (ALA) than olive. ALA is an omega-3 fat that may help lower the risk of heart disease.

But if preliminary studies hold up, ALA may also raise (slightly) the risk of prostate cancer. Right now that's a big if.

"I don't think the data is strong enough for recommendations," says Lichtenstein.

And there are other ways to cut back on ALA. "Red meat and dairy fat are also sources of ALA, and they have been more consistently related to higher prostate cancer risk," says Ed Giovannucci of the Harvard School of Public Health.

Our advice: at home, switch off between canola and olive.

Since roughly 80 percent of the oil used in the U.S. is soy, odds are you already get plenty from salad dressings, mayonnaise, and restaurant foods. You wouldn't want olive oil in your blueberry muffin recipe anyway.

3. Vitamin C prevents colds.

Ever since Linus Pauling, people have rushed for a bottle of vitamin C at the first sniffle. And some take extra C all winter in hopes of keeping germs at bay.

Researchers recently looked carefully at 30 trials that tested the vitamin and colds. Their conclusion: taking high doses (up to 1,000 mg—or one gram—a day) for several winter months didn't ward off those pesky cold germs.[5]

However, vitamin C did appear to shorten colds slightly—by a little less than half a day per cold. On average, the vitamin reduced days of misery by about eight percent, but the results varied widely.

It doesn't hurt to try vitamin C—about 1,000 mg a day—once you feel that sore throat or reach for the tissues. Just don't expect miracles.

4. If your blood sugar, triglycerides, cholesterol, and blood pressure aren't high, don't worry.

Even before you hit "high," you hit trouble.

Your risk of a heart attack, stroke, or diabetes doesn't jump from low to high when your number crosses a sharp cutoff. It's gradual.

That's why experts keep ratcheting down what's "normal." For example:

■ **Blood sugar.** In April 2004, the National Institute of Diabetes & Digestive & Kidney Diseases (NIDDK) announced that 40 percent of U.S. adults have "pre-diabetes," which means their fasting blood sugar is between 100 and 125. (Over 125 is diabetes.) Using the old cutoff (110), only 20 percent of adults had pre-diabetes.

■ **Blood pressure.** In May 2003, the National Heart, Lung, and Blood Institute (NHLBI) declared that an estimated 22 million Americans have pre-hypertension—that is, blood pressure over 120 (systolic) or over 80 (diastolic). (Another 25 percent have hypertension, or high blood pressure, which starts at 140 over 90.)

■ **Triglycerides.** Triglycerides under 200 used to be "normal." Now normal ends at 150, and "borderline high" ranges from 150 to 200, says the NHLBI.

■ **HDL ("good") cholesterol.** The lower your HDL, the higher your risk of heart disease. "Low" used to be 35 or below. Now it's 40 or below (for men) and 50 or below (for women).

■ **LDL ("bad") cholesterol.** A "borderline high" LDL is 130 to 160. But 129 isn't ideal. So NHLBI now makes it clear that only LDLs under 100 are "optimal." An LDL between 100 and 129 is "above optimal."

Why do the numbers keep dropping (or rising for HDL)? Studies show that people in that gray area between "low" and "high" are at risk.

Take blood sugar. "Many people with pre-diabetes go on to develop type 2 diabetes within 10 years," says the NIDDK. But not if they do something about it.

"Research has clearly shown that losing five to seven percent of body weight through diet and increased physical activity can prevent or delay pre-diabetes from progressing to type 2 diabetes," explains NIDDK director Allen Spiegel.

"The emphasis has shifted from treatment to prevention," says Tufts's Alice Lichtenstein. And most people can prevent illness with diet, exercise, or other lifestyle changes.

"We're trying to minimize disease progression without putting everyone on medication," she says.

5. People gain a lot of weight over the holidays.

Office parties, neighborhood gatherings, family celebrations—from Thanksgiving to New Year's Day, most Americans are surrounded by luscious, tempting, irresistible food. So the conventional wisdom—that most of us start the new year about five pounds heavier—seems reasonable.

Reasonable but not necessarily true.

In 2000, researchers tracked 200 people from late September to early March, and, in some cases, into June.[6] On average, they gained only about a pound during the holidays.

But that doesn't mean you can live it up from turkey to eggnog:

■ **You might not lose what you gained.** In the study, most people lost little weight after the holidays, whether they tried to or not. And one pound is half of what the average person gains in a year. Those two pounds may not seem like much, but after 10 years, they could easily move you from trim to chubby.

■ **You may not be average.** Among the overweight or obese participants in the study, 14 percent gained more than five pounds. What's more, the participants may not be typical.

"The study followed employees of the National Institutes of Health, an upscale, professional, health-conscious bunch if ever there was one," notes Susan Roberts of the Human Nutrition Research Center on Aging at Tuffs University.

"Weight gain is a likely consequence of overindulgence," she cautions. "It's always easier to overeat than to lose weight, because our bodies don't seem to count a few thousand extra calories, but start screaming hunger if we cut a few thousand."

6. Antioxidants prevent cancer and heart disease.

It sounded so convincing.

Damage caused by renegade oxygen could trigger cancer, injure arteries, hamper vision, and accelerate aging, said enthusiasts. And antioxidants—like beta-carotene and vitamins C and E—could neutralize the damage before it took hold.

But so far, the best studies—trials that randomly assigned people to take antioxidants or a placebo—have flopped:

■ **Cancer.** In two trials, high doses of beta-carotene raised the risk of lung cancer in smokers. In other studies, the antioxidant had no impact on skin, mouth, or throat cancer.

And when European researchers pooled the results of 14 studies on more than 170,000 people, they found that vitamins A, C, E, and beta-carotene—separately or together—failed to cut the risk of cancers of the colon, pancreas, stomach, or esophagus.[7]

"We could not find evidence that antioxidant supplements can prevent gastrointestinal cancers," the authors concluded.

■ **Heart disease.** "With vitamin E and heart disease, the evidence looked rosy a few years ago," says Meir Stampfer, chairman of the department of epidemiology at the Harvard School of Public Health.

Since then, researchers examined evidence from three trials testing beta-carotene supplements on 70,000 people and five trials testing vitamin E on 29,000 patients at high risk of cardiovascular disease.[8]

"The results of these trials have been disappointing and failed to confirm any protective effect of these vitamins for either cancer or for cardiovascular dis-

ease," wrote Robert Clarke of the Radcliffe Infirmary in Oxford, England.

That's not to say that all antioxidants are useless. "The door isn't closed," says Stampfer. For example, a large trial is still testing whether vitamin E and selenium can prevent prostate cancer.

The mistake, he explains, is to assume that if antioxidants work, it's because they're antioxidants.

"It's a myth that antioxidants are a meaningful category," says Stampfer. "Some, like vitamin C, are antioxidants in one setting and pro-oxidants in others. You have to look at the specifics."

If vitamin E and selenium protect the prostate, it may not be because they're antioxidants. "They may work through different pathways," says Stampfer. "To say that a food is rich in antioxidants is meaningless."

7. A high-fiber diet prevents colon cancer.

"The National Cancer Institute believes eating the right foods may reduce your risk of some kinds of cancer," said the All-Bran label in 1984. "That's why a healthy diet includes high-fiber foods like bran cereals."

Within months, President Reagan underwent surgery for colon cancer. The media advised people to eat more fiber to lower their risk.

But the evidence wasn't as airtight as it sounded.

In 2000, two trials testing fiber-rich diets on precancerous colon polyps came up empty. One found no fewer polyps in roughly 1,000 people who ate a diet rich in fiber (33 grams a day) and fruits and vegetables (6 1/2 servings a day) than in 1,000 people who ate their usual diet (with about 19 grams of fiber) for four years.[9]

A second trial found no fewer polyps in 700 people who ate 14 grams a day of wheat bran fiber than in nearly 600 people who ate only two grams a day of fiber for three years.[10]

It's always possible that the trials didn't last long enough, but many experts have thrown in the towel. "The theory is close to disproved," says Stampfer.

But don't throw out your All-Bran yet, he adds. "People should still eat fiber

because we have strong evidence that it has other benefits."

Among them: "Fiber—especially grain fiber—has been consistently linked to a lower risk of cardiovascular disease," Stampfer explains. Researchers aren't sure how fiber may protect the heart, but the link shows up in study after study.[11]

"And there's no question that fiber decreases the risk of constipation and diverticulitis," he adds. "They're not marquee diseases, but they make people uncomfortable and kill some."

8. Don't drink milk if you have a cold.

"Milk makes mucus," goes the conventional wisdom. Yet few studies have tested milk's effect on cold sufferers. (Okay, so it's not a life-or-death issue that's crying out for research funds.)

However, Australian researchers took up the challenge in 1990.[12] They infected 50 volunteers with a cold virus and asked them to keep track of how much milk or other dairy foods they consumed for 10 days. Meanwhile, all used tissues were weighed to measure nasal secretions.

The results: mucus ranged from zero to one ounce a day, and milk ranged from zero to 11 glasses a day, but one had nothing to do with the other.

It's hard to know how to sort out the good and bad things you hear about dairy these days. Here's a brief rundown:

■ **Weight loss.** "Burn more fat, lose weight," promise the milk ads. "3 servings of dairy a day in a reduced-calorie diet supports weight loss."

In fact, the evidence comes largely from research by Michael Zemel, a University of Tennessee professor. His only published study in humans showed more weight loss in 11 people who had three servings of dairy a day.[13]

But Zemel has a stake in finding that dairy aids weight loss because he has a patent on the claim. (He's already licensed it to Yoplait, the American Dairy Association, and the National Dairy Council.)

Until other researchers get into the act, stay skeptical.

■ **Cancer.** It's not so much dairy, but calcium, that's under scrutiny. So far, it looks like too much calcium—more than 1,500 mg a day—may slightly raise the risk of prostate cancer.[14] That's how much you'd get in a typical diet plus four servings of milk (or yogurt or cheese). However, other studies show that roughly 1,000 mg of calcium or at least one glass of milk a day may cut the risk of colon cancer.[15]

Where does that leave consumers? Women can simply go for the recommended levels (from food and supplements). That's 1,000 mg a day if you're 50 or younger, and 1,200 mg a day if you're over 50. Women have a higher risk of osteoporosis than men anyway.

Men, on the other hand, should try not to exceed the recommended levels. "We know of no benefits at intakes that exceed 1,500 milligrams a day," says Ed Giovannucci of the Harvard School of Public Health.

"So it may be advisable for men to not exceed about 1,000 milligrams of calcium a day." If that seems scary, remember that if calcium raises the risk of prostate cancer, it's not by much.

9. Hamburgers are safe to eat when the meat is no longer pink.

Chicken is safe when the pink is gone, the juices run clear, the leg moves easily in its socket, or the thigh reaches an internal temperature of 180°F (170°F for a breast). That's enough to kill *Salmonella* and *Campylobacter*, the usual poultry contaminants.

But ground beef is a different story. *E. coli* O157:H7 can survive even when the pink is gone and the juices are clear. And you don't want to mess around with O157:H7.

In some people, it can cause severe bloody diarrhea and stomach cramps. They're the lucky ones.

Roughly two to seven percent of infections—often those in the elderly and children under five—lead to hemolytic uremic syndrome. Red blood cells are destroyed, the kidneys fail, and even with intensive care, three to five percent die. (Antibiotics don't help and may even hurt.)

About a third of the survivors have abnormal kidney function many years later, and a few require long-term dialysis. Another eight percent have lifelong complications like high blood pressure, seizures, blindness, or paralysis, or lose part of their bowel.

How can you tell when your burger is done? Use a thermometer to make sure the internal temperature reaches 160°F. (Chain restaurants typically cook burgers enough to kill *E. coli*.)

Beyond burgers, make sure your milk, juice, or apple cider has been pasteurized. Pasteurizing heats beverages enough to kill the *E. coli*. If you're elderly, under age five, have a weak immune system, or simply want to play it safe, skip raw bean or alfalfa sprouts. You can wash other fruits and vegetables, but there's no way (yet) to make sure that sprouts are clean.

10. Being overweight is largely a threat to your heart and risk of diabetes.

Extra pounds can make your heart pound when you exercise. Maybe that's why people remember that being overweight puts a strain on the heart. And many know that the risk of diabetes shoots up with weight gain.

But they tend to forget that obesity can wreak havoc elsewhere. For example, after tobacco smoking, obesity is the principal cause of cancer in the U.S.

"Being heavy or gaining weight as an adult increases the risk for a number of cancers," says Rachel Ballard-Barbash of the National Cancer Institute. "The list includes postmenopausal breast cancer, colorectal cancer, endometrial cancer, esophageal cancer, and kidney cancer."

And it's not just cancer.

"Many people aren't aware that obesity also increases the risk of stroke, hypertension, gastroesophageal reflux disease, gallstones, osteoarthritis, and venous thrombosis—that's when blood clots form in the legs and sometimes travel to the lungs," says JoAnn Manson of Harvard Medical School and Brigham and Women's Hospital in Boston.

What's more, some risks start to climb with just a small spare tire. "Even a weight gain of 15 to 20 pounds during adulthood increases the risk of diabetes, high blood pressure, and coronary heart disease," she adds.

On the flip side, losing 10 to 20 pounds can cut those risks. "If you're overweight, losing even five to 10 percent of your starting weight can significantly improve blood pressure, cholesterol levels, and blood sugar levels," says Manson.

Notes

1. *Breast Cancer Res. Treat. 77:* 171, 2003.
2. *Urology 64:* 510, 2004.
3. *Cancer Epidemiol. Biomarkers Prev. 13:* 644, 2004.
4. *Obstet. Gynecol. 104:* 824, 2004.
5. *Cochrane Database Syst. Rev. 2:* CD000980, 2000.
6. *New Eng. J. Med. 342:* 861, 2000.
7. *Lancet 364:* 1219, 2004.
8. *Cardiovasc. Drugs Ther. 16:* 411, 2002.
9. *New Eng. J. Med. 342:* 1149, 2000.
10. *New Eng. J. Med. 342:* 1156, 2000.
11. *Arch. Intern. Med. 164:* 370, 2004.
12. *Amer. Rev. Respir. Dis. 141:* 352, 1990.
13. *Obes. Res. 12:* 582, 2004.
14. *Cancer Epidemiol. Biomarkers Prev. 12:* 597, 2003.
15. *J. Nat. Cancer Inst. 96:* 1015, 2004.

What Does Science Say You Should Eat?

Most diets aren't realistic or advisable, including the U.S. agriculture department's famous food pyramid. Instead, a Harvard scientist recommends a new way of eating based on the world's largest and longest food study.

By Brad Lemley

America clearly needs dietary guidance.—More than 44 million people are clinically obese compared with 30 million a decade ago, putting them at increased risk for heart disease, stroke, type 2 diabetes, and breast, prostate, and colon cancers. In the meantime, the noun *diet* seems to attract a different adjective every week, including Atkins, Ornish, Cooper, grapefruit, rice, protein, Scarsdale, South Beach, Beverly Hills, Best Chance, Eat Smart, and Miracle, not to mention Help, I'm Southern and I Can't Stop Eating. While some of these plans overlap, others seem to specifically contradict each other, notably the meat-intensive regime of the late Robert Atkins versus the near-vegetarian program of Dean Ornish.—No wonder Americans are tempted to follow Mark Twain's admonition to "eat what you like and let the food fight it out inside." But still, we wonder: Is there really an optimum way to eat?—Although debate rages, academic nutrition researchers have begun to form a consensus around a plan with an important advantage—it is based on a preponderance of sound science. The regime does not as yet have a name, but it might well be called the Willett diet, after its leading proponent, Walter Willett, chairman of the department of nutrition at the Harvard School of Public

Health.—Featuring abundant fruits, vegetables, whole grains, and vegetable oils, as well as optional portions of fish and chicken, Willett's plan resembles the much-touted Mediterranean diet shown in several studies to reduce the risk of heart disease. Nonetheless, Willett resists the comparison. "The Mediterranean diet is specific to a certain climate and culture," he says, adding that by focusing on healthy ingredients rather than specific dishes, "anyone can adapt this plan to his own tastes." The results: stable blood-sugar levels, easier weight control, clearer arteries, and overall better health.

In this case it's hard science, not just opinion. Willett's plan is based on the largest long-term dietary survey ever undertaken: the 121,700-participant Nurses' Health Study, begun in 1976 by Harvard Medical School professor Frank Speizer, with dietary assessments supervised by Willett since 1980. The study isn't just big: Willett carefully crafted it so that he and others could extract specific recommendations about food intake. Participants even surrender blood and toenail samples so that Willett can track absorption of trace elements and other nutrients. If a participant reports a major illness, such as heart attack or cancer, "we write for permission to obtain medi-

cal records for further details," says Willett. To ensure that the data include both sexes and two generations, Willett and several colleagues also launched the Health Professionals Follow-Up Study, which includes 52,000 men, and the Nurses' Health Study II, a survey of 116,000 younger women.

In the past, nutritional scientists have largely relied on studies of animals, small groups of people, and/or petri-dish biochemistry that may not reflect the vagaries of human metabolism, although Willett uses such studies when he deems it appropriate. His access to a unique quarter-million-person pool of humans who carefully track both their diets and their health lends added credibility to his research. "When you put animal, metabolic, and epidemiological studies together and they all point in the same direction, you can be pretty confident about your conclusions," Willett says.

'Nutrition used to be like religion. Everyone said, I have the truth, everyone else is wrong'

While soft-spoken and self-effacing in person, Willett isn't shy about using this formidable database to take on the federal establishment.

WILLETT VS. ORNISH VS. ATKINS

Walter Willett's dietary recommendations are similar in many ways to those advanced by another doctor-nutritionist, Dean Ornish, who pioneered an ultralow-fat, near-vegetarian regime that has been shown to halt or reduce coronary blockage in most heart patients. Both Willett and Ornish emphasize whole grains, fruits, and vegetables, and both minimize animal proteins. But they part ways on fats: Willett recommends replacing saturated fats in the American diet with unsaturated ones, while Ornish suggests sharply cutting fat intake altogether, especially for those at risk for heart disease. "No one has shown that the kind of diet that Walter Willett recommends can reverse heart disease," says Ornish.

For his part, Willett insists that "replacing saturated fats with unsaturated fats is a safe, proven, and delicious way to cut the rates of heart disease." He says the Lyon Diet Heart study, a French trial that tracked heart-attack survivors on an oil-rich Mediterranean diet versus those on the low-fat American Heart Association diet, showed a significant drop in second attacks for the Lyon group. Ornish responds that the drop in deaths in

that study was most likely due to increasing heart-healthy omega-3 fats and decreasing intake of omega-6 fats, saturated fats, animal protein, and cholesterol, not to high overall consumption of fat. Ornish recommends that everyone consume three grams of omega-3 fats daily, either through eating fish or taking supplements.

In contrast with both Willett and Ornish, the late Robert Atkins recommended a meat-intensive, protein-rich regime. "Studies at Duke University, the University of Cincinnati, and the University of Pennsylvania all show that people can lose significant weight, lower their triglycerides, and improve their HDL [high-density lipoprotein] cholesterol levels by consuming protein and limiting carbohydrates," says Stuart Trager, an orthopedic surgeon who assumed the spokesman's mantle for the diet after Atkins's death in April 2003. Trager believes the real strength of the Atkins diet is that "it is something people are willing and able to do."

Willett concedes that Atkins "was really onto something. He believed, correctly, that most people can better control

their weight by reducing the glycemic load of the diet than by other means. But there is evidence that the traditional Atkins diet, which is high in animal fat, is not optimal. There are benefits to having cereal in one's diet. There is relief from constipation, and we do see [in the Nurses' Health Study] some benefit for heart disease and diabetes. This is probably partially from the fiber in whole grains, and also partly from the other minerals and vitamins that come along with whole grains that are in short supply in many people's diets."

While at first blush the three approaches seem sharply divergent, Trager sounds a conciliatory note. "No one has ever bothered to point out that we are compatriots on many points," he says. All three nutritionists share an emphasis on reducing blood-sugar spikes by reducing the glycemic load. Moreover, all three condemn trans fats, white flour, and sugar. "There really is universal agreement that you should cut those things out of your diet," Trager says.
—Brad Lemley

His Healthy Eating Pyramid differs radically from the Food Guide Pyramid pushed by the U.S. Department of Agriculture. "At best, the USDA pyramid offers wishy-washy, scientifically unfounded advice," Willett argues in his book, *Eat, Drink, and Be Healthy: The Harvard Medical School Guide to Healthy Eating.* At worst, he adds, "the misinformation contributes to overweight, poor health, and unnecessary early deaths."

The numbers back him up. Men and women in Willett's studies whose diets most closely paralleled the Healthy Eating Pyramid's guidelines lowered their risk of major chronic disease by 20 percent and 11 percent respectively, according to an article published in the December 2002 issue of *The American Journal of Clinical Nutrition.* That compares with reduced risks of 11 percent and 3 percent for those whose diets most

closely mirrored the USDA pyramid's guidelines.

"Nutrition used to be like religion. Everyone said, 'I have the truth, everyone else is wrong,' and there wasn't much data to refute that," says Willett. "Now we're starting to have a real scientific basis for understanding what you should eat."

JUST INSIDE THE DOOR OF WILLETT'S OFFICE AT the Harvard School of Public Health in Boston sits his bicycle, mud-spattered from his daily commute over the Charles River from his home in Cambridge. Past that, on top of a pile of medical journals, perches a plastic bag full of plump, homegrown cherry tomatoes, a late-season-harvest gift from his administrative assistant. Willett knows good tomatoes. As a member of a fifth-generation Michigan farming family, he paid his undergradu-

ate tuition at Michigan State by raising vegetables, and today he grows "as much as possible" in his tiny urban backyard.

Behind the cluttered desk sits Willett himself, trim, toned, and turned out in a sharp gray suit. "All you have to do is take a look at Walter to see the value of his research. The proof is in the pudding," says David Jenkins, a nutrition researcher at the University of Toronto. Willett vigorously follows his own plan and at age 58 reports that his weight, cholesterol, and triglycerides are all where they should be. He is, in short, the picture of where applied nutritional science might deliver us all, if we had the proper information.

That's the problem. In recent years, Willett says, the American public has been victimized by dodgy advice. Not only has obesity skyrocketed but "the incidence of heart disease is also not going down anymore. It has really stalled."

What happened? In Willett's view, things began to go awry in the mid-1980s, when a National Institutes of Health conference decreed that to prevent heart disease, all Americans except children under 2 years old should reduce their fat intake from 40 percent to 30 percent of their total daily calories. The press touted the recommendation as revealed truth, and the USDA's Food Guide Pyramid, released in 1992, reflects this view, calling for 6 to 11 servings of bread, cereal, rice, and pasta daily, while fats and oils are to be used "sparingly."

Too bad, says Willett. "The low-fat mantra has contributed to obesity. The nutrition community told people they had to worry only about counting fat grams. That encouraged the creation of thousands of low-fat products. I call it 'the SnackWell revolution.'" Blithely consuming low-fat foods full of carbohydrates is a prescription for portliness, says Willett, adding that any farmer knows this. "If you pen up an animal and feed it grain, it will get fat. People are no different."

The problem with overeating refined carbohydrates such as white flour and sucrose (table sugar) is that amylase, an enzyme, quickly converts them into the simple sugar called glucose. That goads the pancreas to overproduce insulin, the substance that conducts glucose into the cells. But excessive sugar is toxic to cells, so after years of glucose and insulin overload, the cells can become insulin resistant and may no longer allow insulin to easily push glucose inside them. That keeps blood glucose levels high, forcing the pancreas to make even more insulin in a desperate attempt to jam the stuff through cell membranes. Willett likens the effect to an overworked, undermaintained pump that eventually wears out. Type 2 diabetes can be one result, but Willett contends that insulin-resistant people who don't develop full-blown diabetes still face significant health risks.

Other researchers agree. Stanford endocrinologist Gerald Reaven coined the term Syndrome X to describe the constellation of health problems that spring from insulin resistance. Until the late 1980s, Reaven says, "the common scientific view was that insulin resistance only mattered if it led all the way to type 2 diabetes. Looking at the data, it's clear that most people who are insulin resistant don't get diabetes but are greatly at risk for coronary heart disease, hypertension, non-alcoholic-type liver disease, polycystic ovary syndrome, and several kinds of cancer."

In the case of heart disease, Reaven says that high blood concentrations of insulin and glucose can damage the endothelium that lines coronary arteries and set the stage for the formation of plaques. "A big problem is the lack of drugs to treat this problem," he adds. "A lot of doctors' education comes from drug companies. They know about cholesterol because everyone is pushing their statin. They know about hypertension because there are multiple hypertensive drugs. But they know a lot less about insulin resistance and its consequences, and that's unfortunate."

Syndrome X, also known as metabolic syndrome or insulin-resistance syndrome, is largely unknown to the public as well. While many people avoid cholesterol and fat-laden foods, few understand the threat posed by carbohydrate excess. That needs to change, says Willett. "Cholesterol is relevant, but the danger is overblown," he says. "Syndrome X is the global public-health problem of the 21st century. Almost certainly the vast majority of Americans have a higher degree of insulin resistance than is optimal."

The Willett plan aims to even out the glucose roller coaster through an emphasis on foods with low glycemic loads—foods that convert to glucose slowly—like whole grains, plant oils, and vegetables. This keeps blood glucose levels relatively constant, sparing the pancreas overwork. Steady blood glucose also helps keep the appetite in check,

which makes maintaining a healthy weight easier, says Willett. So instead of high carb, low fat, one might summarize the Willett plan's directive as good carb, good fat.

"People are being told to reduce fat and eat more carbohydrates. For many people, particularly overweight people with a high degree of insulin resistance, that produces exactly the opposite of what they need," says Willett. Randomized trials, he says, show that people on low-fat diets generally lose two to four pounds after several weeks but then gain back the weight even while continuing the diet. "Most of them would be better off reducing carbs, switching to better carbs, and increasing their intake of healthy fats."

'Instead of high carb, low fat, one might summarize the Willet plan's directive as good carb, good fat'

WILLETT, LIKE VIRTUALLY EVERY OTHER NUTRITION researcher, advises eating vegetables in abundance, consuming alcohol in moderation, and taking a daily multivitamin to cover nutritional gaps. He also touts fish as a source of protein and heart-protective n-3 fatty acids, which are also known as omega-3 acids. (Those who worry about mercury contamination in fish got some good news recently: In one study conducted in the Seychelles, a group of islands in the Indian Ocean, scientists from the University of Rochester Medical Center tracked pregnant women who ate an average of 12 fish meals a week, about 10 times the quantity of fish eaten by the average American. "We've found no evidence that the low levels of mercury in seafood are harmful," said lead author Gary Myers. Moreover, various tests indicated that the women's children suffered no adverse cognitive, behavioral, or neurological effects.)

High on the list of food ingredients Willett counsels avoiding are hydrogenated fats, often referred to

GOOD CARBS/BAD CARBS

The glycemic index (GI) is a way of measuring how quickly the carbohydrate in a given food raises the level of blood sugar. So eating a low-GI food causes a slow, mild rise, while the same quantity of carbohydrate in a high-GI food will trigger a faster, bigger rise. A GI of 55 or less is considered low, 56 to 69 is medium, and 70 or more is high.

But the GI is of limited use in the real world of pears, pork, and pudding because it ignores how much of that food a person eats. A few years ago, Walter Willett pioneered the concept of the glycemic load (GL), a measurement that factors in the quantity of carbohydrates eaten in a single serving of a particular food. The carbohydrates in parsnips, for example, are quickly converted to glucose, so parsnips have a rather high index of 97, plus or minus 19 (the numbers are sometimes imprecise because they are based on feeding foods to test subjects and monitoring their blood-sugar response, which can vary for many reasons). But parsnips have a GL of just 12, because a single 80-gram serving contains a relatively small amount of carbohydrate. A GL of 10 or less is considered low, 11 to 19 is medium, and, 20 or more is high. Consistently eating low-GL foods evens out blood-sugar peaks and valleys, which Willett says helps keep appetite and weight under control. Eating low-GL foods also reduces the risk of developing type 2 diabetes. When Willett says "good carbs," he is essentially referring to fiber-rich, low-GL foods.

Generally, whole grains have lower glycemic loads than refined grains. For example, a 150-gram serving of brown rice has a GL of 18, while the same serving of quick-cooking white rice has a GL of 29. Although the photographs in this story tally the "sugar equivalence" of the carbohydrates in various American foods, the glycemic index and glycemic load of each of these foods needs to be considered as well. The glycemic numbers accompanying the photographs in this article are from Janette Brand-Miller of the University of Sydney, based on a table published in the July 2002 issue of *The American Journal of Clinical Nutrition*. An adaptation of that table can be seen at `diabetes.about.com/library/mendosagi/ngilists.htm`.

—*B. L.*

as trans fats, which are found in shortening, margarine, deep-fried foods, and packaged baked goods. That advice was controversial when Willett published a groundbreaking paper on the subject in 1991, but it has since become close to dogma. "Both controlled-feeding studies that have examined the effects of trans fat on blood cholesterol and epidemiological studies of trans-fat intake in relation to the risk of heart disease and diabetes indicate they are considerably worse than saturated fats," he says.

Daily exercise is essential, Willett adds, and he confirms the often-cited advice that walking is the best choice for many people. The Nurses' Health Study revealed a "very strong link" between walking and protection against heart disease: Women who walked an average of three hours a week were 35 percent less likely to have a heart attack over an eight-year period than those who walked less. It may seem odd that Willett includes exercise in his Healthy Eating Pyramid, but he is adamant that exercise and diet cannot be teased apart. "It doesn't have to be extreme. I run along the Charles for 25 minutes most mornings." A half hour daily of moderate activity offers "impressive health benefits," he says,

but there is "added benefit for greater intensity for longer times."

Willett's more iconoclastic conclusions include the heretical notion that soy—touted as a miracle food that fights cancer, obesity, and virtually every other human ill—may have "a dark side." He points to a British study in which 48 women with suspicious breast lumps were randomly assigned to receive either no supplement or one containing soy isoflavones (a compound in soybeans molecularly similar to estrogen) for 14 days. Those taking the supplement showed substantially more cell growth in the tissue removed than the women who were not taking the soy. Another troubling study showed memory loss and other cognitive declines in elderly Japanese men in Hawaii who stuck to their traditional soy-based diet, as opposed to those who switched to a more of a Western diet. "In moderation, soy is fine," says Willett. "Stuffed into everything, you could get into trouble." And soy isoflavone supplements, he counsels, should be regarded as "totally untested new drugs."

Willett also counsels that dairy products—which supply concentrated calories and saturated fat—are not the best way to get calcium

and that the recommended daily intake of 1,200 milligrams daily for adults over 50 appears to be more than what's needed. His advice: Eat calcium-bearing vegetables, including leafy greens, take calcium supplements if you're a woman, and exercise. "The evidence for physical activity being protective against fractures is huge," he says.

'No research has ever shown that people who eat more eggs have more heart attacks than people who eat fewer eggs'

And he defends eggs. Although cholesterol fears have caused American per capita egg consumption to drop from 400 to 250 per year, "no research has ever shown that people who eat more eggs have more heart attacks than people who eat fewer eggs," Willett says. A 2001 Kansas State University study identified a type of lecithin called phosphatidylcholine in eggs that interferes with cholesterol absorption, which may explain why many studies have found no association between egg intake and blood cholesterol level. If the breakfast menu option is a white-flour bagel or an egg fried in vegetable oil, says Willett, "the egg is the better choice."

Perhaps the most comprehensive studies Willett has assembled compare the health consequences of eating saturated versus unsaturated fat. The term *saturated* means that every available site along each fat molecule's carbon chain is filled with a hydrogen atom; such fats—including butter and animal fat—are solids at room temperature. There are two types of unsaturated fats: monounsaturated fats such as olive oil, which are missing one pair of hydrogen atoms, and polyunsaturated fats such as soy, corn, and canola oils, which lack more than one pair. Both sorts are liquid at room temperature.

Some researchers have questioned whether saturated fat is dangerous. In his book, *The Cholesterol Myths: Exposing the Fallacy That Saturated Fat and Cholesterol Cause Heart Disease*, Swedish physician Uffe Ravnskov asserts that as of 1998, 27 studies on diet and heart disease had been published regarding 34 groups of patients; in 30 of those groups investigators found no difference in animal fat consumption between those who had heart disease and those who did not. "Anyone who reads the literature in this field with an open mind soon discovers that the emperor has no clothes," Ravnskov writes.

Willett turns to his Nurses' Health mega-study for the definitive word. "The amounts of specific fats did make a difference," he says. "Women who ate more unsaturated fat instead of saturated fat had fewer heart problems." Willett calculated that replacing 5 percent of saturated fat calories with unsaturated would cut the risk of heart attack or death from heart disease by 40 percent. Other studies—notably the French Lyon Diet Heart study, begun in 1988—show a similar correlation.

A HEALTHY DIET PLAN IS WORTHLESS IF PEOPLE won't stick to it, and Susan Roberts, director of the energy metabolism laboratory at Tufts University, contends that Willett's regimen is too severe. "Most people would say his recommendations are healthy but that other, less difficult diets are healthy too," she says.

Difficult is in the palate of the eater. The last half of Willett's book aims to dispel any taint of Calvinism with recipes that verge on the sybaritic, including pork tenderloin with pistachio-gremolata crust, chicken enchilada casserole, and grilled salmon steaks with papaya-mint salsa. On the other hand, some resolve might be required to soldier through a few of the other dishes listed there, including hearty oat-wheat berry bread or the onion-crusted tofu-steak sandwich. But most people, Willett believes, can summon the willpower to substitute whole-wheat flour for white and plant oils for shortening or lard, and eat less sugar overall. "I think what I suggest is not severely restrictive, because it can be achieved mainly by substitution," rather than slavishly following recipes, Willett says. In any case, "it does not mean you cannot eat any of those foods but rather that they should be de-emphasized."

So take heart. Even Willett has a little chocolate now and then.

From *Discover*, February 2004, pp. 43-49. Copyright © 2004 by Brad Lemley. Reprinted by permission of the author.

UNIT 4
Exercise and Weight Management

Unit Selections

Key Points to Consider

- How can exercise affect mental health and mental abilities?

- How important is exercise to achieving optimal health? Explain.

- Why should exercise be included in any weight control program?

- What advice would you give to someone who was considering going on the low carbohydrate diet to lose weight?

- How do the three components to the Female Athlete Triad affect health status?

- How do you feel about people who are overweight? Has your weight ever been a problem for you? If so, what have you done about it?

- Do you exercise on a regular basis? If not, why not? What would it take to get you exercising on a regular basis?

- Do you believe that stretching before exercise will prevent injury? Why?

- Should obesity be classified as a disease rather than a lack of willpower?

- What role does volumetrics play in weight management?

Student Website
www.mhcls.com/online

Internet References
Further information regarding these websites may be found in this book's preface or online.

American Society of Exercise Physiologists (ASEP)
http://www.asep.org
Cyberdiet
http://www.cyberdiet.com/reg/index.html
National Eating Disorders Association
http://www.nationaleatingdisorders.org
Shape Up America!
http://www.shapeup.org

Recently, a new set of guidelines, dubbed "Exercise Lite," has been issued by the U.S. Centers for Disease Control and Prevention in conjunction with the American College of Sports Medicine. These guidelines call for 30 minutes of exercise, 5 days a week, which can be spread over the course of a day. The primary focus of this approach to exercise is improving health, not athletic performance. Examples of activities that qualify under the new guidelines are walking your dog, playing tag with your kids, scrubbing floors, washing your car, mowing the lawn, weeding your garden, and having sex. From a practical standpoint, this approach to fitness will likely motivate many more people to become active and stay active. Remember, since the benefits of exercise can take weeks or even months before they become apparent, it is very important to choose an exercise program that you enjoy so that you will stick with it. While a good diet cannot overcome lack of exercise, exercise can overcome a less than optimal diet. Exercise not only makes people physically healthier, it may also keep their brains healthy. While the connection hasn't been proven, there is evidence that regular workouts may cause the brain to better process and store information —that results in a smarter brain.

While exercise and a nutritious diet can keep people fit and healthy, many Americans are not heeding this advice. For the first time in our history, the average American is now overweight when judged according to standard height/weight tables. In addition, more than 25 percent of Americans are clinically obese, and the numbers appear to be growing. Why is this happening, given the prevailing attitude that Americans have toward fat? One theory that is currently gaining support suggests that while Americans have cut back on their consumption of fatty snacks and deserts, they have actually increased their total caloric intake by failing to limit their consumption of carbohydrates. The underlying philosophy goes something like this: fat calories make you fat, but you can eat as many carbohydrates as you want and not gain weight. The truth is that all calories count when it comes to weight gain, and if cutting back on fat calories prevents you from feeling satiated you will naturally eat more to achieve that feeling. While this position seems reasonable enough, some groups, most notably supporters of the Atkins diet, have suggested that eating a high-fat diet will actually help people lose weight because of fat's high satiety value in conjunction with the formation of ketones (which suppress appetite). "The Skinny on Popular Diets" claims that counting carbohydrates without attending to the calories may tempt dieters to eat more, particularly new low-carb snack foods. The original low-carb diets such as Atkins probably worked because they were monotonous and people ultimately ate fewer calories. With a huge array of low-carb, high-calorie foods now available, dieters may end up eating more calories and not lose weight. The article also addresses other diets and rates their effectiveness.

America's preoccupation with body weight has given rise to a billion-dollar industry. When asked why people go on diets, the predominant answer is for social reasons such as appearance and group acceptance, rather than concerns regarding health. Why do diets and diet aids fail? One of the major reasons lies in the mind-set of the dieter. Many dieters do not fully understand the biological and behavioral aspects of weight loss, and consequently they have unrealistic expectations regarding the process. In "Why We're Losing the War Against Obesity," the causes related to the rise in overweight and obesity are addressed.

Being overweight not only causes health problems; it also carries with it a social stigma. Overweight people are often thought of as weak-willed individuals with little or no self-respect. The notion that weight-control problems are the result of personality defects is being challenged by new research findings. Evidence is mounting that suggests that physiological and hereditary factors may play as great a role in obesity as do behavioral and environmental factors. Researchers now believe that genetics dictate the base number of fat cells an individual will have, as well as the location and distribution of these cells within the body. The study of fat metabolism has provided additional clues as to why weight control is so difficult. These metabolic studies have found that the body seems to have a "setpoint," or desired weight, and it will defend this weight through alterations in basal metabolic rate and fat-cell activity. While this process is thought to be an adaptive throwback to

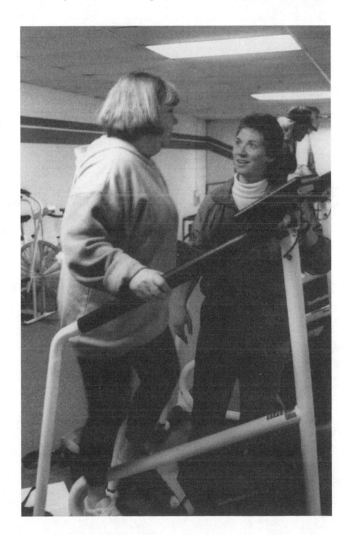

primitive times when food supplies were uncertain, today, with our abundant food supply, this mechanism only contributes to the problem of weight control.

It should be apparent by now that weight control is both an attitudinal and a lifestyle issue. Fortunately, a new, more rational approach to the problem of weight control is emerging. This approach is based on the premise that you can be perfectly healthy and look good without being pencil-thin. The primary focus of this approach to weight management is the attainment of your body's "natural ideal weight" and not some idealized, fanciful notion of what you would like to weigh. Unfortunately, for many female athletes, the desire to have a perfect body has led some to develop eating disorders that can lead to osteoporosis. In "The Female Triad," authors Lola Ramos and Gregory Welch discuss a condition that affects female athletes who eat too little and exercise too much. The concept of achieving your natural ideal body weight suggests that we need to take a more realistic approach to both fitness and weight control and serves to remind us that a healthy lifestyle is based on the concepts of balance and moderation.

Sweating Makes You Smart

Exercise doesn't just make you look and feel better—it also keeps your brain young and strong. A good workout may be as good for your mind as it is for your muscles.

By Chris Jozefowicz

John Lavery is a rower. Whether cutting through green water under a clear blue sky or sliding past wet black rocks under a light snow, Lavery is usually out on the Potomac River six days a week, as long as the water is free of ice. Last year he covered more than 1,500 miles of river in his thin racing boats. It's an impressive feat for any athlete—but John Lavery is also 73 years old.

Lavery first put oar to water when he was 57, to fight becoming a "blob," he says. His goal was to keep his body toned. But as he perfected his technique, he relished the sense of mastery he achieved, what he calls his "Zen zone." Although Lavery was looking to help his body through exercise, he was probably keeping his brain in top shape as well. Now, at an age when some of his friends are beginning to slip into mental decline, Lavery feels pretty good. "This is not an ego statement," he says, "but most people think I am at least ten years younger than I am."

It turns out that the brain-body connection is more powerful than anyone thought. Shaking a leg (or curling a bicep) doesn't just make you stronger, healthier and better-looking—it also helps your brain shrug off damage and the effects of aging.

Thanks to brain-imaging studies in humans and neurochemical studies in animals, scientists have found evidence that exercise actually makes a stronger brain. Physical exertion induces the cells in the brain to reinforce old connections between neurons and to forge new connections. This denser neuron network is better able to process and store information, essentially resulting in a smarter brain.

Best of all, exercisers may not need the endurance of an ironman—or even a John Lavery, for that matter—to benefit. For older people in particular, even a moderate program of exercise can boost brain health and cognition.

Much of this new research focuses on a protein called BDNF, for "brain-derived neurotrophic factor." This chemical, which helps nerve cells grow and connect, is important for fetal development. But it turns out to be critical in the adult brain, as well.

The benefits of BDNF are broad. Rats with boosted BDNF in their brains navigate mazes faster than cage mates with lower levels. Brain injuries in the high-BDNF animals heal faster. Data even suggest that an increase in BDNF helps rats avoid a type of behavior that is considered to be the rodent equivalent of depression.

How does the chemical work? Vassilis Koliatsos, a psychiatrist at Johns Hopkins University in Maryland who has studied BDNF for more than a decade, says the molecule actually helps rewire the brain. BDNF is one of the tools a brain uses to turn life experiences into long-lasting changes, influencing everything from memory to mood. "Learning is taking signals that come in from your senses and embedding them into brain anatomy," he says. BDNF, which helps build the nervous system, seems to play an important role.

Even better, researchers have learned that boosting this beneficial brain chemical may be simple to do: Scores of studies during the last decade show that short stints of exercise increase BDNF in the brains of animals. In rat studies conducted by Fernando Gomez-Pinilla and his colleagues at UCLA, even a few minutes of swimming raised levels of BDNF.

The dynamics of BDNF are harder to study in people, but researchers have been able to use imaging techniques to show that exercise helps human brains. Using magnetic resonance imaging, which allows the living brain to be visualized, University of Illinois at Urbana-Champaign researchers Arthur Kramer and Stanley Colcombe have found that exercise postpones the effects of aging.

Everyone's brain loses nerve tissue as it ages, beginning in the third decade of life. "[Aging] sort of damages the brain as you go along," says Colcombe. But people who exercise lose brain tissue more slowly. In early 2003, Kramer and Colcombe demonstrated that athletic older adults had denser brains than their inactive counterparts, suggesting that workouts protected their brains.

Colcombe and Kramer think that exercise does more than simply preserve brain tissue—it can also improve thinking. In a recent comparison of 18 studies, inactive older adults who began an exercise routine got significantly better at cognitive tests that measured skills such as planning and paying attention.

Gym-phobes take note: The kind of exercise that makes a difference is not hard to tackle.

Gym-phobes take note: The kind of exercise that makes a difference in these studies is not hard to tackle. In Kramer and Colcombe's research, subjects work up from a slow 15-minute walk to a brisk 45-minute jaunt. They follow this regimen three days a week for six months. "It's not like people are running marathons here," Kramer says.

So far, Kramer's research has focused on adults who are 55 and older. He doesn't believe that working out will transform smart young people into geniuses—but he does think that athletic activity helps sharpen the brain over the long term.

"There isn't much cumulative decline in brain function and cognitive condition when you're 20," Kramer says, "so there's less room for improvement." Still, young exercisers can expect to see some benefits, such as an improved ability to handle complex cognitive tasks and the knowledge that their brains are probably somewhat protected. "I think you get long-term benefits that accrue as you age," he says.

Since diet and exercise are so often connected, Gomez-Pinilla and colleagues have broadened their studies to find out how other aspects of the couch-potato lifestyle might influence brain health. In 2003, they found that rats who were fed lots of saturated fats and sugar—such as the bacon-cheeseburger-and-extra-large-Coke diet that many Americans love—had less BDNF in the brain and did not recover as well from brain injuries. In his latest research, which has not yet been published, Gomez-Pinilla finds that, in contrast, a healthy diet high in omega-3 fatty acids like fish oils increases BDNF in rats.

Direct connections between BDNF, physical exercise and brain health haven't been proven in humans, so Gomez-Pinilla and a colleague, Paul Vespa, have launched a new project to study BDNF in exercising people. In the meantime, given the other benefits of exercise, the smart thinking seems to be with athletes like John Lavery. Although he wasn't so concerned with his mental health when he began, he gets more out of his workouts than he expected. "It's greater than just exercise," he says. "There is a great psychic reward."

Chris Jozefowicz is a New York City-based writer.

The skinny on popular diets

Bestselling diet plans don't necessarily work any better than do-it-yourself programs.

If losing weight was one of your New Year's resolutions and you have already quit your diet, don't despair. Many off-the-shelf diets come with the seeds of failure—restriction, deprivation, hunger, and cravings—already planted.

Finding an effective eating strategy is serious business if you are considerably overweight and are interested in improving your long-term health. Halting any further weight gain and gradually shedding pounds can have beneficial effects on blood pressure, cholesterol, diabetes, your risk of having a heart attack or stroke, joint pain, and the energy and ability to do everyday activities.

What you *really* need is a plan you can stick with for many, many moons. It should be as good for your heart, bones, colon, and psyche as it is for your waistline. It should offer plenty of tasty and healthy choices, banish few foods, and not require an extensive and expensive list of groceries or supplements.

Let's use this yardstick as a way to measure some of the popular diet books.

Low carbs

The most popular diets today are those preaching the carbs-are-bad gospel. Once seen as the go-to foods for weight loss, carbohydrates such as bread, pasta, and rice are now reviled as dietary demons, thanks to the **Atkins, South Beach,** and other low-carb diets. Avoiding carbohy-

drates, so the thinking goes, forces the body to burn fat.

Does this theory translate into actual weight loss? Yes and no—it depends on the individual and the time period. Some people lose a substantial amount of weight on a low-carb diet, while others lose little and some actually gain weight. And for those who lose, the effects typically aren't permanent. After a few months, weight loss tends to slow and reverse, just as happens with most other diet types.

Bottom line: Low carb diets work for some people and not others. There's no evidence that their short-term effects produce long-term weight loss, while the added expense could lighten your wallet. Equally important, we know little about the long-term health effects of high-protein, high-fat, low-carb diets.

Low fat

Once the main strategy for losing weight, low-fat diets have been elbowed aside by the low-carb frenzy. That's not necessarily a bad thing, since neither of the two foundations on which low-fat diets were built—fat makes you fat, and fat is bad for the heart—are very solid. Healthy fats can actually promote weight loss, while some fats are good for the heart and eliminating them from the diet can cause problems.

Scores of low-fat diets have been promoted over the years. One of the best known is Dr. Dean Ornish's *Eat More, Weigh Less* plan. Since fat con-

tains 9 calories per gram while carbohydrates contain 4, you can theoretically double your food intake without taking in more calories by cutting back on fatty foods and eating more that are full of carbohydrates, especially water-rich fruits and vegetables.

Keep in mind that the Ornish plan doesn't stop at a whole-grain, vegetarian, very-low-fat (less than 10% of calories from fat) diet, but also includes exercise, stress management, and group support.

Bottom line: Low-fat diets have unquestionably helped some people lose weight and keep it off. They've been dismal failures for others, in part because they tend to be less filling, less flavorful, and all around less satisfying than other eating strategies. They also tend to be fairly restrictive about food choices, which can limit your options when dining out.

Correct carbs

Diets such as *Sugar Busters!* and the *Glucose Revolution* don't ban carbohydrates. Instead, they embrace "correct" carbs while shunning "harmful" ones. In a nutshell, this means eating plenty of fruits, vegetables, and whole grains, and cutting back or cutting out refined sugars (white sugar, high-fructose corn syrup, honey, molasses, etc.) and processed grains.

Right-carb diets rely heavily on the glycemic index and glycemic load (see the December 2002 *Heart*

Letter). In theory, foods with a low glycemic load generate small but steady increases in blood sugar that help stave off hunger. In contrast, the rapid increases in blood sugar and insulin that follow consumption of foods with a high glycemic load are followed by equally steep drops that soon get your internal hunger alarm ringing.

Bottom line: In general, right-carb diets promote healthy eating by focusing on fruits, vegetables, and whole grains. But you don't really need to rely on the sometimes contradictory glycemic index and glycemic load tables to tell you that. Plans that prohibit refined sugars also make dieting and healthy eating more complicated than it needs to be. Refined sugars aren't toxic; they just add unnecessary calories.

Perfect proportions and careful combinations

Several popular diets sell the idea that specific proportions of nutrients or certain combinations of foods are essential to weight loss. If you want to enter *The Zone*, you must create meals and snacks that contain 9 grams of carbohydrate for every 7 grams of protein and 1.5 grams of fat (40% carbohydrate, 30% fat, and 30% protein).

The *Eat Right 4 Your Type* diet promotes the wholly unscientific idea that your blood type determines what you should eat, along with how you should exercise, what supplements you need, and what type of personality you have. Following it isn't easy, since you must remember lists of good and bad foods. It isn't balanced, something you can tell from the long list of recommended supplements. And it makes it hard to prepare meals for a family with several different blood types.

Bottom line: Proper proportions or correct combinations force you to focus on what you are eating, which helps most people eat less each day. That's where any weight loss from these diets comes from, *not* from any

nutritional or physiologic secrets the diet developers have uncovered.

Does density matter?

According to the *Volumetrics* plan, focusing on foods that fill the belly without adding too many calories will help you shed pounds. Foods with a high water content, such as fruits, vegetables, low-fat milk, cooked grains, beans, soups, and stews, get the thumbs up, while high-fat foods like potato chips get the thumbs down, as do dry, calorie-dense ones like pretzels, crackers, and fat-free cookies.

Bottom line: This strategy helps people lose weight the same way most other diets do—it narrows your choices so you take in fewer calories each day. Whether it has a long-term role for weight control isn't known.

Behavior change

Some people use food for comfort and overeat in response to sadness, loneliness, depression, or any number of other triggers. Breaking an unhealthy relationship with food can help such individuals lose weight. That's where *Dr. Phil's Ultimate Weight Solution, the Automatic Diet*, and others come in.

Dr. Phil offers "seven keys to permanent weight loss"—right thinking, healing feelings, a no-fail environment, mastery over food and impulse eating, intentional exercise, a circle of support, and what Dr. Phil calls high-response cost, high-yield nutrition. The plan offers little advice about nutrition. The Automatic Diet uses behavior modification techniques to reprogram the patterns that work against healthy eating.

Bottom line: If you think that your habits, behaviors, and relationships with other people and with food promote poor eating habits or influence your ability to lose weight or maintain a steady weight, then a behavioral approach makes sense. Combining it with a healthy eating pattern based on sound nutrition would be even better.

The evidence

Given the sheer number of diets promoted over the years and Americans' long-standing interest in losing weight, it's appalling how little solid information we have on effective strategies for weight loss.

Surveys of people who have successfully lost weight and kept it off, conducted by the National Weight Control Registry and *Consumer Reports,* reveal that most did it on their own without resorting to commercial weight loss programs. They tend to chalk up their successes to—drumroll, please—eating less and exercising more. The latest news from the Registry indicates that participants report taking in an average of 1,800 calories a day and burning an average of 400 calories a day in physical activity, the equivalent of about an hour of brisk walking.

Interestingly, the Registry participants tended to rely on low-fat diets, while the *Consumer Reports* group relied mostly on low-carb diets.

Another line of evidence about effective weight-loss strategies comes from a few carefully controlled trials in which obese volunteers were blindly assigned to either a standard low-fat diet or a low-carb, high-protein diet. Overall, these trials showed that a low-carb, high-protein diet leads to quicker weight loss than a low-fat diet. In the few studies that lasted for a year, though, weight loss was about the same *regardless of diet type*. These studies focused primarily on weight, and were too short to track other important consequences of diet, such as heart disease, diabetes, bone strength, and cancer.

The overall results mask some startling individual differences. In one trial, on both low-carb and low-fat diets, some people lost weight while others gained. In the low-fat group, the range was from 53 pounds lost to 31 pounds gained. In the low-carb group, it was from 65 pounds lost to 18 gained.

The take-home lesson is that it is okay to experiment on yourself. If you give a diet your best shot and it doesn't work, maybe it wasn't the right one for you, your metabolism, or your situation. Don't get too discouraged or beat yourself up because a diet that "worked for everybody" didn't pay off for you. Try another.

Do it yourself

You could also strike out on your own, like thousands of successful dieters before you. You can build your own plan by choosing the smart parts of the diets discussed here.

Or you could try a healthy eating plan based on the best science available, like the one that Dr. Walter Willett, a member of the *Heart Letter* editorial board, and his colleagues have developed. Its elements include moderation (portion control); eating more fruits and vegetables; cutting back on unhealthy saturated and trans fats and including more healthy unsaturated fats; eating more whole grains and less refined grain; and choosing healthy sources of protein, such as fish, poultry, beans, and nuts.

An overall approach to healthy eating like this one will do more for you in the long term than a diet based on certain foods. One problem with these is that people often think they can eat all they want of the "right foods."

Dr. Willett's book, *Eat, Drink, and Be Healthy,* offers a road map for this strategy.

The Female Triad

By Lola Ramos and
Gregory L. Welch, M.S.

In the past 30 years the opportunities for adolescent girls and young adult women to participate in all levels of sports competition have increased tremendously. This is certainly a positive direction for women because with increased physical activity comes associated wellness benefits. Chronic physiological adaptation to exercise training is well documented in regard to improved cardiovascular efficiency, muscular strength, self-esteem and overall body image (Wilmore and Costill 1999).

In addition to women who train at a competitive level, many non-competitive women exercise vigorously as well. It is not just that they train at high intensities but that their ambition to train surpasses that of individuals who are more moderate in their exercise programs. This mindset is such that training becomes a lifestyle philosophy as well as a passion. While this is generally an admirable trait, it is not without significant risk. For example, "over training" injuries in the form of muscular strain, tendonitis and stress fractures will likely occur to many individuals who overprioritize their workouts at the expense of sufficient recovery and nutrition. Specifically for young women, there is an even greater health concern that far outweighs typical "overuse syndrome"—the female triad. If not dealt with appropriately, the female triad can damage women's wellness throughout their lives.

Defining the Female Triad

The female triad is a combination of three coexistent conditions associated with exercise training: disordered eating, amenorrhea and osteoporosis (Hobart and Smucker 2000). Originally termed "female athlete triad," the name was derived at a meeting led by members of the American College of Sports Medicine in the early 1990s (Yeager et al. 1993). Papanek (2003) reports that the meeting was called in response to the alarming increase in stress fracture rates, documented decreases in bone mineral density and menstrual dysfunction in otherwise healthy female athletes. Furthermore, the depiction of the triad as a triangle was developed to demonstrate the interrelationship between the three disorders normally considered independent medical conditions.

Over the last decade, the triad's definition has evolved to be more precise about the involvement of related clinical conditions. Anorexia nervosa (AN) and bulimia nervosa (BN) are the most common clinical disorders. A third category for eating disorders not otherwise specified (EDNOS) was created in an effort to expand treatment access for patients at high risk for an eating disorder (Papanek 2003). In other words, an athlete who falls short in meeting the criteria for AN or BN could still be recognized as needing treatment by being placed in the EDNOS category. *See Table 1.*

However, not all restrictive eating behaviors necessarily reach the clinical level (Beals and Manore 2000). Even with the addition of the EDNOS category, female athletes with the triad display a wide range of food-related pathologies. Therefore, the term "eating disorder" was found to be too restrictive and replaced by "disordered eating" to include the various forms of aberrant eating behaviors that disrupt caloric balance (Papanek 2003). Common disordered eating patterns exhibited by female athletes include food restriction, prolonged fasting as well as abuse of diet pills, diuretics and laxatives (Donaldson 2003).

Eumenorrheic or regular menstrual cycles are defined as regular flow occurring every 21 to 45 days, with 10 to 13 cycles per year, and oligomenorrhea refers to three to six cycles occurring per year (Rome 2003). Marshal (1994) classifies amenorrhea as primary or secondary and defines them as follows: primary amenorrhea or delayed menarche is defined as not having experienced a single menstrual cycle by the age of 16 and secondary amenorrhea is the absence of menses for six months or a length of time equivalent to at least three of the woman's previous menstrual cycle lengths. The main difference is that in secondary amenorrhea, at least one menstrual period has occurred. Physiologically, this means all parts of the reproductive axis (i.e., hypothalamus, pituitary, ovaries and uterus) worked together once, but for some reason, this integrative function has changed (Papanek 2003).

Osteoporosis is a systemic, skeletal disease characterized by low bone density and microarchitectural deterioration of bone tissue, with a consequent increase in bone fragility and fracture susceptibility (O'brien 2001). To clar-

Table 1. Diagnostic criteria and warning signs for eating disorders

	DIAGNOSTIC CRITERIA	WARNING SIGNS AND SYMPTOMS
Anorexia Nervosa (AN)	1. Refusal to maintain body weight at or above 85 percent of normal weight for age and height 2. Intense fear of gaining weight or becoming fat, even though underweight 3. Disturbance in the way in which one's body weight or shape is experienced, undue influence of body weight or shape on self-evaluation or denial of the seriousness of current low body weight 4. Amenorrhea	1. Fat and muscle atrophy 2. Dry hair and skin 3. Cold, discolored hands and feet 4. Decreased body temperature 5. Lightheadedness 6. Decreased ability to concentrate 7. Bradycardia (i.e., slowness of the heartbeat, so that the pulse rate is less than 60 per minute) 8. Past history of physical or sexual abuse
Bulimia Nervosa (BN)	1. Recurrent episodes of binge eating 2. Sense of lack of control over eating during the episode (e.g., feeling that one cannot stop eating or control what or how much one is eating) 3. Recurrent inappropriate compensatory behavior to prevent weight gain (e.g., diuretics, enemas, self-induced vomiting, misuse of laxatives or other medications, fasting or excessive exercise) 4. The binge eating and inappropriate compensatory behaviors occur, on average, at least twice a week for three months 5. Self-evaluation is unduly influenced by body shape and weight 6. The disturbance does not occur exclusively during episodes of anorexia nervosa	1. Swollen parotid glands 2. Chest pain, sore throat 3. Fatigue, abdominal pain 4. Diarrhea or constipation 5. Menstrual irregularities 6. Callous formation or scars on knuckles
Eating Disorder Not Otherwise Specified (EDNOS)	1. For females, all of the criteria for AN are met except the individual has regular menses 2. All criteria for AN are met except that, despite significant weight loss, the person's current weight is in the normal range 3. All the criteria for BN are met except that the binge eating and inappropriate compensatory mechanisms occur at a frequency of less than two per week for a duration of less than three months	4. Regular use of inappropriate compensatory behavior by an individual of normal body weight after eating small amounts of food (e.g., self-induced vomiting after consumption of two cookies) 5. Repeatedly chewing, but not swallowing, and spitting out large amounts of food 6. Binge-eating disorder: recurrent episodes of binge eating in the absence of the regular use of inappropriate compensatory behaviors characteristic of BN

ify, the term osteoporosis, as referred to in this writing, is actually secondary osteoporosis because it is caused or exacerbated by other disorders (Stein and Shane 2003). Additionally, osteopenia, which is abnormally low bone density and believed to be an osteoporosis precursor (Nelson 2000), has also been included when identifying the female triad syndrome. Amenorrheic adolescent athletes do not acquire proper bone mass and, thus, will be osteopenic in their early adult years (Elford and Spence 2002).

Disordered Eating

Society has done a great disservice to adolescent females by perpetuating the "ideal" body image. For young women, this can intensify the pursuit of a thin physique at a time when nutrition plays a key role in proper growth and development. According to a 1997 Youth Risk Behavior Surveillance Survey, 34 percent of adolescent females were likely to consider themselves "too fat" and, therefore, limited their dietary intake (Kann et al. 1998). Hobart and Smucker (2000) add that many factors may create poor self-image and pathogenic weight-control behaviors in female athletes. Likewise, frequent weigh-ins, punitive consequences for weight gain, pressure to "win at all costs," an overly controlling parent or coach and social isolation caused by intensive sports involvement may increase a female athlete's risk of disordered eating behavior.

Disordered eating occurs in 5 percent of the general population (Donaldson 2003), but affects as many as two thirds of young female athletes (Nativ et al. 1994). According to Gidwani and Rome (1997), 32 percent of female athletes, at all levels of competition, practice pathogenic behavior for weight control. Rosen and Hough (1988) reported disordered eating behavior in 15 to 62 percent of female college athletes. Even before the triad was officially recognized as a distinct syndrome, Calabrese (1985) performed a study with collegiate gymnasts and discovered 62 percent displayed some type of disordered eating—26 percent vomited on a daily basis, 24 percent used diet pills, 12 percent fasted and 75 percent had been told by their coaches that they weighed too much. Disordered eating behavior is believed to contribute to a disruption in the hypothalamic-gonadal axis, resulting in amenorrhea (Donaldson 2003).

The Interrelationship of the Triad

The three components of the female triad—disordered eating, amenorrhea and osteoporosis—pose serious health concerns for young athletic women. Shafer and Irwin (1991) state that the adolescent growth spurt accounts for approximately 25 percent of adult height and 50 percent of adult weight. Additionally, girls develop reproductive capacity during this time and dieting behaviors and nutrition can have an enormous impact on their gynecologic health (Seidenfeld and Rickert 2001).

While they can all occur independently, the interrelationship between the three parts of the triad is such that one component will affect another. In order to under-stand the physiological beginning of this syndrome, one must first realize that, in addition to the calories required for basal metabolic rate and physical activity, calories are required for menstruation, building and repairing muscle, healing and, in younger athletes, growth (Papanek 2003). The pathophysiology of the triad can be explained by a caloric deficit which disrupts the release of gonadotropin-releasing hormone, resulting in low levels of gonadotropins and secondarily reduced levels of estrogen and progesterone, leading to amenorrhea and osteopenia (Elford and Spence 2002).

Disordered eating behavior affects the number of calories available for normal life function. Manore (1999) states that any athlete, regardless of size, who consumes less than 1,800 calories per day is unable to meet caloric and nutrient requirements. Furthermore, a female athlete exercising 10 to 20 hours per week requires at least 2,200 to 2,500 calories per day to maintain body weight.

Negative Caloric Balance and Amenorrhea

Dueck, et al., (1996) reported that the average difference between amenorrheic and eumenorrheic athletes was only a caloric balance deficit of 250 calories per day. Many athletes do not realize the nutritional demands of their sports and, thus, it is this disordered eating that causes a negative caloric balance leading to amenorrhea (Papanek 2003). Even as early as 1981, Frisch, et al., found that amenorrheic competitive runners had an average intake of 1,700 calories per day, whereas eumenorrheic runners consumed 2,200 calories per day.

In addition to a caloric deficit due to disordered eating, physical training intensity plays an important role in the triad syndrome. Even if caloric deprivation does not occur through disordered eating, negative caloric imbalance can result from failing to support the training regimen with adequate recovery. Primary and secondary amenorrhea can occur in the context of eating disorders or intense athletics (Rome 2003). DiPietro and Stachenfeld support this by adding that a chronic negative energy balance, being underweight and exercise stress are important elements in the pathway to amenorrhea (1997). Cobb, et al., (2003) write that female athletes with disordered eating may limit their calorie and/or fat intakes but maintain high training levels, often resulting in a state of chronic energy deficit. Athletic amenorrhea occurs more frequently in activities such as running, ballet and gymnastics, in which intense physical training is combined with the desire to maintain a lean build (Warren 1980).

Osteoporosis and Negative Caloric Balance

Bones require a normal level of systemic hormones, adequate caloric intake (including protein, calcium and vitamin D, in particular) and regular, weight-bearing exercise throughout life (O'brien 2001). Exercise's effects on the growing skeleton are complex and influenced by many factors, including the nature and intensity of the activity, skeleton area primarily involved, body weight and dietary calcium intake (Stein and Shane 2003). Although moderate exercise protects against osteoporosis, too little or excessive exercise may actually cause it (O'brien 2001).

> "In general, women struggle with the perception of the 'perfect body image' society has unfairly placed upon them. Regardless of the circumstances, we as health care providers, coaches and parents are ultimately responsible for protecting the wellness of the young women in our care. Therefore, we must provide a proper wellness environment by nurturing sound physical training and nutritional habits."

The minimum daily calcium requirement is 1,300 milligrams for people ages 11 to 23. Unfortunately, 85 percent of adolescent females do not consume this amount (National Institutes of Health and Child Development Publication 2001). Attitudes about their bodies during puberty can contribute to the dietary changes adolescent females make. This can lead to possible chronic dieting disorders, resulting in low bone mass and a risk for osteoporotic fractures later in life (Ali and Siktberg 1996).

Osteoporosis is a prevalent AN complication. In fact, the duration of AN is a predictor of low bone mineral density because the longer the illness lasts, the greater bone mineral density is reduced (Mehler 2003). For example, more than 50 percent of female patients with AN develop osteoporosis (Treasure and Surpell 2001). Miller and Klibanski (1999) add that the lack of nutrition is so severe in anorexics that an increased osteoporosis risk may exist due to associated endocrine abnormalities, including estrogen deficiency.

Amenorrhea and Osteoporosis

Continuing the triad syndrome's assault on the female athlete's wellness is the relationship between the absence of menses and bone deterioration. Some athletes see amenorrhea as a sign of appropriate training levels, while others regard it as a great solution to a monthly inconvenience (National Institutes of Health 2003). There is a prevailing myth in women's athletics that equates a disrupted menstrual cycle with the appropriate level of elite training (Papanek 2003). Mickelsfield, et al., (1995) state that amenorrheic/oligomenorrheic athletes on average have lower bone mineral density than eumenorrheic controls. Stein and Shane (2003) agree that low bone min-

eral density is a consequence of exercise-induced amenorrhea. Osteopenia or significantly reduced bone mass occurring with prolonged loss of menses has been associated with an increased risk of stress fractures (Mansfield and Emans 1993).

Summary

The female triad is a unique phenomenon that does not occur overnight but rather appears to gradually infiltrate female adolescents' lifestyle. Under intense pressure from parents, coaches teammates and often themselves, many young women begin to fall into patterns of disordered eating and/or overintense caloric expenditure without the support of adequate rest and nutrition. The triad is especially troubling due to the fact that, while each affliction can occur independently, they often are interrelated by a chain reaction. Amenorrhea/oligomenorrhea is likely to follow the caloric imbalance, which leads to osteopenia and ultimately osteoporosis. This downward spiral can result in termination of an athletic career as well as a chronically unhealthy adult life.

Identification of the triad can be difficult. When confronted by family, friends, coaches and physicians about their eating behavior, athletes can be anywhere from elusive in their explanation to perfectly convincing that nothing is wrong. Although it is more common to find this syndrome affecting athletic women, it is certainly not exclusive to this population. In general, women struggle with the perception of the "perfect body image" society has unfairly placed upon them. Regardless of the circumstances, we as health care providers, coaches and parents are ultimately responsible for protecting the wellness of the young women in our care. Therefore, we must provide a proper wellness environment by nurturing sound physical training and nutritional habits.

References

Ali, N. and Siktberg, L. "Osteoporosis prevention in female adolescents: Calcium intake and exercise participation," *Pediatr. Nurs.* 1996, 27 (2), 132-9.

Beals, K.A. and Manore, M.M. "Behavioral, psychological and physical characteristics of female athletes with subclinical eating disorders." *Int. J. Sports Nutr. Exerc. Metab.*, 2000, 10, 128-43.

Calabrese, L.H. "Nutritional and medical aspects of gymnastics." *Clin. Sports Med.*, 1985, 4, 23-37.

Cobb, K.L., et al. "Disordered eating, menstrual irregularity, and bone mineral density in female runners." *Med. Sci. Sports Exerc.*, 2003, 35 (5), 711-9.

DiPietro, L. and Stachenfeld, N.S. "The female athletic triad: American College of Sports Medicine position." *Med. Sci. Sports Exerc.*, 1997, 29, I-IX.

Donaldson, M.C. "The female athlete triad: A growing health concern." *Orthop. Nurs.*, 2003, 22 (5), 322-3.

Dueck, C.A., Manore, M.M. and Matt, K.S. "Role of energy balance in athletic menstrual dysfunction." *Int. J. Sports Nutr.*, 1996, 6, 165-190.

Elford, K.J. and Spence, J.E.H. "The forgotten female: Pediatric and adolescent gynecological concerns and their reproductive consequences." *J. Pediatr. Adolesc. Gynecol.*, 2002, 15 (2), 83-105.

Frisch, R.E., Gotz-Welbergen, A.V. and McArthur, J.W. "Delayed menarche and amenorrhea of college athletes in relation to age of onset of training." *JAMA*, 1981, 246, 1559.

Gidwani, G. and Rome, E. "Eating Disorders." *Clin. Obstet. Gynaecol.*, 1997, 40 (3), 601.

Hobart, J. and Smucker, D. "The female triad." *Am. Fam. Physician*, 2000, 61, 3357-64, 3367.

Kann, L., et al. "Youth risk behavior surveillance-United States, 1997." *MMWR*, 1998, 47 (SS-3), 1-89.

Manore, M.M. "Nutritional needs of the female athlete." *Clin. Sports Med.*, 1999, 18, 549-63.

Mansfield, M.J. and Emans, S.J. "Growth in female gymnasts: Should training decrease puberty?" *J. Pediatr.*, 1993, 122, 237-40.

Marshal, L.A. "Clinical evaluation of amenorrhea in active and athletic women." *Clin. Sports Med.*, 1994, 13, 371-87.

Mehler, P.S. "Osteoporosis in anorexia nervosa: Prevention and treatment." *Int. J. Eat. Disord.*, 2003, 33 (2), 113-26.

Mickelsfield, L.K., et al. "Bone mineral density in mature, premenopausal ultramarathon runners." *Med. Sci. Sports Exerc.*, 1995, 27, 688-96.

Miller, K.K. and Klibanski, A. "Amenorrheic bone loss." *J. Clin. Endocrinol. Metab.*, 1999, 84, 1775-83.

National Institutes of Health. "Fitness and Bone Health: The skeletal risk of overtraining." *National Resource Center*, 2003, Bethesda, Maryland.

National Institutes of Health and Child Development Publication. "Why milk matters now for children and teens under childhood adolescent nutrition." January 2001, no. 00-4864.

Nativ, A., et al. "The female athlete triad." *Clin. Sports Med.*, 1994, 13, 405-18.

Nelson, M. *Strong Women, Strong Bones.* New York: G.P Putnam's and Sons, 2000.

O'brien, M. "Exercise and osteoporosis." *Ir. J. Med. Sci.*, 2001, 170 (1), 58-62.

Papanek, P.E. "The female athlete triad: An emerging role for physical therapy." *J. Orthop. Sports Phys. Ther.*, 2003, 33 (10), 594-614.

Rome, E.S. "Eating disorders." *Obs. Gyn. Clin.*, 2003, 30 (2), 353-77.

Rosen, L.W. and Hough, D.O. "Pathogenic weight-control behaviors of female college gymnasts." *Phys. Sports Med.*, 1988, 16, 140-3.

Seidenfeld, M.D. and Rickert, V.I. "Impact of anorexia, bulimia and obesity on the gynecologic health of adolescents." *Am. Fam. Physician*, 2001, 64 (3), 445-50.

Shafer, M.B. and Irwin, C.E. "The adolescent patient." In Rudolf A. M., ed. *Rudolf's Pediatrics.* 19th ed. Norwalk: Appleton & Lange, 1991: 39.

Stein, E. and Shane, E. "Secondary osteoporosis." *Endocrinol. Metab. Clin.*, 2003, 32 (1) 889-92.

Treasure, J. and Serpell, L. "Osteoporosis in young people. Research and treatment in eating disorders." *Psychiatr. Clin. North Am.*, 2001, 24 (2), 359-70.

Warren, M.P. "The effects of exercise on pubertal progression and reproductive function in girls." *J. Clin. Endocrinol. Metab.*, 1980, 51, 1150.

Wilmore, J.H. and Costill, D.L. *Physiology of Sport and Exercise.* Champaign: Human Kinetics, 1999.

Yeager, K.K., et al. "The female athlete triad: disordered eating, amenorrhea, osteoporosis." *Med. Sci. Sports and Exerc.*, 1999, 25: 775-7.

Lola Ramos is pursuing her bachelor's degree in kinesiology and health promotion at California State University, Fullerton. She has recently completed an academic internship through the SpeciFit Foundation.

Gregory L. Welch, M.S., is an exercise physiologist and president of SpeciFit, An Agency of Wellness and Competitive Performance Enhancement, located in Seal Beach, California. He is also founder and CEO of the SpeciFit Foundation, a non-profit entity providing wellness concepts for adolescent women. Welch has published several articles regarding wellness of older adults and through his foundation has added adolescent women to the category of special populations. He can be reached at (562) 431-5206 and www.specifit.com.

Stretching...
...out?

Stephen B. Thacker, MD, isn't used to getting hate mail. As director of the epidemiology program office at the Centers for Disease Control and Prevention (CDC) in Atlanta, Thacker spends most of his time assessing research, evaluating its implications for policy, and writing the occasional paper. So he was taken aback this year when, as lead author of a meta-analysis of studies on the impact of stretching on injury risk,[1] he started getting flamed.

People who advocate stretching were outraged at the paper's conclusion that stretching appeared to be neither particularly helpful nor harmful, according to Thacker. On the other side were those who felt the CDC had gone weak in the knees and should have slammed the practice.

"At CDC we encourage physical activity," Thacker said. "We want people to do things that have been documented to prevent injury, which includes interventions that improve balance, strength, and conditioning. We just don't want people depending on stretching, thinking they'll be all right."

Healthy skepticism

Even defining stretching can be complex, because physical therapists and trainers promote different approaches depending on their own preferences, experience, and perceived needs of the athlete (see table, page 22).

Thacker's paper makes clear why athletes and performers should be skeptical of stretching's alleged benefits. For example, several investigators found little evidence to support injury prevention by stretching immediately before or after events, and determined that the practice may negatively affect performance."[2-5]

Other studies have found that stretching decreases muscle strength for anywhere from 10 minutes to 24 hours,[6,7]—a drop that increases injury risk in itself—and that passive stretching adversely affects jumping ability and plantar flexion.[8,9] Increased flexibility also appears to decrease running economy and peak performance.[10-12]

Duane Knudson, PhD, a professor of biomechanics at Chico State University in Chico, CA, has conducted extensive research into stretching and comes down on the side of the naysayers, even though several of his own studies suggest that stretching has little effect one way or the other.[14-16] Knudson raised questions about the purported merits of stretching in a 1999 paper in the *Journal of Physical Education, Recreation & Dance*, as well.[17] There he pointed out the difference between static flexibility—measured by the limits of joint motion—versus dynamic flexibility, which refers to how quickly resistance (tension) increases in stretched muscles.

Regular stretching does increase static flexibility, which is important in activities such as dance or gymnastics, where performers exceed normal motion ranges. However, the gain may be due more to increased "stretch tolerance," or the ability to be comfortable in those extended ranges, than to actual decreases in muscle stiffness, Knudson reported.

He also noted that the literature doesn't support the notion that increases in static flexibility prevent injury. For one thing, more mobile joints tend to be less stable, and the most flexible athletes have higher injury rates.[18] Some stretching techniques may also increase risk by stretching ligaments or creating hazardous loading patterns. And no research has documented ranges of motion related to minimized injury risk.

Although little is known about the long-term effects of stretching on dynamic flexibility, it does affect a muscle's viscoelastic properties in the short run. What remains unclear is whether this is beneficial, neutral, or harmful. Overall, Knudson concluded, "light to moderate muscle actions of gradually increasing intensity are more appropriate than stretching as warm-up activities for most sports." He added, however, that for those who need a range of motion beyond the norm—gymnasts, dancers, or divers—stretching during the warm-up may be necessary.

"I'm generally of the belief that unless you're doing a sport where you need a lot of flexibility—or you're a very inflexible person—you don't need to stretch," Knudson said recently. "There is just an overwhelming amount of evidence that you make yourself weaker."

Eccentrics Stand out

Other researchers have had similar results but are somewhat more equivocal in their conclusions. Joel Cramer, PhD, assistant professor of kinesiology at the University of Texas at Arlington, has investigated the effects of static stretching on the vastus lateralis and rectus femoris, two muscles in the quadriceps group,[19,20]

"We found that static stretching seems to decrease the muscles ability to produce force at both slow and fast velocities," Cramer said.

According to new data he and his team presented in June at the annual meeting of the American College of Sports Medicine, the acute effects of static stretching may be mode-specific, affecting isometric and concentric force production, but not eccentric force production.[21] (Eccentric force would be, for example, extending the arm while holding a barbell; concentric force would be raising the barbell to the shoulder; isometric force would be holding it in place.)

"We know that there is this decrease in concentric and isometric force production as a result of static stretching," Cramer added, "but what we really want to know is why."

The question arises due to the intriguing discovery that stretching one leg weakens both, implying that more than mechanical forces ate at play. One theory is that a central nervous system mechanism is invoked.

Cramer doesn't feel as if he has enough information to recommend sweeping changes in training methods, regardless.

"Our studies suggest that these decreases in force production are so small that this may be a nonissue in actual practice," he said. "This fall were going to conduct a longer study to see if regular static stretching (versus preexercise stretching alone) may avoid some of these deleterious effects."

Different approaches

Ian Shrier, MD, PhD, a past president of the Canadian Academy of Sport Medicine and currently director of the epidemiology consultation service at the Sir Mortimer B. Davis Jewish General Hospital in Montreal, has earned a reputation for speaking bluntly about the issue.

"Most people believe that if you stretch immediately before exercise, it prevents injury and improves your performance," Shrier said. "Both of those are wrong. Lots of studies show that stretching right before exercise decreases the amount of force you can produce and how high you can jump."

Though it doesn't seem to have much effect on running speed, he added.

In a 2000 article in the *British Journal of Sports Medicine* concluding that preexercise stretching didn't prevent injury unless it was combined with an overall warm-up,[23] Shrier made several key points. For one, most injuries occur during eccentric contractions rather than concentric ones—and eccentric actions typically cause damage within the normal ROM, suggesting that stretching isn't likely to prevent such injuries. He also pointed out that stretching often increases pain tolerance, which in itself can increase injury risk for the simple reason that athletes may not be aware when they're hurting themselves.

But Shrier acknowledged that when stretching is done as part of a comprehensive program, the situation changes.

"Where most people mess up is by lumping stretching before exercise with stretching in general," he said. "If you stretch regularly, but not immediately before exercise, you actually increase your force, increase the amount you jump, and increase your speed. My guess is that if you stretch three or four times a week, you'll see benefits, and I personally believe that in the future people will say that it prevents injury—though the jury's out on that."

Fitting the stretch to the activity

It's illustrative of the tenor of the broader argument that Malachy McHugh, PhD, claims friendship with Shrier, then laughingly claims to disagree with most of what Shrier says, then proceeds to agree with him on several issues including this last one.

McHugh, director of research at the Nicholas Institute of Sports Medicine and Athletic Trauma at Lenox Hill Hospital in New York, has published several studies of the effects of stretching on muscle elasticity. One found that muscle stiffness may be a risk factor for postexercise damage,[24] but others have suggested that the relationship of flexibility to performance may depend on which sport is studied.[25]

Nevertheless, McHugh thinks preexercise stretching is valuable as part of an overall warm-up. He noted that most people stretch to avoid muscle strains, and that little research has focused on its effects in sports with a high incidence of strains, such as soccer or football.

The rationale for strain prevention is that stretching makes the muscle more compliant, he said, which has implications for force production and injury prevention.

"We think a more compliant muscle has a greater functional range of motion, meaning the longer muscle should be able to produce more force," he said. "Usually at longer muscle lengths you lose strength because there is less overlap of your cross-bridges—the force-generating part of the muscle. But if you make a muscle a little more compliant, you can get more cross-bridge overlap and generate more force at the longer length. The muscles

STRETCHING METHODS	
METHOD	DESCRIPTION
Passive	Slow, sustained muscle lengthening with a partner
Static	Slow, sustained muscle lengthening held by subject for 15 to 60 seconds
Isometric	Static stretching against an immobile force
Ballistic	Rapid lengthening of the muscle using bouncing movements (now largely discredited due to increased injury risk)
Dynamic	Use of an antagonist muscle to help stretch another (e.g., activating the quadriceps to help stretch the hamstrings)
PNF*	Stretching with or without a partner by contracting, then relaxing, the muscle to be lengthened

*Proprioceptive neuromuscular facilitation
Source: Adapted from reference 1, with changes based on information from other sources.

adapt rapidly, which is why a workout that makes you sore one week doesn't do so the next."

McHugh also offered an intriguing theory about the nature of strength loss after an acute bout of stretching. In some spots, such as sprinting, athletes must push their muscles almost to the point of failure.

"Maximal performance and injury risk might be complementary," he said. "The safety window might get smaller and smaller. As a result, if there's a small decrease in the amount of force you can produce, it might have a protective effect."

However, viewed in the context of reports from Cramer (that static stretching doesn't reduce eccentric force production) and Shrier (that most injuries occur during eccentric contractions), McHugh may need some evidence to back this up.

Overall, McHugh believes that the activity should determine the flexibility required—and that in many cases, stretching in some form is essential.

"In a lot of sports, dance and gymnastics in particular, you have to have the range of motion to perform your task," he said. "If dancers don't warm up and stretch, they won't be able to get their bodies into the positions required. Hurdlers have to have flexible hamstrings or they're not getting over the hurdle. But for a long-distance runner, tighter hamstrings are actually beneficial. A lot of other sports fall in between, and that's where the controversy lies."

Another kind of performance

When it comes to activities such as dance, performance doesn't just mean power and speed, of course; it carries connotations of artistry. And in this, consensus emerges among the factions.

"Say a ballet dancer has a vertical jump of 23 inches," Shrier said. "If she stretches before her performance and it drops to 22 inches, nobody in the audience is going to notice. But she might feel that it is easier, less strenuous, and

that she can hold her form longer. So even though she isn't jumping as high, her performance is actually better. And though I don't think stretching needs to be part of most warm-ups, the rest of warm-up is extremely important. I'm not saying the ballerina should go out there cold."

Ruth Solomon agrees. Professor emeritus at the University of California, Santa Cruz, Solomon has been a dancer and dance trainer all of her professional life. She has published dozens of books, monographs, and journal articles about training and injury prevention, and is a member of the board of the International Association for Dance Medicine & Science.

She is often shocked when she walks into dance studios to teach for the first time and sees dancers stretching on a cold floor. "I say, 'Please don't do that!' and explain that we'll stretch in the middle and at the end of class," she said.

According to Solomon, stretching must be an integral part of the warm-up process.

"As long as the blood is coursing through the body, the oxygen is flowing through the muscles, and the muscles are warm—then you can stretch," she said. "But not before. If you don't stretch and strengthen together, you'll have a weak muscle. The strength must balance the stretch if you wait to control your movements."

Solomon explained that dancers are at risk for injury partly because dance demands such extended ranges of motion. Moreover, ballet dancers typically do exercises such as *développés* and *grand battements* that develop their quadriceps, but may neglect the hamstrings. The resulting strength imbalance puts extra stress on the knee joint.

"If the muscles are really stretched out, the ligaments may not be able to protect the joints," she said. "So you get unstable joints, particularly knees, and you may get hyperextension and ligament tears." Proprioceptive neuromuscular facilitation stretches are now favored in the dance community because they both strengthen and lengthen muscles, Solomon said.

A holistic view

Because dancers do get injured, however, its helpful to have physical therapists available who understand the injuries, how best to rehab them, and how to prevent recurrence. Rocky Botnstein, PT, was a dancer for 25 years before going into practice at Westside Dance Physical Therapy in New York.

Although Bornstein understands the necessity of isolating muscle groups to measure biomechanical forces, as in the studies described earlier, from a practical perspective she must consider her patients more holistically.

"Dancers tend to have a lot of laxity in their joints, a lot of range of motion, so in some cases strengthening may be more of an issue than stretching," she said. "If you have a joint that is not biomechanically lined up, the muscles that move it will be working overtime to compensate. Stretching the muscle without addressing the joint won't help."

For Bornstein, it's also critical to address how certain muscle groups affect the whole body. These data are typically missing from clinical trials because they are hard to measure, but perplexing results such as those reported by Knudson (where complex motions seemed to nullify the weakening effects of stretching) or by Cramer (where unilateral stretching had bilateral effects) highlight the issue's importance.

"Muscle lengths affect other joints in the body," Bornstein said. "People with short hamstrings who don't stretch them are going to break down somewhere else, probably in the lower back. We stretch our pectorals not just to lengthen them, but to alleviate upper back or cervical strain. It's allowing joints to move in the best way possible—and that's not necessarily the joint directly attached to the muscle."

Consensus begins to emerge when it comes to long-term stretching regimens.

"Dancers should stretch when their bodies are warm," Bornstein said. "That would not be right before you go out to perform. For that, you want to increase your circulation, be warm and ready and viable. Afterward, when the muscle has been worked really hard, is a better time to stretch,"

As noted, Shrier supports this notion.

"Think of stretching like weight training," he said. "If you do it regularly, you get stronger. It's just that nobody does an exhausting workout right before they compete."

"I think he's exactly right," Knudson said when told of this remark. "Studies of strength and weight training in combination with stretching show that stretching doesn't diminish the effects. Some people who stretched did a little better."

It's apparent that the extent to which stretching is incorporated into warm-ups will depend on the individual and the activity, but it's reassuring to know that professional opinions may be converging. And who knows?—as time goes on, Stephen Thacker at the CDC may even get a little less hate mail.

Cary Groner is a freelance writer based in Northern California.

References are available online at www.biomech.com

EAT MORE WEIGH LESS

THE ANSWER MAY LIE IN THE NEW SCIENCE OF 'VOLUMETRICS'

Amanda Spake

Three young women scurry back and forth from the stainless steel counters to the big walk-in refrigerator, loading plates, written instructions, and questionnaires on trays in this commercial-style kitchen. But this is not like any other restaurant kitchen. The staff members not only prepare the food; they carefully weigh, measure, and record the food before it's served. They also weigh and measure what diners leave on their plates.

> **BARBARA ROLLS**
>
> **Her "kitchen" at Pennsylvania State University also serves as her Volumetrics laboratory.**

The adjoining dining room is also not typical. There are 16 individual cubicles separated by short walls and long, blue curtains, rather like the instant-photo booths once found in variety stores. Buffet tables are set up where dishes are kept hot. Small, unobtrusive video cameras record food selections at the buffet and the eating habits of diners inside the booths, all of it broadcast to monitors in the kitchen and in some of the offices surrounding the dining room.

Welcome to Pennsylvania State University's Laboratory for the Study of Human Ingestive Behavior, one of the world's most sophisticated centers for the study of what and how humans eat. The queen of this quirky culinary empire is Barbara Rolls, professor and Guthrie chair in nutrition at the university. For nearly three decades, Rolls, 60, has researched food choices, portion sizes, the caloric or energy density of foods, and myriad other factors that influence the human appetite and what satisfies it.

Most recently, the lab has been studying the impact of energy or calorie density—that is, the number of calories in a given weight of food—on satiety and weight control. Rolls calls this research "Volumetrics," and her new book, *The Volumetrics Eating Plan,* arrives in bookstores this week. Part weight-control program, part cookbook, it is an effort to put into practical form a lifetime of study on why people eat what they do and

how to satisfy the human biological drive for abundant food while achieving a healthy weight.

IN MANY WAYS, THE THEORY REPRESENTS THE ULTIMATE "VALUE MEAL": EAT MORE FOR LESS.

It was Rolls who realized that satiety, or the sensation of fullness, is "food specific." That is, when people are full of one food, they can still eat another—an explanation, says Rolls, "for why you always have room for dessert." She was among the first to notice that humans eat about the same weight or volume of food every day but not the same calories, a notion now accepted by nutrition scientists.

Supersize. Yet she also discovered an apparent contradiction: When food portions are "supersized," people eat more. Adults offered four different portions of macaroni and cheese at her lab ate 30 percent more calories when given the largest portion, compared with the smallest. Fewer than half noticed any difference in the serving sizes. Likewise, in Rolls's sandwich experiments, men and women were served 6-, 8-, 10-, and 12-inch submarine sandwiches. When given the 12-inch sub, women ate 31 percent more calories and men 56 percent more—compared with those given the 6-inch sub. Asked to rate their fullness after lunch, diners reported little difference whether they had eaten the larger or smaller sub. In a two-day study, portion sizes were increased for some dishes by as much as 100 percent, and people continued to eat more over both days. "As to why people respond this way, I don't know, but that is part of what we're working on," Rolls says. "Clearly, visual and cognitive cues are important."

What has become clear from her Volumetrics studies is that the key to weight management lies in "food choices that help you feel full with fewer calories." The absence of satiety is one reason most "diets" don't work very well or for very long. "Satiety is the missing ingredient in weight management," Rolls writes, and she's impatient with those who say the nation's obesity epidemic can be reversed by "telling people to eat less. People need to eat *more* low-energy-dense food, such as fruits and vegetables, so they get a satisfying amount of food and enough calories." This view is echoed in the 2005 Dietary Guidelines for Americans. And studies show that encouraging overweight families, for example, to eat more fruits and vegetables results in greater weight loss than telling them not to eat foods high in fat and sugar. "Emphasizing what people *can* eat rather than what they should not eat seems more sustainable," says Rolls.

In her lab, she tested these theories recently in the first year-long clinical trial of Volumetrics, involving 97 obese women. One group was given Volumetrics ideas and encouraged to eat more fruits, vegetables, soups, whole grains, and legumes. The other group received more traditional and negative messages about restricting fat and portion sizes. Neither group counted calories or fat grams, yet both groups showed a similar reduction in fat intake, and both groups lost weight. "The low-energy-density diet group ate a greater weight of food over a year but lost more body weight—about 20 pounds," says Rolls. The group given negative messages, to eat less fat and smaller portions, lost about 15 pounds. While the 33 percent greater amount of weight lost by the Volumetrics group may not have made anybody skinny, the group also ate more fruits and vegetables—five servings a day compared with 3.5—and a diet lower in energy density and richer in important nutrients.

While the trial is encouraging, Rolls is the first to say that it's small. Volumetrics needs to be tested at a number of medical centers, among more participants, and over a longer time. "There is so much research money going into diets that change the proportion of macronutrients [fat, protein, and carbohydrates]," says Rolls. "Yet what we're advocating will lead people to follow the new dietary guidelines and optimize not only weight but nutritional status as well."

In many ways, the theory represents the ultimate "value meal": Eat more for less. The secret ingredients that make foods less energy dense are water and fiber, which explains why most vegetables are among the lowest-energy-dense foods available, while vegetable oils, with all the water and fiber removed, are the highest. The principle becomes obvious when thinking of fruit: One hundred calories of grapes represents a great deal more food in terms of weight and volume, and is more filling, than 100 calories of raisins, or dried grapes. The same is true for nearly any dish. The drier the food, the higher its energy density. Potato chips (dry and cooked in vegetable oil) are five times as energy dense as a baked potato. Pasta, which absorbs water as it cooks, is about half as energy dense as Italian bread, even though the ingredients are similar. Adding water or water-rich foods, like vegetables, and using oils and energy-dense ingredients sparingly lower the density of most dishes, allowing larger portions and increasing satiety.

VEGGIES OR JUNK?

Nothing wrong with a few chips now and then, but the fiber and water in veggies will leave you far more satisfied.

The formula. Energy density is easy to calculate from a food label. Just divide the calories in one serving by its weight in grams, and you have the energy density of the food. To use Volumetrics for weight control, Rolls recommends making up a large portion of the diet with foods that have fewer calories in a serving than their weight in grams, resulting in energy densities below 1 (most fruits, vegetables, and low-fat dairy products). Also good are foods with calories equal to or slightly greater than their weight, or an energy density of 1 to 2 (beans, fish, chicken without fat or skin, potatoes, pasta, rice, low-fat salad dressings). Foods that have two or more times as many calories as their weight (ice cream, beef, french fries, cheese, pretzels, full-fat salad dressings, chips, cookies, bacon, oils) need to be controlled.

The Volumetrics principles are also useful for lowering the caloric density of whole meals. Rolls demonstrated the concept in her salad studies. Different groups of diners ate different sizes of salads with different energy densities. High-density salads had full-fat dressing and cheese, for example, while low-density salads were vegetables with fat-free dressing. She found that the diners who ate the large, low-density salads before a pasta entree ate about 100 fewer calories of pasta and 12 percent fewer calories for the meal. By contrast, the high-density salads increased the total calories by 17 percent. In a similar study of 200 overweight individuals on a weight-loss diet, those who ate soup as a snack twice a day lost 50 percent more weight than dieters snacking on dry, low-fat, calorie-dense foods, like pretzels or baked chips.

"We're being urged to manage calories," says Rolls. "So Volumetrics gives people a way to do that without having to count calories. If people understand where the calories are in foods, they can go for lower calories, lower density, and bigger portions of foods." Portion size and energy density independently contribute to the total calories of a meal, says Rolls, which is why restaurant eating is such a waist-expanding experience—energy density is high, and portions are large. "When people really get the energy-density message, they can accommodate in their diet some high-energy-dense foods in moderation," says Rolls. "But it's all trade-offs: You can eat a lot more apples than apple pie, but if you really want that piece of apple pie, it's better to accommodate it."

Food family. Rolls comes from a family fascinated by food. Her great-grandparents were farmers. Her grandfather, a professor at Cornell University, helped establish the New York agricultural extension program. Rolls grew up in Adelphi, Md., outside Washington, D.C., where her father spent most of his career at the U.S. Department of Agriculture. Her mother was a teacher and homemaker who struggled with food choices and weight control. "She was obese," Rolls says, "and she died of obesity-related illnesses—diabetes and cardiovascular disease."

A premed student at the University of Pennsylvania, Rolls graduated in biology and secured a fellowship to Cambridge University in England. She stayed in England, became a research fellow in experimental psychology and nutrition, and married Edmund Rolls, a professor of experimental psychology at Oxford. Her first studies of satiety were in the early 1980s. "My ex-husband was doing some neurophysiology experiments and found that cells in the brain stopped firing when we reached satiety with a certain kind of food but started firing again when we eat another food. This was fascinating because it meant that satiety is not global. It can be specific to the food or type of food you have been eating. People tire of salty or spicy foods and like the change to the sweet taste. So, when we have a variety of foods, we eat more."

Spice of life. In a series of experiments, Rolls looked at how variety influences the amount of food people eat. Students fed four courses at a meal ate 60 percent more than when they were served just one of the foods. When student nurses were offered sandwiches for lunch with either one filling or four different fillings, they ate 33 percent more food when offered the variety. Even the shape of food affects how much people eat: Volunteers ate 15 percent more pasta when served three different shapes than when served only one. "This is why it's important to have on hand a variety of low-energy-dense foods [oranges, pears, apples, carrots, celery, salad greens, soup, stew]. Otherwise, we eat high-density foods that are all too readily available [chips, crackers, cookies, pizza, fast-food burgers, and fries] because we want variety."

Rolls divorced and came back to the United States in 1984 with her two daughters, Juliet and Melissa, to an associate professorship in psychiatry at Johns Hopkins School of Medicine. "Members of the department were interested in the role gut hormones play in satiety," she says. She became a full professor in 1991 and made the move to Pennsylvania State in 1992 when the university offered her the directorship of the school's new Laboratory for the Study of Human Ingestive Behavior.

SALAD SOLUTION

A large, low-fat salad before the main course reduces the amount of calories people eat during the entire meal.

"I spent the 1990s comparing proportions of carbohydrate and fat because that's where the action was," she says, meaning the research money. "But we really weren't finding much difference in the effect of fat or carbohydrates on the total calories people ate. So, I noticed that people were eating the same weight or volume of food. I remember going to meetings where everybody was talking about the right proportion of fat or protein in the diet, and I'd say, 'Look at the weight of the food people are eating! It's the same, whether it's high in fat or carbohydrates.' See, we all thought people were eating for calories, the same number of calories per day. But they weren't. They were eating for the same weight or volume of food." The idea of Volumetrics was born.

Much nutritional research still focuses on macronutrients, or the ratio of fat, protein, and carbohydrate in the diet. Clinical studies on the effectiveness of low-carbohydrate versus low-fat diets for weight loss are still underway, but so far most show similar outcomes and modest long-term results. In fact, much of the public remains confused about these seemingly contradictory diet strategies, in part, as Rolls puts it, "because there has really been a lot of controversy in the field over fat. Understanding energy density resolves a lot of these issues." Both high-fat foods and foods high in refined carbohydrates are energy dense and make weight control difficult.

One of the first studies on this subject was done not by Rolls but by researchers at the University of Alabama in 1983, who found that people on a low-energy-dense diet reached satiety with about half the calories of those on a high-density diet. Rolls uses the study in her presentations and laments that the researchers didn't continue it. But that article and Rolls's subsequent studies began to influence those working in the weight-loss trenches. "I was in private practice at that time," says James J. Kenney, nutritionist at the Pritikin Longevity Center. "I had this one woman who wasn't losing weight on a low-fat diet. I started looking at what she was eating, and everything was dry: dried fruit, dried cereal, dry crackers, energy-dense foods." When she switched to soups, salads, fresh fruit, and vegetables, her weight dropped.

Once at Pritikin, Kenney suggested the center change its emphasis from the low-fat regimen that the program had been founded upon to one emphasizing a lower-caloric-density approach. Kenney was fearful that the wave of low-fat but high-energy-dense cookies, crackers, and snack foods hitting the market would lead to more obesity and confuse the public about the usefulness of reducing fat calories. "And that's just what happened," he says. "In the 1990s, we saw Americans gaining weight like never before. … The public has been oblivious to the very important role calorie density plays in how full people feel when they eat a set amount of calories."

Of course, a small group of elite dieters who attend some of the premier weight-control centers have been schooled in energy density. At the Duke Diet and Fitness Center, as at Pritikin, nutrition manager Elisabetta Politi has been using an energy-density approach for a few years. "I think Barbara Rolls has a great theory, and there is a lot of interest in it," says Politi. "We take advantage of what she's found in what we do here. We start with a big salad, soup, smaller servings of protein and higher-density foods; and our clients feel satisfied on 1,200 or 1,300 calories a day." Likewise, Brian Zehetner, the lead nutritionist at Canyon Ranch SpaClub at the Venetian in Las Vegas, says, "We promote foods that are high in fiber and water. They add bulk, but it's not calorie-containing bulk. So theoretically, you can decrease your calorie intake and eat more food while eating low-energy-dense foods compared to eating high-energy-dense foods." Rolls wants Volumetrics to be accepted by a wider audience, however. She's now on the board of the Jenny Craig weight-loss program, and she notes that Weight Watchers seems to be incorporating aspects of Volumetrics as well, though she quibbles with both of these programs.

Paradigm. If the majority of the public, outside of a few weight-control programs, has been oblivious to the role energy density could play in cleaning up the American diet, so have many nutritional scientists. "This is a paradigm shift," agrees Gary Foster, clinical director of the Weight and Eating Disorders Program at the University of Pennsylvania School of Medicine. Volumetrics is "an overarching concept, less based on macronutrients, though clearly, high-fat foods have higher energy density. It's a more unifying approach to diet, and there are data to support it." The downside, Foster says, is that energy density is not listed on food labels. Rolls hopes that will change: "If we had an energy-density number on food labels, it would give people an immediate way to compare foods and the calories in a portion."

"My sense is people are becoming disenchanted with a low-carbohydrate diet, which is a high-energy-dense diet," says Columbia University's Xavier Pi-Sunyer, a member of the dietary guidelines advisory committee and director of the Obesity Research Center at St. Luke's-Roosevelt Hospital Center. "So this would be a return to a lower-energy-density diet. And that is in line with the new guidelines."

THIS EXPLAINS WHY YOU ALWAYS HAVE ROOM FOR DESSERT.

The grocery bill for a week of Volumetrics meals may be higher, says Adam Drewnowski, director of the Nutritional Sciences Program at the University of Washington. "On a per-calorie basis, fruits, vegetables, fish, lean protein, and low-fat dairy products are more expensive sources of pure calories. But we spend so little on food and so much on our cellphones; it really should be the other way around." Drewnowski is an advocate of a diet based on its nutrient density. "But Barbara and I end up in the same place—eating more fruits, vegetables, whole grains, water, and fiber-rich foods, which are nutrient dense."

Foster, Drewnowski, and Pi-Sunyer, like Rolls herself, would like to see Volumetrics and the energy-density concept fully evaluated in long-term clinical trials. "Let's roll this out now to three or four different centers," says Foster, "and see how it works for 300 to 400 people."

A longtime practitioner of Volumetrics, Rolls herself is slim. She swims every day in a lap pool at her house on a mountaintop near the university, walks on campus, takes the stairs instead of the elevator, and encourages people to use step counters to monitor their activity. A past president of the North American Association for the Study of Obesity, Rolls is no ascetic, however. She loves good food, and as she puts it, "I save my juice calories for wine." She and her partner of seven years, Charles Brueggbors, an architect turned foodie, developed the recipes in the book. Brueggbors came to a Volumetrics diet before he met Rolls, after consulting a dietitian some 15 years ago when he developed hypertension and a spare tire. "I still want chips; I still want sausage," Brueggbors says. "But I've learned to like the fresh veggies and low-fat foods, too. And so now I have chips, but I get a bowl, put in a small amount, and when it's gone, I just don't go back."

It's lunchtime, and the first volunteer diner enters the laboratory and is seated in a curtained booth. He's told he may take his plate to the buffet, get as much as he wants, and go back as often as he wants for any of the four dishes: a chicken and noodle casserole; a creamy, green bean and fried onion dish; a broccoli salad; and whipped sweet potatoes. Most diet programs recommend using a small plate to reduce calories in a meal. "We're not finding it's true," says Rolls. "People just go back for more."

Rolls watches on a video monitor as the man makes his way to the buffet table for the third time, piling the noodle casserole and the green bean and onion rings concoction onto his small plate. "Look at that," Rolls laments. "He's not even touching the broccoli salad."

Clearly, we have a long way to go.

Why We're **Losing** the War Against
Obesity

About two-thirds of all adult Americans are fat, but what's alarming is that more children and teenagers are overweight, and as they grow up, their health problems will have huge repercussions for our society.

Louise Witt

The first time Krista Pournaras, 16, remembers dieting was when she was 6 years old. She was gaining weight like "mad," packing on 30 pounds in one year alone. By second grade, it was obvious Pournaras was fat. That's when her mother Lynn Katekovich, a nurse, took her to a pediatrician, who put the young girl on a strict diet that didn't allow any between-meal snacks, not even an apple.

That diet didn't work. Neither did the others. Pournaras went on low-fat diets, she tried Weight Watchers, she even took diet pills. She'd bike around the neighborhood, go to the gym and swim at the local YMCA. Pournaras would lose a few pounds, but then she'd gain them back or gain even more. This year, when Pournaras, who stands slightly taller then 5'2", started her junior year at the local vo-tech in Conway, Pa., north of Pittsburgh, she weighed 245 pounds. She couldn't play with her dogs without becoming short of breath and feeling achy. This summer Pournaras discovered her weight had seriously affected her health: She had high blood pressure and elevated insulin levels, putting her at risk for Type 2 diabetes, and Polycystic Ovarian Syndrome, a condition in which a female has heightened levels of testosterone.

After Katekovich, who owns a medical staffing company, found out her daughter was likely to develop heart disease and diabetes, she cried. That's when she decided to talk to her about having bariatric surgery. Katekovich and her two sisters had had the drastic procedure in January 2003. Since then, the 44-year-old Katekovich, who had weighed 264, has lost 100 pounds. With bariatric surgery the stomach is reduced by 90 percent—to the size of the top joint of the thumb—and the large intestines

are bypassed. On Nov. 12, Dr. Philip Schauer, director of Bariatric Surgery at Magee Women's Hospital in Pittsburgh, operated on Pournaras.

"I was against the surgery," Pournaras says. "But my mom and Dr. Schauer talked to me and said that if I didn't do something about my health, I'd die much younger, younger than usual. I want to be happier about myself and not have as many health problems."

Getting Worse Faster

Pournaras's extreme solution may be unusual, but her weight problem isn't. About 9 million children and adolescents in the U.S. are overweight or obese. That's roughly 15 percent of the children and adolescents between the ages of 6 and 19 who are overweight or obese, according to the latest data compiled during 1999 and 2000 by the Centers for Disease Control and Preventions National Center for Health Statistics. Health officials and physicians blame children's poor eating habits—having supersized portions of junk food and sweetened soft drinks—and physical inactivity, such as watching TV; playing video games or clicking away on PCs, instead of playing. Just take a look at the numbers from a little more than 30 years earlier to see how rapidly children's health has deteriorated: In a similar CDC survey taken from 1971 to 1974, 4 percent of children between the ages of 6 and 11 were overweight or obese, and 6 percent of adolescents between the ages of 12 and 19 were overweight or obese.

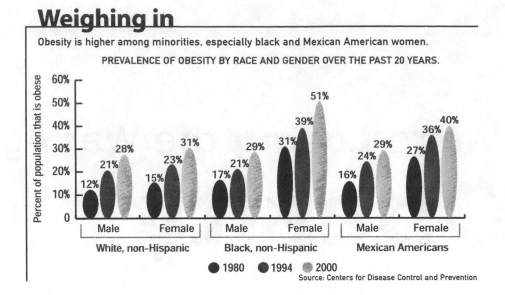

Weighing in

Obesity is higher among minorities, especially black and Mexican American women.

PREVALENCE OF OBESITY BY RACE AND GENDER OVER THE PAST 20 YEARS.

● 1980   ● 1994   ● 2000

Source: Centers for Disease Control and Prevention

And, the nation's obesity problem will only worsen. As today's young people grow older, it's estimated that 3 in 4 overweight children will become fat adults and will suffer from obesity-related diseases at earlier ages than previous generations. Already, about two-thirds of all adults are overweight and about 31 percent of those are considered obese. Generally, if someone weighs more than 30 pounds above his ideal weight, then he's considered obese. The CDC considers someone overweight if his body mass index, or BMI, a calculation based on height and weight, is more than 25. If a person's BMI is over 30, then he is considered obese. Health officials have now deemed obesity in America a health epidemic.

By 2010, only six years away, about 40 percent of all adult Americans, or 68 million, will be obese. If trends continue, almost every single American will be overweight, or obese, (except the few that are genetically prone to have higher metabolisms) by 2040, says John Foreyt, director of Behavioral Medicine Research Center at Baylor College of Medicine in Houston. "It may happen more quickly," he says. "Twenty years ago, it was unusual to see a 300-pound person in my clinic, now we see it all the time. And it used to be we'd see obesity only in adults, but now we see it in children. This may be the first generation of children who will die before their parents."

Foreyt based his projections on data collected from the CDC's Health and Nutritional Examination Surveys, which record actual weights and heights of Americans surveyed, showing that the U.S. population has become much heavier in the past 20 years. In 1980, 46 percent of the adult population was overweight or obese. In 1990, 56 percent was overweight or obese. In 2000, the percent jumped to 64.5 percent. That's 1 percentage point gain a year. Foreyt says part of the problem is that Americans eat 200 more calories a day than they did 10 years ago. Over a year, those extra calories add up to 20 pounds.

Efforts to Reverse Trend

In an effort to slow the rate of increase in obesity, and maybe even reverse the trend, the U.S. Surgeon General's office requested $125 million in the 2004 budget to expand the Healthier US Initiative, a campaign President George W. Bush announced in June 2002 to encourage Americans to eat healthier and exercise more. The 2003 budget was $25 million. In November, the Surgeon General teamed up with the American Academy of Pediatrics, Nike Inc. and McNeil Nutritionals, maker of Splenda artificial sweetner, to launch Shaping America's Youth. Initially, this program intends to find out the scope of children's weight problems and identify community resources available to help them.

"It's an extraordinary project because there are children out there who are sedentary and who eat indiscriminately," says Dr. Richard H. Carmona, the U.S. Surgeon General. "When [these children] are middle-aged and overweight, or obese, they will have Type 2 diabetes, hypertension and cardiovascular disease. We're making an unhealthy society for our children. We have to break that cycle; it affects all of us."

Costs add up

It's difficult to put a price tag on what it costs people who are overweight to live in a society that values thinness and fitness. What's the price of a chubby teenager who is so fearful of being mocked by classmates that he decides not to go college? Yet, for more tangible expenses, the CDC estimates that in 2000, the latest figures available, obesity cost $117 billion: $56 billion in lost productivity and $61 billion in medical treatments. About 300,000 deaths a year are attributed to obesity-related diseases. "That's approaching the costs for treating people with tobacco-related diseases," says Mary Kay Sones, a spokesperson with the CDC's National Center for Chronic Disease Prevention and Health Promotion in Atlanta.

It's a Big Country

The maps compare obesity levels across the country in 1991 and today. It seems Colorado residents have been watching their weight, while Midwesterners and Southerners have been spreading out.

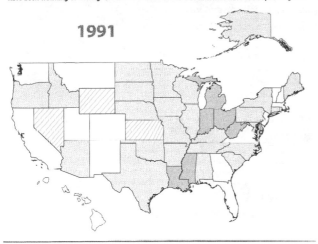

1991

Obesity Index
Percentage of adult population that is obese, by state.

- ○ 8%–10%
- ○ 11%–14%
- ○ 15%–17%
- ● 18%–20%
- ● 21%–23%
- ● 24%–26%
- ○ Data not available

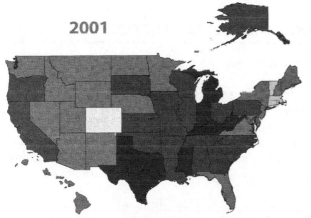

2001

Source: National Center for Chronic Disease Prevention and Health Promotion. Map created using ESRI ArcView 8.3

That may be an underestimate, because obesity has so many ramifications. It contributes to higher incidences of cancer, specifically kidney cancer, and orthopedic complications, due to the excess stress on bones and cartilage. Diabetes alone costs about $130 billion a year. The disease can cause blindness, kidney failure, strokes and heart disease. It's estimated that diabetes shortens a person's life by 10 to 15 years. Dr. K.M. Venkat Narayan, chief of the CDC's diabetes epidemiology section, says the disease "has a high impact economically and in terms of suffering" for the patients.

The CDC estimates that 1 American in 3 born in 2000 will develop Type 2 diabetes, as they grow older; some while they're still young. In the past, people weren't usually diagnosed with the disease until they were in their 50s or 60s. If obesity trends continue, Narayan projects that in 50 years 28 million Americans will have diabetes, up from 17 million in 2003.

Ronald Sturm, an economist at Rand Corp., a think tank in Santa Monica, Calif., says the number of severely obese people is increasing at an even higher rate. To be considered severely obese a person has to have a BMI of 40 or higher. In 1986, 1 in 200 were considered severely obese. In 2000, that increased to 1 in 50. An average adult male would be roughly 100 pounds more than his ideal weight. For instance, a man who is 5'10" would weigh more than 300 pounds, and a woman who is 5'4" would be more than 250 pounds. Sturm, who studied people between the ages of 50 and 60, projects that by 2020, more than half of men will be obese and about a quarter of those will be severely obese.

Sturm estimates that in 2003 medical costs for an obese man who is 50 years old are $1,000 more a year than they are for a similarly aged man of normal weight. Costs for a severely obese man would be $10,000 more. Sturm figures the costs would be slightly less for severely obese women: about $7,000 a year. That's not even taking into consideration more pricey measures. Bariatric surgery, for instance, costs about $25,000.

Ed Bernstein, executive director of the North American Association for the Study of Obesity in Silver Springs, Md., wants patients' who are under a doctor's care to be reimbursed for weight-loss costs. Currently, patients pay for their treatments, but then they can deduct those expenses from their federal income taxes. "We ridicule people for their health problem," Bernstein says. "We wouldn't do that for someone with diabetes, cancer or heart disease, but we do that with people who are obese....Your body fights you very hard when you try to lose weight. People do it; there are a few success stories. We're learning about what helps keep weight off, but it's not simple."

Who's responsible anyway?

Weight gain seems to be a simple calculation: more calories are consumed than are burned. But it's more complicated. Genes aren't solely responsible for the increase in obesity, but they do play a role. Forty percent of people's weight problems can be blamed on their genes, says Patrick O'Neil, a psychologist and director of the Weight Management Center at the Medical University of South Carolina in Charleston. That's because Homo sapiens evolved under conditions, requiring vigorous physical activity at a time when food supplies were uncertain.

"We're programmed to be able to store energy from our earlier days," O'Neil says. "As far as evolution goes, it's only yesterday that human beings have been on the planet." Today, Americans have ready access to tasty, cheap, high-caloric food. And in our modern society, we're less active. We drive instead of walking. We use a remote to change our TV channels instead of getting up to switch them. And we buy our food in supermarkets rather than hunt animals or raise crops. As he says, "Genes load the gun and the environment pulls the trigger."

Scientific studies suggest that many modern conveniences and luxuries lead to obesity, especially in children. One showed that school-age children who drank sweetened soft drinks had a total energy intake 10 percent higher than those who did not. Fast food is also thought to contribute to obesity because it

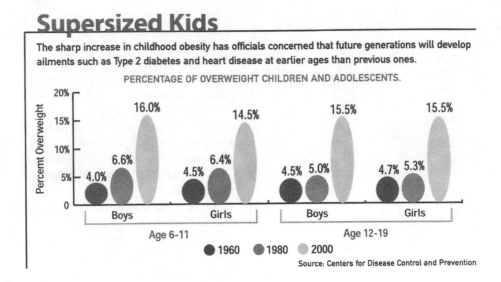

Supersized Kids

The sharp increase in childhood obesity has officials concerned that future generations will develop ailments such as Type 2 diabetes and heart disease at earlier ages than previous ones.

PERCENTAGE OF OVERWEIGHT CHILDREN AND ADOLESCENTS.

● 1960 ● 1980 ◯ 2000

Source: Centers for Disease Control and Prevention

tends to be high in saturated and trans fat—which increases LDL cholesterol, or bad cholesterol—high in sugar and served in large portions. Fast food also tends to be low in dietary fiber, nutrients and antioxidants.

Local efforts in schools

Faced with the burgeoning number of overweight students, state and local government have begun their own initiatives. Two of the nation's largest public school systems, New York City and Los Angeles, banned soda vending during school hours. (The L.A. ban becomes effective January 2004.) New York went a step further, prohibiting snack-food vending machines in schools and reducing the fat content in the school cafeteria food. In October, the L.A. school district followed, banning fried chips, candy and other junk foods from vending machines. The plan also calls on school administrators to end contracts with vendors who sell pizzas and burgers at some institutions.

Last summer, South Carolina started the South Carolina Nutrition Research Consortium, pooling the resources of Clemson University, the University of South Carolina and the Medical University in Charleston to tackle the state's growing overweight population. Almost 22 percent of the state's residents are obese, according to CDC data. "We were concerned about being a chubby state," says Peter Kent, a spokesman for Clemson University. "We're a state at risk."

Surgeon General Carmona says he would like food producers to assume a greater role in fighting obesity. He'd like them to make the nutritional contents of their products more available to consumers, make sure animals are raised under healthy conditions, promote healthy eating messages and offer healthier food options. Suing companies isn't the answer, he says. In 2002, two obese teenagers sued McDonald's, blaming the chain's poor labeling of the nutritional and caloric content in its fast food for their weight gain. The lawsuit was thrown out.

"Rather than make an enemy of corporate America, let's talk to them," Carmona says. "Let's make them part of the solution, rather than the problem."

Food marketers respond

Indeed, food companies have been taking steps to promote healthier eating habits. Kraft Foods Inc., maker of Oscar Mayer cold cuts, Velveeta and Oreo cookies, launched a global anti-obesity effort in July, which calls for smaller portion sizes and improving the nutritional content of some Kraft products. It also includes ending marketing in schools and setting up guidelines for marketing aimed at children. (A San Francisco man dropped a lawsuit last year against Kraft, after it agreed to reduce trans fat in Oreos.)

Recently, Pizza Hut added low-fat items and salads to its menu. Dubbed Fit 'N' Delicious, the pizzas have 25 percent less fat and 30 percent fewer calories. Ruby Tuesday, a restaurant chain, changed its cooking oil from soybean to canola and introduced a low-carbohydrate menu. Burger King began offering salads and a new low-fat chicken sandwich, and KFC has a low-fat barbecue sandwich.

Liz Castells-Heard, president of Castells & Asociados Advertising in Los Angeles, says she used reports on the alarming number of overweight Hispanic youngsters to convince McDonald's to reach out to Hispanic customers with healthier menu items in its California and Texas markets. As a result, Castells-Heard says, the fast-food giant developed three new salads, a veggie burger, a chicken sandwich on whole wheat bread and yogurt parfaits.

Castells-Heard approached McDonald's after noticing that a higher number of Hispanics, especially youngsters, were overweight or obese than the overall U.S. population. According to the NCHS, 27.3 percent of Mexican American boys between the ages of 6 and 11 are overweight, compared with 12 percent of white non-Hispanic boys of the same age. For Mexican American males between 12 and 19 years old, 27.5 percent are

Pound for Pound

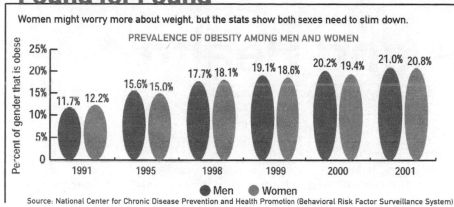

Women might worry more about weight, but the stats show both sexes need to slim down.

PREVALENCE OF OBESITY AMONG MEN AND WOMEN

Year	Men	Women
1991	11.7%	12.2%
1995	15.6%	15.0%
1998	17.7%	18.1%
1999	19.1%	18.6%
2000	20.2%	19.4%
2001	21.0%	20.8%

Source: National Center for Chronic Disease Prevention and Health Promotion (Behavioral Risk Factor Surveillance System)

overweight, compared with 12.8 percent of white non-Hispanics males in that age group. For Mexican American girls between the ages of 6 and 11, 19.6 percent are considered overweight. For Mexican American females between 12 and 19, about 19.4 percent are considered overweight, compared with 12.4 percent of their white non-Hispanic counterparts. "It's part of the Hispanic culture," says Castells-Heard. "They don't have that obsession that younger females have about getting so skinny, or being anorexic or bulimic—that's the good news. The bad news is that we have a higher rate of obesity."

Yet, Americans think that they are slimming down. In its latest survey, released in October, Port Washington, N.Y.-based NPD Group found that Americans said they weren't gaining weight. Of the 5,000 people in the study, 55 percent said they were overweight, compared with 56 percent the year before. "I've never seen that," said Harry Balzer, NPD's vice president, in a statement. "Looks like we're focusing on health again, a return to the '80s. People are interested in a balanced diet; they ate more fruits and vegetables last year than the year before and snacked less in the evening."

NPD survey's respondents were more concerned with fat, cholesterol, sugar and food additives. Thirty-five percent said they plan nutritious meals, up from 32 percent in 2001. And 66 percent said they were strenuously exercising at least once a week, up from 63 percent in 2002. Fifty-three percent said they check food labels to avoid harmful substances, that's up from 51 percent in 2002. But Belzer added: "The question is which trends are the beginning of a new direction and which are short-term disruptions."

Tougher measures needed

The nation's anti-smoking campaign may be an indication of how hard it is to change people's lifestyles. The Surgeon General warned about the dangers of cigarette smoking in 1964.

"Forty years down the line and we're still seeing 440,000 smoking-related deaths a year," says Dr. Carmona. "Obesity kills over 300,000. So, it's rapidly catching up and becoming the fastest growing killer of Americans. It will eclipse smoking in the near future. People are used to eating a certain way from their family and friends. We're talking about changing American culture. It's not cool to be the Marlboro man, but look how long it took us to get to that point."

Kelly D. Brownell, director of the Yale Center for Eating and Weight Disorders, doesn't think the Surgeon General's new anti-obesity program goes far enough. Americans have been bombarded with public service messages to eat healthier and exercise more for years with disappointing results. Brownell, coauthor of *Food Fight* (Contemporary Books, 2003) about America's food industry and the growing prevalence of obesity, thinks banning soft drinks and fast food in schools is a step in the right direction. But he says food advertising geared toward children must change. The average child is inundated with ads for fast food, candy, sugared cereals and soft drinks. "If parents ate every meal with their children and persuaded them to eat healthier, then that would be 1,000 messages for the parents and 10,000 for them," he says. "The advertisers have Britney Spears, Shaquille O'Neal and Beyonce Knowles. It's not a fair contest."

Brownell thinks food and drink ads marketed toward children will eventually change, just as cigarette ads did. "Our nation is quick to respond when it feels children are being victimized and American children are suffering in record numbers with poor diets and physical inactivity," he says.

For some children, these changes can't come soon enough. After her bariatric surgery in November, Krista Pournaras hopes her life will improve. She thinks that she will be a better student when she is thinner, because she won't be afraid to participate in class discussions. Pournaras thinks other obese teens could benefit from this surgery. "I figure if this can help me, and make me happier, why not help other adolescents?

Reprinted by permission of Advertising Age's *American Demographics*, December 2003/January 2004, pp. 27-31. Copyright © 2004 by Crain Communications Inc.

UNIT 5

Drugs and Health

Unit Selections

Key Points to Consider

- Should Americans be legally permitted to buy prescription drugs from Canada?

- How should athletes who abuse enhancement drugs be punished? How should professional sports teams prevent the use of these drugs among athletes?

- Do you think America has a drug problem? Defend your answer.

- Why do teenagers use drugs despite the messages they've heard from DARE and "Just Say No"?

Student Website

www.mhcls.com/online

Internet References

Further information regarding these websites may be found in this book's preface or online.

Food and Drug Administration (FDA)
  http://www.fda.gov/

National Institute on Drug Abuse (NIDA)
  http://165.112.78.61

Prescription Drugs: The Issue
  http://www.opensecrets.org/news/drug/

As a culture, Americans have come to rely on drugs—not only as a treatment for disease but also—as an aid for living normal, productive lives. This view of drugs has fostered both a casual attitude regarding their use and a tremendous drug abuse problem. Drug use and abuse has become so widespread that there is no way to describe the typical drug abuser.

There is no simple explanation for why America has become a drug-taking culture, but there is certainly evidence to suggest some of the factors that have contributed to this development. From the time that we are children, we are constantly bombarded by advertisements about how certain drugs can make us feel and look better. While most of these ads deal with proprietary drugs, the belief is created that drugs are a legitimate and effective way to help us cope with everyday problems. Certainly drugs can have a profound effect on how we feel and act, but research has also demonstrated that our mind plays a major role in the healing process.

Growing up, most of us probably had a medicine cabinet full of over-the-counter (OTC) drugs, freely dispensed to family members to treat a variety of ailments. This familiarity with OTC drugs, coupled with rising health-care costs, has prompted many people to diagnose and medicate themselves with OTC medications without sufficient knowledge of their possible side effects. While most of these preparations have little potential for abuse, that does not mean that they are innocuous. Generally speaking, OTC drugs are relatively safe if taken at the recommended dosage by healthy people, but the risk of dangerous side effects rises sharply when people exceed the recommended dosage. Another potential danger associated with the use of OTC drugs is the drug interactions that can occur when they are taken in conjunction with prescription medications. The gravest danger associated with the use of OTC drugs is that an individual may use them to control symptoms of an underlying disease and thus prevent its early diagnosis and treatment. The issue of high prescription drug costs is addressed in "The New Drug War." Due to rising drug costs, many Americans are seeking out lower prices in Canada. Pharmaceutical companies are against this practice while many politicians seek to legalize Canadian drug purchases.

Another category of over the counter medications, herbal preparations, has become extremely popular. They include approximately 750 substances such as herbal teas and other products of botanical origin that are believed to have medicinal properties. Many have been used for centuries with no ill effects, but others have questionable safety records. One drug with a checkered history is the herb ephedra, used in over-the-counter weight control products sold in pharmacies, mall kiosks, and via the Internet. The recent death of 23 year old Baltimore Orioles pitcher Steve Bechler in February 2003, attributed to the use of ephedra, brought attention to the risks of the herb. Soon after Bechler's death, minor league baseball banned the herb, joining other sports organization that had already banned its use. Health officials caution consumers against the use of the drug, especially if it's combined with other stimulants such as caffeine, or if strenuous exercise is involved. In the article, "Sports and Drugs," Kenneth Jost discusses the dangers of sports enhancing drugs. Other dangerous supplements are addressed in "Dangerous Supplements Still at Large."

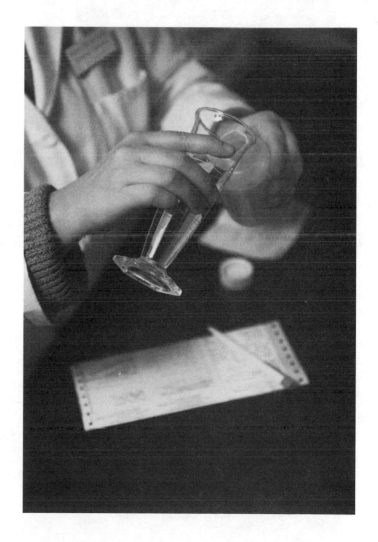

As a culture, we have grown up believing that there is, or should be, a drug to treat any malady or discomfort that befalls us. Would we have a drug problem if there were no demand for drugs? One drug that is used widely in the U.S. is marijuana. Despite drug education that discourages its use, marijuana is still a popular drug on high school and college campuses and among many adults. In "Just Say No Again: The Old Failures of New and Improved Anti-Drug Education," Renee Moilanen compares various drug education programs including DARE, Just Say No, and others.

The New Drug War

Pharmaceutical companies need profits to develop new drugs.
Patients need pills that they can afford. Their interests are colliding at the Canadian border.

BY ROGER PARLOFF

Four years ago, on the frozen prairies of Manitoba, two young pharmacists, working independently, founded a billion-dollar industry. In the process they created a quandary for global health-care policy, a hot-button issue for this year's U.S. presidential race, and a potential diplomatic crisis for Canada and the U.S.

It all started in Minnedosa (pop. 2,426), about two hours west of Winnipeg and three hours north of the North Dakota line—when the roads are passable. Freshly graduated pharmacist Andrew Strempler, then 25, noticed that prices of Nicorette gum were much lower in Canada than in the U.S. So he began selling it to Americans over eBay. (Nicorette does not require a prescription.) Soon he set up a website. Within three months, Strempler recalls, his sales had gone from about one box a week to 150 per *day*. His distributor informed him that he was selling more Nicorette than any drugstore in Canada.

At just about the same time, Winnipeg pharmacist Daren Jorgenson began selling glucose-monitoring equipment over the Internet. Jorgenson had first checked with U.S. officials to make sure that the sales were legal, which they were. But while making his inquiries, Jorgenson says, he came across a U.S. Food and Drug Administration official, whom he identifies only as "Tom." Tom told Jorgenson that what he *really* ought to be selling over the Internet was prescription drugs, because that's where the price disparity was greatest—about 30% to 80% on brand-name drugs—and where the demand was most urgent.

"I didn't think I could," says Jorgenson in an interview, alluding to U.S. laws generally forbidding the importation of pharmaceuticals except by manufacturers. But then Tom told him about the FDA's "personal use" policy. Jorgenson understood him to say that Americans were allowed to bring in a small supply of drugs (no more than three months' worth) for their own use.

Unquestionably, for many years busloads of American seniors lucky enough to live near the border have been crossing into Canada to buy cheap drugs with the tacit indulgence of U.S. Customs and the FDA. Nevertheless, the

FDA says today that its "personal importation" policy has never actually authorized those bus trips, let alone what Jorgenson was contemplating. (The written policy countenances only noncommercial importation under defined circumstances, such as when drugs are prescribed in another country and equivalent drugs are unavailable in the U.S.)

By March 2000, after consulting with lawyers who could find no *Canadian* laws against selling prescription drugs to American customers, Jorgenson launched CanadaMeds.com. Strempler followed suit with RxNorth.com.

The business idea worked. Over the next three years, RxNorth's sales multiplied 20-fold, from $3.2 million (all figures are in U.S. dollars) in 2001 to about $70 million in 2003. Strempler's Minnedosa facility now employs about 200 people. "We employ 10% of the population," he says. "The other 90% are unemployable, because they're retired." Though Strempler has a matter-of-fact, understated manner, he wears a gem-studded ring the size of a PDA.

Meanwhile, Jorgenson's CanadaMeds and a second Internet pharmacy he subsequently set up *each* sold about $70 million last year. Revenue for the whole industry—there are now 64 Internet pharmacies in Manitoba and maybe 75 more scattered across the rest of Canada—was about $800 million in 2003.

Strempler and Jorgenson are two brass knuckles on Adam Smith's invisible hand, which is now battering away at the fragile lattice of geographic price disparities that overlays the global pharmaceutical market. Though that structure evolved for complex reasons, the fundamentals are simple. Most Western nations other than the U.S. regulate the price of prescription drugs, either through direct price controls or through other government-driven cost-containment schemes. In Canada, for instance, a federal board effectively sets ceilings on the prices of patented drugs, while each province exerts further downward pressure by creating formularies and capping reimbursements under its social insurance plan. (It is only brand-name drugs that are cheaper in Canada; generics actually cost less in the U.S. because of greater competition.) Though Canada's regulated prices exceed the manufacturers'

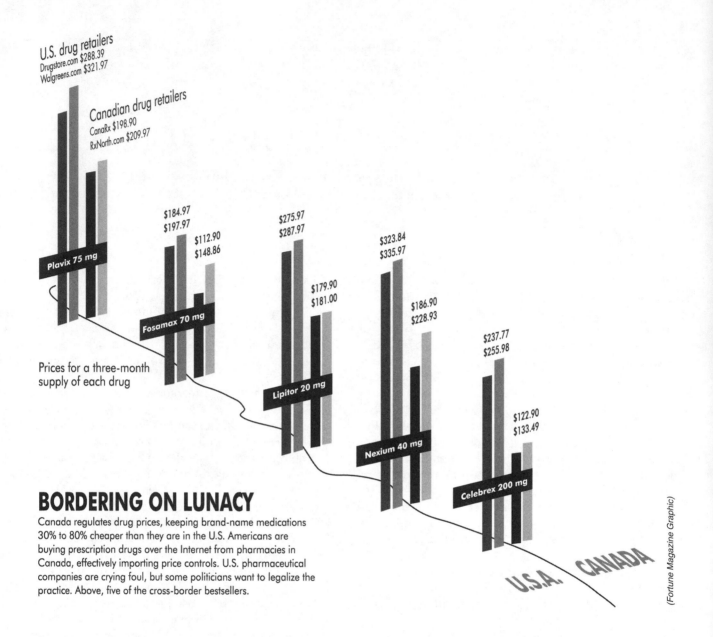

U.S. drug retailers
Drugstore.com $288.39
Walgreens.com $321.97

Canadian drug retailers
CanaRx $198.90
RxNorth.com $209.97

Plavix 75 mg

$184.97
$197.97
$112.90
$148.86

Fosamax 70 mg

Prices for a three-month
supply of each drug

$275.97
$287.97
$179.90
$181.00

Lipitor 20 mg

$323.84
$335.97
$186.90
$228.93

Nexium 40 mg

$237.77
$255.98
$122.90
$133.49

Celebrex 200 mg

BORDERING ON LUNACY

Canada regulates drug prices, keeping brand-name medications
30% to 80% cheaper than they are in the U.S. Americans are
buying prescription drugs over the Internet from pharmacies in
Canada, effectively importing price controls. U.S. pharmaceutical
companies are crying foul, but some politicians want to legalize the
practice. Above, five of the cross-border bestsellers.

U.S.A. CANADA

(Fortune Magazine Graphic)

rather trivial costs of making the pills, the companies claim that they do not begin to pay for the enormous R&D expenditures necessary to develop an innovative drug in the lab and see it through the years of animal testing and clinical trials needed to gain FDA approval. That process can often take as long as 12 years and cost as much as $802 million per drug that makes it to market, one academic study estimates. The manufacturers maintain that they must recover high returns where they can—i.e., the U.S.—to encourage the R&D that sustains the industry and benefits mankind. Greed might be a factor too.

The pressure is growing daily on U.S. politicians to alter that odd global price structure—in which the rest of the world seems to catch a free ride on the backs of American seniors. Expenditures on retail prescription drugs in America—$162 billion in 2002—now account for 10.5% of the nation's total health-care costs, which, in turn, consume 14.9% of the GDP. Prescription-drug expenditures

are the fastest-growing piece of the health-care pie, having risen at a 15.6% annual rate from 2000 to 2002. As Americans live longer, as miracle drugs become an ever more crucial component of health care, as Medicare expands to encompass prescription-drug coverage, and as the baby-boom generation marches toward retirement, prognosticators can agree on only one proposition: Something's got to give.

You'll be hearing more about those issues in the coming weeks too, because Democrats believe President Bush is vulnerable on his pro-industry health-care stances. In the Democratic reply to the State of the Union address, Senator Tom Daschle urged legalization of Canadian drugs—as have all the Democratic presidential candidates.

But it's not just Democrats who are clamoring for legalization. For many of the 43 million Americans—including 40% of all seniors—who have no prescription-drug insurance, Canadian prices are a godsend. These Americans can't afford to heed safety warnings from FDA officials or lectures from economists about R&D incentivization. For them the new, gap-ridden Medicare prescription-drug benefit is unlikely to diminish the allure of Canadian drugs, even once it kicks in, in 2006. (No one knows yet if the government's discount drug card program, which launches in April, will afford greater benefits than existing discount cards, which have failed to deter seniors from exploring the Canadian option.)

More important, seniors aren't the only Americans who have come to see Canadian drugs as a quick fix. Elected state officials of both parties are looking north for relief from their own groaning budget crises. While Canadian Internet pharmacies currently account for a tiny percentage of the U.S. pharmaceutical market, that situation will change quickly if the officials have anything to say about it.

"We pay about $600 million just through Medicaid for pharmaceutical products," says Minnesota attorney general Mike Hatch. "We can save $300 million by using a Canadian-style system. Then add in the state employees—which is huge. We're talking real dollars here." (The Pharmaceutical Research and Manufacturers Association—known as PhRMA—claims that Hatch's savings calculations are outlandishly inflated.) In late January, Minnesota's Republican governor, Tim Pawlenty, added a page to his official website telling Minnesotans how to order drugs from Canada and also recommending specific Canadian Internet pharmacies. Asked in the past about the FDA's safety concerns, Pawlenty has famously responded, "Show me the dead Canadians."

Notwithstanding PhRMA's notorious clout in Washington—the association and its members reportedly spent $139.1 million on lobbying during the first six months of 2003—national policymakers are also sharply split on the legalization issue. To be sure, most pro-corporate conservatives oppose importation, which they see as a way of importing foreign price controls into this country, undermining R&D. That is the view held by, for instance, the *Wall Street Journal* editorial board, certain American Enterprise Institute commentators, free-market icon Milton Friedman, and Republican Senators Bill Frist and Orrin Hatch.

Seniors aren't the only ones who want Canadian drugs. State officials see them as a way to alleviate the pain of swelling budget crises.

But many libertarian conservatives come down in favor of legalization, which they see as a way of destroying foreign price controls and finally forcing other nations to shoulder their fair share of R&D costs. How would that happen? They theorize that once the manufacturers realize that they can no longer rely on American consumers to pay for R&D, they'll force Canada and Europe to relax the limits on prices—on pain of cutting off those nations' drug supplies. Partisans of that theory include Cato Institute economists Roger Pilon and Edward Crane, and Republican Congressmen Dan Burton of Indiana, Jeff Flake of Arizona, and Gil Gutknecht of Minnesota. In fact, because Canada is so small a market, Cato types favor importation from other countries as well, including all the European Union countries. As sometimes happens, the libertarians are aligned with liberal Democrats on this issue. The day after President Bush signed the new Medicare law, Senators Daschle and Ted Kennedy each introduced bills that would, among other things, legalize importation from Canada.

What's most troubling about the drug-importation conundrum is that when you survey the chessboard and try to anticipate each player's future moves, most paths seem to lead to cataclysm. As ever more Americans turn to Canada for brand-name drugs, the manufacturers will limit Canada's supply—as at least six have already started doing. If the constriction in Canadian supply cuts off American seniors' lifeline to affordable drugs, state attorneys general may sue manufacturers alleging a collusive boycott—as Minnesota's Hatch is already threatening to do.

Meanwhile, manufacturers will start raising their Canadian prices—as at least four have done. Canadian price regulators will try to block those hikes—as Quebec is now trying to do. If manufacturers can't raise Canadian prices, they'll clamp down further on Canadian supply, creating shortages. If drug shortages threaten Canadians' health, Canada may cease honoring manufacturers' patents. And if Canada stops honoring U.S. patents, the U.S. might bring a complaint against Canada before the World Trade Organization. Or invade.

But we're getting ahead of ourselves.

When he launched CanadaMeds, Jorgenson placed a small ad in the *Grand Forks* (North Dakota) Herald. "I got a lot of reaction from regulatory bodies," he recalls. "Yours called ours." The Manitoba Pharmaceutical Association was very dubious about what Jorgenson was doing. "Whereas historically the pharmaceutical association inspected once or twice a year, we were getting inspected on a daily basis, seven days a week," he says. "We had search warrants issued against our premises. They took up vanloads of stuff and scoured through it for months and months."

Internet pharmacies raise two obvious regulatory issues, one small and one big. The small one concerns the mechanics of prescription-filling. Jorgenson, Strempler, and all genuine, licensed Canadian pharmacies require U.S. customers to provide short medical histories and to mail or fax a U.S. prescription for each drug sought. But Canadian law bars Canadian pharmacists from filling U.S. prescriptions. So the Internet pharmacies typically fax the U.S. patient's medical history and prescription to a Canadian doctor. The Canadian doctor reviews them, writes a Canadian prescription, and faxes that back to the pharmacy to fill. The problem is that the provincial regulatory bodies for doctors all take the position that it is a substandard practice for doctors to write prescriptions for patients they've never examined. Pharmaceutical regulators, in turn, are reluctant to let pharmacists run businesses predicated on substandard medical practices.

Then there is the bigger issue. Because pharmaceuticals are easy to counterfeit or dilute or sell past their expiration dates or damage through improper storage, Canada and the U.S. each use very similar "closed" systems of regulation. Deploying both federal and local authorities, each country oversees every step in the supply chain as a drug makes its way from manufacturer to wholesaler to retailer to patient. Though the manufacturing plants are often outside either the U.S. or Canada, each country's federal regulators—the FDA and Health Canada's equivalent agency—inspect those facilities and set up paper trails to ensure that the drugs pass through a seamless pipeline from that point forward. Regulators in each country get nervous when the pipeline is breached by an international transaction, since neither country has authority to inspect facilities or subpoena information across the border. Accordingly, the FDA and nearly every U.S. state board of pharmacy has denounced Canadian Internet pharmacies as unsafe; Health Canada has also acknowledged that it cannot guarantee the safety of drugs sent to America.

After Springfield, Mass., signed up for Canadian drugs, all hell broke loose.

On the other hand, Health Canada has not tried to shut down the traffic, which it regards as fundamentally a U.S. issue. Moreover, its officials have taken offense at the FDA's sometimes broad-brush denigrations of Canadian pharmacies as a buyer-beware market. "We have no evidence at this time, in the context of Internet pharmacies, that there are unsafe products going to the United States," said assistant deputy health minister Diane Gorman last November, after a tense meeting with FDA commissioner Mark McClellan in Toronto. "It's very clear that Canada's safety record is second to none internationally," she pointedly added.

In fact, the FDA has hyped aspects of the safety threat. The agency periodically performs "blitz" inspections of drug packages entering the U.S. through the mail, for instance, and then reports that alarmingly high percentages of the packages seized—about 87% last November, for instance—contained drugs "unapproved" by the FDA. Photos are displayed of pills wrapped in baggies and bottles labeled in Chinese.

The phrase "unapproved drug" may be a bit misleading. In FDA parlance, a drug is unapproved if it is improperly labeled, and Canadian drugs are, by definition, improperly labeled. A Canadian box of Lipitor may be "unapproved" for no other reason than that it bears a Health Canada identification number instead of an FDA identification number. Canadian drugs also seldom carry precisely the same litany of small-print warnings that the FDA requires. In its public pronouncements the FDA doesn't distinguish between packages sent by licensed Canadian pharmacies—Manitoba's regulators require that return addresses be clearly displayed—and those sent, say, anonymously. The latter could come from any of the many illegitimate operators that advertise by spam, require no prescriptions, and claim to be Canadian but often aren't. Obviously, when people order V1AGR@ or VAL[I]UM from anonymous spammers, Lord knows what they receive in return. Licensed Canadian mail-order pharmacies cannot sell controlled substances like Valium at all. They primarily deal in long-term "maintenance" drugs—Plavix, Lipitor, and the like—rather than drugs that treat acute conditions. They typically send drugs to U.S. customers in the same sealed containers in which the manufacturers originally sent the drugs to Canadian wholesalers. In this respect, containers from licensed Canadian Internet pharmacies are arguably less likely to have counterfeit pills in them than ones from the U.S., where pills are often repackaged multiple times in their trek from the factory.

Notwithstanding serious misgivings, the Manitoba regulators have so far permitted the industry to survive—and, indeed, thrive. But as with many gray-market activities, thriving presents its own perils. If Canadian pharmacies were to begin selling too much of their supply to Americans, they could create shortages for Canadians. At that point Health Canada might abandon its neutrality toward the industry and shut it down—possibly overnight. Consequently, the industry is now divided against itself.

"We need to be prudent and responsible so that we don't jeopardize the drug supply," says Dave MacKay, who represents one side of the schism. He heads the Canadian International Pharmacy Association, or CIPA, a group of about 35 of the largest Internet pharmacies. MacKay supports the creation of websites, like Governor Pawlenty's, that assuage Americans' safety concerns by effectively accrediting legitimate Canadian pharmacies. But MacKay believes that his industry should not start entering into contracts with American municipalities or states. "We just cannot sustain that kind of volume," he says. "It's not a problem for one state. But as soon as one state sets the precedent, it's going to be 20 or 30 states. And if it's California or New York, we're gonna be dead in the water, because there's more Californians than there are Canadians."

But not everyone shares MacKay's commitment to prudence.

When Tony Howard, who runs CanaRx.com, picks me up in a slush-encrusted Chevy van at the Detroit Metro airport in mid-January, I am surprised. I had assumed he'd send a chauffeur to take me to his office across the river in Windsor, Ontario. That's because I'd been told that Howard can't enter the U.S. any more for fear of being sued by the FDA—or maybe even arrested.

Howard received two warning letters from the FDA last fall advising him that CanaRx's operations violated the Federal Food, Drug, and Cosmetic Act and "present a significant risk to public health." Nevertheless, it is definitely Howard himself—cheerful, jokey, disheveled, logorrheic, intense—at the wheel. He immediately launches into a monologue without the formality of any questions having been posed. Just before entering the tunnel to Windsor, he stops at the Detroit post office and picks up a handful of prescription orders from a P.O. box he keeps there. He stopped listing this U.S. address on his website after the FDA sent its first warning letter last September, but some of Howard's longtime customers still don't know about the change.

The FDA opposes the trade, but it hasn't filed suits against any mayors or retirees—guaranteed PR fiascoes.

Though he presents like Buddy Hackett, Howard, 54, is a bit of a crusader. He grew up in Windsor but has had homes on both sides of the border and thinks of himself as a North American, he says. About ten years ago, after an early heart attack, he sold his Windsor insurance consulting firm and retired. He and his wife spent much of their time in Florida and Phoenix, and many of the people they befriended were much older. After one asked him to buy drugs for her in Canada, he found out about the enormous price disparities. Outraged by those inequities, he and what are now his partners—his wife, two doctors, and a pharmacist—decided to take action.

They're not in it for the money, Howard claims: "We're all well-off individuals. We want to change the laws, not build an empire." Their goal is to shame the U.S. government into forcing drug companies to lower their American prices. If he succeeds, of course, he'll put the whole Canadian Internet pharmacy industry out of business—including himself. He says he doesn't care. "I've put in all this time without any pay"—he claims to have recovered no profits for himself so far—"to be that one person who can say, 'I was there, and I helped.' It will affect so many Americans."

Accordingly, Howard, who is not a pharmacist, declines to play by MacKay's rules. Howard tries to sign up American towns, cities, states, unions, seniors' groups, and corporations, offering to supply Canadian drugs to their employees, retirees, prisoners—whomever! He has set up a network of Canadian pharmacies—mainly con-

ventional brick-and-mortar types—that have agreed to sell through him at a single low price, which is often even lower than those of the Internet pharmacies. In 2002, Howard sold his house in Florida—"My lawyers told me to divest of all U.S. property," he explains—and in July 2003 he went operational with his first client: Springfield, Mass.

Springfield's then mayor, Michael Albano, had seen the town's prescription-drug bills double since he took office in 1996. When he heard about Howard's operation, he traveled to Windsor and visited several pharmacies in the CanaRx network. In March he tried out the service on his own family and, happy with the results, chose to offer it to all Springfield's municipal employees and retirees. (The program is voluntary, in that nobody has to get his drugs through CanaRx; if an enrollee chooses to, however, the city agrees to cover his or her whole co-pay.) Albano says that about 3,300 Springfielders had used the program by the time his term as mayor expired in December, saving the city about $1 million. (Albano's successor has continued the program.)

Just as MacKay feared, once the Springfield precedent was set, Albano, Howard, and MacKay himself were deluged with inquiries. City officials from Miami, Seattle, Burlington, Vt., Boston, and Brockton, Mass., contacted them, as did state officials from Illinois, Minnesota, Iowa, Wisconsin, Michigan, North Dakota, Utah, West Virginia, New Hampshire, Rhode Island, and, yes, California. Illinois governor Rod Blagojevich's staff published an 85-page study last October setting forth a proposal that it claimed could safely provide Canadian drugs to state employees and retirees while saving the state as much as $56 million a year. He and Minnesota governor Pawlenty are hosting a national governors' summit on the topic in Washington, D.C., on Feb. 24.

So far, most officials have proved more cautious than Albano. Only Montgomery, Ala., and Westchester County, N.Y., are known to have actually followed Springfield's example, though Boston mayor Thomas Menino has vowed to launch a program by July. (Howard claims that he is already doing business with two other U.S. municipalities—as well as with two American unions and five corporations—but declines to name them, saying that they prefer to remain "under the radar.")

Since the arrival of Springfield-style operations, the FDA's rhetoric has grown more bellicose, and the agency has begun suing American intermediaries that try to profit from the trade. Last November the agency shut down Rx Depot—an Oklahoma chain of 85 storefronts that were connecting American seniors to Canadian pharmacies—and in January it sent a warning letter to Expedite-Rx, a Texas intermediary that helps the city of Montgomery get its supply.

Notwithstanding the earlier warnings to CanaRx, Howard's ensconcement across the border appears to be sheltering him. To this point, the FDA has also shied away from the ugly spectacle of suits against American mayors, municipal employees, or retirees—guaranteed PR fiascoes.

With neither Health Canada nor the FDA shutting down the cross-border traffic, pharmaceutical companies have taken matters into their own hands. In January 2003, GlaxoSmithKline's Canadian unit advised distributors that they were contractually barred from selling to pharmacies that resell to U.S. customers, demanded to see their sales records, and warned that violators would be cut off from all future GSK products. Subsequently Astra-Zeneca, Wyeth, Eli Lilly, Pfizer, and Novartis have taken steps to clamp down on supply. GSK, Lilly, Pfizer, and Bayer have also begun raising their Canadian prices.

In press releases each company has usually stressed the FDA's safety concerns as the driving motivation for making certain that their drugs are not resold to Americans. But professor Richard Epstein, a law and economics professor at the University of Chicago Law School, speculates that the companies are also delivering a different message. The message is addressed to Canada, he says, and goes like this: "Look, this is your population. This is your utilization. We'll sell you enough to satisfy that population. You want to resell to the United States? Kill your own people."

If helping those in need stalls delivery of new drugs to the next generation, have we acted morally?

Shortly after GSK began its crackdown, Minnesota attorney general Hatch issued civil subpoenas to the company, stating that he was launching an investigation into a possible collusive boycott by pharmaceutical manufacturers against Canadian pharmacies that sell to U.S. seniors. Hatch says he infers collusion from the close proximity in timing among the six companies' actions, and he claims that such a boycott would violate state antitrust laws.

If the reader is puzzled, so was GSK. Its lawyers protested to a Minnesota judge in October that Hatch's subpoenas were "predicated on the remarkable proposition that actions by GSK ... to prevent the illegal importation of drugs from Canada into the United States can somehow give rise to liability under Minnesota's state antitrust laws." Hatch replies in an interview: "There are court cases that say you can't even boycott an *illegal* activity." In any event, he maintains, personal-use importation is legal, given the FDA's "long track record of permitting it."

Though Hatch's theories may sound aggressive, he's evidently not the only official propounding them. He's leading a multistate working group of 24 attorneys general focused on the issues, he says. In December the group submitted a letter to the Minnesota court urging enforcement of Hatch's subpoenas to GSK.

Will Hatch go after other drug companies too? "First, we want to get an order in this case," he says. "Probably nanoseconds after that order is issued, there will be [subpoenas] served on the others as well."

Though Strempler of RxNorth says he's been able to fill all his orders despite the supply crackdown, he's feeling the pinch financially. Suppliers that used to send him shipments on credit now require payment up-front, he says, and he has had to beef up inventory to ensure the continuity of his deliveries. MacKay admits that some Canadian pharmacists are even considering connecting their customers to pharmacies in other countries, like New Zealand, should the Canadian supply dry up. He hopes, he says, that CIPA members will be "transparent" with customers if they resort to such measures.

At one level the notion of legalizing the importation of prescription drugs is absurd on its face. If Canada's or any other nation's price regulations are a good idea, we should adopt such regulations here—not go through the Rube Goldberg mechanism of funneling all our drugs through a price-regulated foreign country.

But while importation may be an ideological dodge for some politicians—a way of getting the short-term benefits of price controls without admitting that's what they're doing—it's more than that. For other, more principled and more nervy people, importation is a high-stakes poker game. They hope it will force foreign countries to lift their price controls on pain of losing their drug supplies.

For most people, though, that's not what importation is about either. "It's a manifestation of an anger within the U.S.—almost like a temper tantrum," says Uwe Reinhardt, a health-care economist at Princeton University. "To my mind, the proper solution would be for Congress to make sure that every American has financial access to the drugs that are beneficial to them, through either their own insurance or subsidized insurance. And once that has been achieved, you can then talk about what prices for drugs should be paid."

But the second step turns out to be exceedingly difficult, he acknowledges, especially for those patented drugs that have unique and indispensable therapeutic benefits. For such drugs, he observes, "the drug manufacturers can in theory charge whatever the hell they like."

And beyond that challenge lie more intractable enigmas. If our efforts to help those now in need end up stalling the delivery of new miracle drugs to the next generation, have we acted morally? What do we do when compassion in the short term causes suffering in the long term? Do we save one life today at the cost of two tomorrow?

The politicians will assure us that no such harsh choices are required. But what else would the say?

Sports and Drugs

Kenneth Jost

THE ISSUES

Tim Montgomery's career has slowed considerably since the evening in Paris two years ago when he blazed to a record-setting 9.78 seconds in the 100-meter dash and earned the title of "world's fastest man."[1]

Today, however, Montgomery's future as an international track star is uncertain. On July 11 he failed to make the Olympic team. Moreover, the 29-year-old South Carolinian is one of several top U.S. track athletes who could be banned from competition for life for alleged use of illegal performance-enhancing drugs.

The charges enveloping Montgomery and the other track stars threaten not only their individual careers but also the United States' chances in the upcoming Olympic Games, set to open in Athens, Greece, on Aug. 13. The growing scandal over pharmaceutically pumped-up athletes—perhaps the largest in U.S. sports history—extends into professional baseball, possibly implicating, among others, Barry Bonds, the hulking San Francisco Giants outfielder who hit a record 73 homers in 2002.

The athletes involved all publicly dispute the accusations, but the controversy underscores the undeniable fact that drugs have become a major part of elite athletic competition. A significant but unknown number of Olympic hopefuls in the United States and elsewhere, as well as many collegiate and other professional athletes, use chemical substances to increase strength and stamina beyond what they can achieve by nutrition and training alone.[2]

"It's human nature to obtain an edge, whether in combat, in business or in sports," says Charles Yesalis, a professor of health and human development at Pennsylvania State University and a leading expert on—and opponent of—performance-enhancing drugs.

Through the years, athletes have sought that edge from a variety of stimulants ranging from caffeine and brandy to heroin and cocaine. But the isolation of the male hormone testosterone in the 1930s paved the way for more sophisticated chemical agents known as anabolic ("tissue-building") steroids.

Steroids produce masculinizing effects comparable to those from naturally occurring testosterone. The resulting increase in muscle mass may be a boon for weightlifters, football players or athletes in track and field throwing events. But steroids also produce undesirable side effects. Some, such as acne and increased body hair, are largely cosmetic. Others are more serious, including tumors and cancer in the liver, increased cholesterol levels and—in some men—shrunken testicles. Women who use steroids see many of the same effects, along with a deeper voice and—in some cases—an enlarged clitoris.

However, the medical effects of steroids are not fully researched, and some athletes and a handful of vocal critics of anti-drug enforcement efforts in sports dispute the health risks claimed by opponents or say they can be minimized. But their use in athletic competition has been widely viewed as unseemly at best ever since the practice first came to widespread attention in the 1960s.

Nonetheless, as the monetary and other rewards of elite competition have increased over the years, steroids have tempted many top-ranking athletes. "The pressure on people to try different things is very high," says William Roberts, an associate professor at the University of Minnesota's St. John's Hospital and president of the American College of Sports Medicine. "The difference between first and fifth place is the difference between fame and money and relative anonymity."

National and international sports federations and professional sports leagues were slow to respond to mounting evidence that steroid use has been increasing since the 1970s. In 1999, however, an international conference of governments and sports organizations led to the writing of a world "anti-doping" code that calls for a two-year suspension in most cases for athletes found to have used banned drugs. The conference also led to the creation of the independent World Anti-Doping Agency (WADA) to police the practice in international competitions, including the Olympics.*

---

* The term "doping" has been used to denote use of performance-enhancing drugs in sports at least since the 1930s. Some critics of anti-doping policies maintain the term is inherently pejorative and improperly skews the debate over the issue.

The charges against Montgomery and other U.S. track stars have been brought by WADA's counterpart in the United States: the U.S. Anti-Doping Agency (USADA). The agency sent letters on June 8 to Montgomery and three other Olympic hopefuls: sprinters Chryste Gaines, Michelle Collins and Alvin Harrison. The agency also has confirmed that it is investigating sprinter Marion Jones, a five-time Olympic gold medallist and Montgomery's live-in girlfriend.

The evidence against the athletes—not officially disclosed as of early July—appears to come from business records seized in a September 2003 raid by federal and state authorities on a San Francisco-area sports lab, the Bay Area Laboratory Cooperative (BALCO), run by sports nutritionist Victor Conte.[3] Federal authorities acted after USADA tipped them off to the existence of a new so-called designer drug—tetrahydrogestrinone or THG—similar to previously known steroids but altered slightly to avoid detection.

USADA itself had been tipped off by a then unidentified track coach, who sent the anti-doping agency a syringe in June containing the new steroid and named Conte as the source.[4] Conte's past clients include Bonds, who has tried unsuccessfully to dispel suspicions that his bulked-up physique and increased home run output in recent years are signs of steroid use.

The raids touched off a succession of high-profile events, including testimony before a federal grand jury by Bonds and many other well-known athletes and an eventual indictment of Conte and three others announced on Feb. 12 by Attorney General John Ashcroft. "This is not just a call to action," Ashcroft said. "It is a call to the values that make our nation and its people strong and free."[*]

Even before the BALCO investigation, Major League Baseball (MLB) was under pressure to more vigorously curb what several players publicly described as widespread use of steroids. President Bush added to the pressure in his State of the Union address on Jan. 20 by calling on "football, baseball and other sports" to "get rid of steroids now."

For years, the Major League Baseball Players Association had resisted drug testing, but the union agreed in 2002 to a year of anonymous random tests. If more than 5 percent of the samples tested positive, the agreement called for once-a-year testing of players by name. In fact, between 5 and 7 percent of the 2003 samples tested positive, so the league began testing all players by name this year.[5]

For Montgomery and the other track stars, USADA's allegations came at the worst of times—as they prepared for the U.S. Olympic trials in Sacramento, Calif., in mid-July. Montgomery and Jones both continued their training even as they and their lawyers publicly battled the accusations. "Tim's position is he's never done anything wrong, he's never failed any drug test, he'll be found not guilty," says his spokesman, Dan Goldberg.

Jones similarly insists on her innocence and is challenging USADA either to bring charges or drop the matter. "At this point, USADA ought to make clear that it doesn't have sufficient evidence, and that should be the end of the matter," says her attorney, Joseph Burton.

Despite the public denials, the *San Francisco Chronicle* reported in late June that Montgomery—in his federal grand jury testimony in November, given under a grant of immunity—acknowledged having used performance-enhancing drugs in the past. He also testified that Conte had admitted supplying steroids to Bonds, according to the *Chronicle*, which did not disclose its sources. Montgomery's lawyer declined to comment, and both Conte and Bonds angrily denied the accusations.[6]

For their part, USADA officials insist the procedures are fair. "Any suggestion that the USADA process compromises any athlete's rights or is unfair is a blatant distortion of the truth," says Legal Director Travis Tygart. As for speeding up action on Jones' case, Tygart says it would be "shortsighted" to rush the agency's review process "just to meet a competition deadline."

Whatever the outcome of the BALCO investigation, anti-doping officials acknowledge they face an uphill battle in trying to stay ahead of pharmacological advances. Some banned substances—such as human growth hormone (HGH)—cannot be detected under current technology, and new drugs such as THG are designed to escape detection. Moreover, looming on the horizon is the possibility of so-called gene doping—manipulation of an athlete's genes—to improve performance.

As the debate over performance-enhancing drugs continues, here are some of the major questions being considered:

Does the use of performance-enhancing drugs hurt athletes and competitive sports?

Baseball fans were held spellbound in the late summer of 1998 as two of the game's leading sluggers—Mark McGwire and Sammy Sosa—chased one of the game's most daunting records: Roger Maris' mark of 61 home runs set nearly four decades earlier, in 1961. By the end of the season, the St. Louis Cardinals' first-baseman and Chicago Cubs' outfielder had both eclipsed the previous record, with Sosa at 66 and McGwire on top with a stunning 70 homers for the year.

As the home-run chase intensified, however, sports reporters noticed that the longtime power hitter had bottles of a dietary supplement called androstenedione—andro for short—in his locker. Questioned, McGwire openly acknowledged taking andro—a manufactured drug that

---

[*] The 42-count indictment charged Conte and three others with conspiracy to give athletes illegal steroids and prescription drugs. The other defendants are BALCO Vice President James Valente; Bonds' personal trainer Greg Anderson; and Remi Korchemny, a San Francisco Bay-area track coach.

the body converts into testosterone. Andro, which was legal for baseball players at the time, had already been banned in other sports—including football, collegiate athletics and the Olympics.

The disclosure stirred a debate over the legitimacy of McGwire's feat. Some critics suggested that the eventual record needed to be marked with a doubt-casting asterisk.[7] Most fans, however, appeared uninterested. And, tellingly, the sale of andro shot up thanks to the publicity.

Bowing to the controversy, MLB finally banned androstenedione on April 12, 2004.

The episode illuminates the opposing views about performance-enhancing drugs in sports. Many fans may share the discomfort of anti-doping advocates who say that drugs tarnish the mythic purity of sports. "The public likes to have a clean game," says Don Catlin, director of the Olympic drug-testing laboratory at the University of California at Los Angeles. "They like it to be fair and square."

But many fans also revel in the enhanced power, speed or endurance that steroids or other performance-enhancing drugs help make possible. "They love to see big, strong guys hit home runs," says Norman Fost, a professor of pediatrics at the University of Wisconsin Medical School and the most vocal academic opponent of anti-doping policies.

Fost has argued—all but alone in the United States—that anti-doping officials and advocates rely for their case on a fictitious image of pure athletic competition and exaggerated warnings of the health consequences of performance-enhancing drugs. He says they have been aided by compliant reporters who have conveyed those views to the public with little analysis and few doubts. "I can't think of a single subject that involves ethical and medical issues that's been so one-sided" in the media, Fost says.[8]

Anti-doping officials, however, insist that performance-enhancing drugs hurt not only the image of competitive sport but the athletes as well. And steroid use by professional and Olympic athletes encourages young people to try them as well, they argue. "It's clearly something that's infiltrated its way down to grade school and up," says Gary I. Wadler, a professor at New York University Medical School and a member of WADA.

Medical authorities generally say that—for otherwise healthy people—steroids have few if any clinical benefits and produce serious side effects, even if not completely documented. Steroids increase cholesterol levels and, by implication, the risk of heart disease, they say. Oral steroids—though not the more common injected versions—also appear to be associated with liver cancer, they say. Anecdotal evidence suggests that steroids can produce hyper-aggressiveness in some users—so-called 'roid rage. And, for young people, steroids cause bones to stop growing, effectively stunting growth.

However, anti-doping officials say some of the dangers are unproven and many exaggerated. "There's no study that steroids cause heart attacks," says Larry Bowers, USADA's senior managing director for technical and information resources.

Yesalis, who has chided the media for "sensationalizing" the dangers from steroids, adds, "That doesn't mean there aren't potentially serious consequences."

Fost, however, says the dangers are greatly exaggerated. "There is a nearly uniform claim as to steroids that they're very dangerous, they can cause death, cancer, heart attacks," he says. "None of that is supported by any medical evidence, or at least it's widely exaggerated."

But Fost agrees with anti-doping advocates on the risks steroids pose to young people. In fact, he favors continuing the ban for anyone under 18, pointing out that the most common use of steroids among young people is not by athletes but by body-builders. "It's middle- and high-school kids who want to look like Arnold Schwarzenegger," he says.

For adults, however, Fost says steroids and other performance-enhancing drugs should be legal, and deciding whether to use them should be left up to the individual athlete. "There's not a single athlete in any competitive sport who's just running on his or her natural ability," he says. "Why pick steroids to be concerned about?"

Steroids, Fost says, are conceptually indistinguishable from other man-made aids, such as fiberglass pole-vaulting poles or super-efficient swimsuits. As for the health consequences, Fost says many sports—from gymnastics to football—involve the risk of injury. "It's morally incoherent to prohibit adult athletes from risking harming themselves," he says.

Anti-doping advocates vigorously rebut Fost's arguments. "Why don't you legalize all these drugs?" asks Marc Safran, director of sports medicine at the University of California at San Francisco. "The winner would be the person who comes closer to risking their life."

Yesalis adds that performance-enhancing drugs take away a real but intangible part of the enduring appeal of sport. "You do not need drugs to have a sense of fulfillment, to feel that you've left it all on the field," Yesalis says. "[Drugs have] taken something that God has given us—love of game and sport—and perverted us."

Is drug testing effective?

The controversy swirling around Montgomery, Jones and the other U.S. track stars stems not from failed drug tests but from a cloak-and-dagger story initiated by an anonymous tipster and a team of chemical sleuths. The newly discovered steroid THG was decoded by chemists at the Olympic drug-testing laboratory at UCLA from a sample delivered to USADA anonymously by someone who identified himself as a track and field coach.

Lab chief Catlin says it took three months of chemical testing to crack the code of the new steroid and develop a test to detect it—a chastening reminder of the difficulties of policing performance-enhancing drugs. "There are always new drugs moving in and the old ones moving out," he says.[9]

Cracking Down on Steroids

With the exception of the National Hockey League, major professional and college sports organizations test and penalize for steroid use.

National Football League

Testing: Random testing during the season; all players tested twice in the off-season and once in the preseason.

Penalties: 1st positive test—four-game suspension
        2nd—six-game suspension
        3rd—one-year suspension

Major League Baseball

Testing: Unannounced testing of all players once during the season, with a follow-up test five to seven days later.

Penalties: 1st positive test—mandatory drug-treatment program
        2nd—15-day suspension or up to a $10,000 fine
        3rd—25-day suspension or up to a $25,000
        4th—50-day suspension or up to a $50,000 fine
        5th—one-year suspension or up to a $100,000 fine

National Basketball Association

Testing: For first-year players, once during training camp and three times in regular season; for veterans, once during training camp.

Penalties: 1st positive test—five-game suspension
        2nd—10-game suspension
        3rd—25-game suspension

National Hockey League

Testing: None   **Penalties:** None

National Collegiate Athletic Association

Testing: Random August-to-June testing for Division I and II football and Division 1 track and field; random testing for all competitors in Division I, II and III championships and Division I-A postseason bowl games

Penalties: loss of one year of eligibility

Drug testing—which involves chemical analysis of athletes' urine or blood samples—has been the principal tool for anti-doping enforcement since its introduction in the 1950s.[10] Drug testing snared its first Olympic medallist in 1972, when the teenage American swimmer Rick DeMont had to relinquish his gold medal after testing positive for the stimulant ephedrine, an ingredient in a prescription asthma medication he was taking. Then in 1984, Finnish runner Martti Vainio lost the silver medal he had won in the 10,000-meter race after testing positive for banned substances, and Canadian sprinter Ben Johnson was stripped of his gold medal in 1988 after testing positive for steroids.

The apparent simplicity and certainty of drug-test results, however, masks the complexity and uncertainty of the actual process. Testing is expensive—as much as $500 to $1,000 or more per test. Testing is susceptible to error, cover-up or even sabotage. And, testing can be circumvented.

Athletes can sometimes escape detection at scheduled tests by halting the use of any banned substances beforehand. They also use more ingenious subterfuges. For instance, NFL players have been known to "borrow" urine specimens from someone else, hide the urine vial inside their athletic supporters and then—shielded by a partition—provide the examiner with the clean samples.[11]

Such problems lead many anti-doping advocates to dismiss drug testing as a failure. "The drug testing system has loopholes big enough that I could navigate an Abrams tank through it," Yesalis says. "It's been a colossal flop. I don't know what other enterprise that has such a poor performance rating would still be in business."

Meanwhile, drug tests have yet to be developed for some banned substances—notably, the synthetic human growth hormone (HGH) and erythropoietin (EPO), a hormone that stimulates production of oxygen-carrying red blood cells, which aid athletes in such endurance sports as cycling or marathons. And sports chemists are constantly developing new substances, such as THG, to evade detection.

"As long as there are people willing to cheat, there will be drugs that are undetectable," says Minnesota's Roberts. "This THG thing would never have come to light except that somebody blew the whistle."

Anti-doping critic Fost agrees. "The drugmakers and the athletes have kept ahead of the testers," he says. The inevitable futility of the effort is another reason to legalize performance-enhancing drugs, Fost suggests.

Moreover, legalizing the drugs would better protect athletes' health, he argues. "As long as they're banned, there will be people trying to avoid detection, and they'll have to do it underground," he says. "They'll be using drugs that won't be adequately tested or subject to [federal] oversight. The worst thing about the THG scandal is that anyone using it has no way of knowing what they're using."

Anti-doping officials acknowledge the difficulties but insist that testing is only one part of the overall effort to keep drugs out of sports. "What we're after is deterrence—not necessarily catching people and sanctioning them but deterring them from using drugs in the first place," USADA's Bowers says. "One of the tools we have for that is testing. We're better now than we were three years ago, and we're capable of seeing more things now than we were three years ago."

"You can't say that testing is going to stamp out drugs," says David Howman, WADA's director general. "You have to have effective education programs. We far prefer to be a preventive body than to be a detection body."

Are penalties for using performance-enhancing drugs stiff enough?

Anti-doping advocates achieved an important breakthrough in 1999 when an international conference of sports organizations and governments agreed to prescribe two-year suspensions for athletes' first doping violation and lifetime bans for a second offense. But U.S. Olympic sprinting champion Maurice Greene advocates even tougher penalties.

"There is no room in our sport for drug cheaters whatsoever," Greene said. "I don't think a year ban or a two-year ban is enough. I think it should be a life ban, if you get caught even once."[12]

USA Track & Field voted last Dec. 7, 2003, to impose a lifetime ban for first-time steroid offenses. It has not yet been implemented, pending a determination that it does not violate the Amateur Sports Act.

Greene's outburst may not have been solely about anti-doping policies. He and Montgomery have a history of bad relations: It was Greene's record of 9.79 seconds in the 100-meter dash that Montgomery clipped in 2002. Greene—who has three of the four fastest times in the event—likes to remind listeners that Montgomery set his mark with a tailwind right at the limit allowed for official records.[13]

Whatever Greene's motivation, some experts agree that a lifetime ban for a first doping violation is worth considering. "If you don't have very stiff penalties, you're not going to deter a lot of people," says the University of California's Safran. "A lifetime ban if you get caught would definitely get people to think twice about it."

But a lifetime ban might be too stringent to be enforceable, Bowers warns. "I'm not sure that we could get people to sanction athletes for life, particularly if that's their livelihood," he says. "If there's a repeat performance or lack of change in behavior after a first time, then I would support a lifetime ban."

In fact, the World Doping Code does allow reduced penalties for unintentional violations for banned substances found in generally available medicinal products. An athlete can also escape penalty by showing that he or she "bears no fault or negligence for the violation."

For his part, Catlin says improved detection is more important than stiffened penalties. "There's enough punishment. A two-year penalty, that's strong enough," he says.

The debate over penalties is most squarely joined today regarding Major League Baseball. The penalties established this season as a result of the 2003 testing include, for a first offense, mandatory referral to treatment and counseling. For a second offense, the player would be suspended for 15 days; only after a fifth offense would a player be suspended for as long as a year. Fines also escalate—to as much as $100,000 for a fifth offense.

Wadler calls the MLB penalties "woefully inadequate," noting that on a first offense, the only response is " 'Go see a doctor.' "

For its part, the league is trying to reopen labor negotiations to provide for stiffer punishment. "The commissioner has been saying he'd like to see immediate discipline in the Major League policy," says Rob Manfred, MLB's executive vice president for labor relations.

But baseball association President Don Fehr insists mandatory treatment actually aids subsequent detection and prevention. " 'Go see a doctor' began with a premise: If you test positive . . . there are going to be a lot more tests for you," Fehr says. "The likelihood of the conduct recurring diminishes very greatly."

On the other hand, legalization advocates see no reason for any penalties for using performance-enhancing drugs. "Athletes ought to be able to use them . . . under the supervision of a sports expert after careful clinical trials showing the benefits and risks," Fost says.

But Minnesota's Roberts says that if performance-enhancing drugs were legal, all athletes would feel pressured to use them. "If you're caught, you should be penalized and penalized to the point that it's not worth getting caught," Roberts says. "And if you're caught twice, you should be penalized for life. I would like for athletes to be able to compete without having to use them. A zero-tolerance policy would make that less likely."

Footnotes

1. See Tim Layden, "The New 100m World Record: 9.78 Seconds," *Sports Illustrated*, Sept. 23, 2002, p. 50.
2. See Richard L. Worsnop, "Athletes and Drugs," *The CQ Researcher*, July 26, 1991, pp. 513-536.
3. For background, see Mark Fainaru-Wada and Lance Williams, "How the Doping Scandal Unfolded," *The San Francisco Chronicle*, Dec. 21, 2003, p. B1. See also Jere Longman and Ford Fessenden, "Rivals Turn to Tattling in Steroids Case Involving Top Athletes," *The New York Times*, April 11, 2004, sec. 8, p. 1.
4. *The San Jose Mercury News* identified Trevor Graham, who once coached both Jones and Montgomery, as the source. See Elliott Almond, et al., "Feud lit fuse on Balco scandal; Track Coach Sent Smoking-Gun Syringe Filled With THG to Anti-Doping Agency," *San Jose Mercury News*, July 4, 2004, p. A1.
5. Jack Curry and Jere Longman, "Results of Steroid Testing Spur Baseball to Set Tougher Rules," *The New York Times*, Nov. 14, 2003.
6. See Mark Fainaru-Wada and Lance Williams, "Sprinter Admitted Use of BALCO 'Magic Potion'," *The San Francisco Chronicle*, June 24, 2004, p. A1; Lance Williams and Mark Fainaru-Wada, "Track Star's Testimony Linked Bonds to Steroid Use," *ibid.*, p. A16.
7. For contrasting views, see Jack McCallum, "Swallow This Pill," *Sports Illustrated*, Aug. 31, 1998, p. 17; and Philip M. Boffey, "Post-Season Thoughts on McGwire's Pills," *The New York Times*, Sept. 30, 1998, p. A16.
8. For a British academic who takes a similar view, see Ellis Cashmore, "Stop Testing and Legalise All Drugs," *The Observer*, Oct. 26, 2003, p. 9. Cashmore is a professor of culture, media and sport at Staffordshire University.
9. For a detailed account, see Jere Longman and Joe Drape, "Decoding a Steroid: Hunches, Sweat, Vindication," *The New York Times*, Nov. 2, 2003, sec. 1, p. 1.
10. Background drawn from Jim Ferstle, "Evolution and Politics of Drug Testing," in Charles E. Yesalis (ed.), *Anabolic Steroids in Sport and Exercise* (2d ed.), 2000, pp. 363-413.
11. See Mike Freeman, "N.F.L. Is Told How Players Cheat on Drug Tests," *The New York Times*, Aug. 5, 1993, p. B2.
12. Liz Robbins, "Greene Supports Lifetime Bans," *The New York Times*, May 18, 2004, p. D2.
13. See Mike DeArmond, "Back Up to Speed: Greene Ran Into Some Injury Problems, but He's Ready to Go for More Gold," *The Kansas City Star*, May 18, 2004, p. C3.

Just Say No Again

The old failures of new and improved anti-drug education

Renee Moilanen

I'm at the February 2001 Teens at the Table conference, a feel-good event sponsored by a coalition of Los Angeles youth organizations and high schools. It's designed to boost self-esteem and teach teenagers how to make smart decisions. In one of the sessions, a group of students is about to learn how easy it is to stay off drugs. It doesn't require anything as lame as red ribbons or "Just Say No" chants. It just takes knowing what constitutes a healthy decision—one that is all your own—coupled with a little real-life practice.

The kids test their skills with a role-playing skit. The scenario: Two girls are walking home from a party late at night when a car full of boys pulls up to offer them a ride. "The boys have been drinking and smoking," the script reads. "Trouble is imminent."

Here is where the teenagers are supposed to call on their newfound decision making skills in choosing whether to get into the car. They're asked to think about their options, weigh the consequences, and decide what to do based on what would be best for them—no judgments, no right or wrong, none of that thoughtless Just Say No stuff from the 1980s and early '90s. Today's drug prevention lessons, scientifically crafted and tested, are supposed to be all about teaching teenagers how to make choices, not telling them what to do; respecting their autonomy, not treating them like ventriloquist's dummies.

So the teenagers choose. If they don't get into the car, they walk home and everything is fine. But if they do ...

Boys: Hop in girls!

(Eventually the boys get out of hand and come on to the girls.)

Girls: Stop it!

Boys: Come on, it will be fun!

Girls: No!

(Car accident.)

The teachers say there's a choice here, but these kids aren't stupid. They can stay out of the car and live, or get in the car and die. So ... just say no.

Dare to Keep Your Kids off DARE

That three-word mantra "Just Say No" became a national punch line for a reason: It didn't keep kids away from drugs. Drug use among teenagers dropped steadily from the early 1980s until 1992, mirroring a decline in drug use among adults. But this downward trend began before the anti-drug curricula developed in the 1980s, exemplified by Drug Abuse Resistance Education (DARE), could have had any impact. The drop was detected in surveys of students who had never heard of DARE or Just Say No. And by the early 1990s, when students who were exposed to DARE and similar programs in grade school and middle school reached their late teens, drug use among teenagers was going up again. In the 2002 Monitoring the Future Study, 53 percent of high school seniors said they had used illegal drugs, compared to 41 percent in 1992. Past-month use rose from 14 percent to 25 percent during the same period.

Meanwhile, the leading model for drug education in the United States has been DARE, which brings police officers into elementary and middle school classrooms to warn kids away from drugs. DARE claims to teach kids how to resist peer pressure and say no to drugs through skits, cartoons, and hypothetical situations. Founded by Los Angeles Police Chief Daryl Gates in 1983 and organized as a nonprofit corporation (DARE America) in 1987, DARE is still used in around three-quarters of the nation's school districts. At the annual DARE Officers Association Dinner a few years ago, Bill Clinton's drug czar, Barry McCaffrey, declared that "DARE knows what needs to be done to reduce drug use among children, and you are doing it—successfully." But as McCaffrey should have known, the effectiveness of DARE has never been demonstrated, a fact DARE America itself implicitly conceded when it announced, half a year after the drug czar's praise, that it was revamping its program.

During the last decade DARE has been widely criticized as unproven and unsophisticated. In one of the most damning studies, published in 1999, a team of researchers at the University of Kentucky found that 10 years after receiving the anti-drug lessons, former DARE students were no different from non-DARE students in terms of drug use, drug attitudes, or self-esteem. "This report adds to the accumulating literature on DARE's lack of efficacy in preventing or reducing substance use," the researchers noted. In a 2003 report, the General Accounting Office reviewed six long-term evaluations of DARE and concluded that there were "no significant differences in illicit drug use between students who received DARE ... and students who did not." The surgeon general, the National Academy of Sciences, and the U.S. Department of Education also have declared DARE ineffective.

Determined not to repeat past mistakes and prodded by a federal government that lately has been demanding accountability in education, teachers today are turning to prevention programs backed by "scientifically based" claims of effectiveness. In 1998 the Department of Education, concerned that money was being wasted on a mish-mash of ineffective programs, decided to fund only those proven by "scientifically based research" to reduce or prevent drug use. Testimonials and we-think-it's-working assurances like those cited by DARE would no longer pass muster. Every prevention program now needed hard numbers, objective experiments, and independently reviewed conclusions based on long-term follow-ups to prove they worked.

In 2000 the Department of Education convened an expert panel that judged nine prevention programs "exemplary" for their proven effectiveness and 33 others "promising." Comprised mostly of educators and health professionals, the panel gave the "exemplary" or "promising" nod only to programs backed by at least one scientific evaluation of effectiveness (DARE did not make the cut). Schools using programs that were not on the list would risk losing their slice of the Department of Education's $635 million drug prevention budget. In 2001 President George W. Bush included the "scientifically based research" criterion for drug education in his No Child Left Behind Act, signing into law what had previously been only administrative practice.

But the officially endorsed alternatives to DARE aren't necessarily better. Once you remove the shiny packaging and discard the "new and improved" labels, you'll find a product that's disappointingly familiar. The main thing that has changed is the rhetoric. Instead of "Just Say No," you'll hear, "Use your refusal skills." The new programs encourage teachers to go beyond telling kids that drug use is bad. Instead, they tell teenagers to "use your decision making skills" to make "healthy life choices." Since drugs aren't healthy, the choice is obvious: Just say no.

The persistence of this theme is no accident. Prevention programs can get the federal government's stamp of approval only if they deliver "a clear and consistent message that the illegal use of drugs" is "wrong and harm-ful." But this abstinence-only message leaves teenagers ill-equipped to avoid drug-related hazards if they do decide to experiment.

After examining some of the new anti-drug curricula and watching a sampling of them in action, I strongly doubt these programs are winning many hearts and minds.

The Class Struggle Against Drugs

In September 2001, I join a class of middle schoolers in the upscale Los Angeles suburb of Palos Verdes Estates as they run through a series of hypothetical scenarios ostensibly designed to put their decision making skills to work. The program, called Skills for Adolescence, is used in about 10 percent of the nation's 92,000 K–12 schools. The curriculum, which the Department of Education deems "promising," "teaches the social competency skills young adolescents need for positive development," according to program literature.

Clustered into small groups, each student fingers a wallet-size blue card. The card—titled "Will it lead to trouble?"—lists the five questions adolescents should ask themselves when confronted with a difficult choice. It's laminated, presumably so teenagers can keep it in their back pockets and whip it out whenever they're faced with a tough decision and need a quick reminder about how to make one.

If the answer to any of these questions is yes, the students are supposed to say no: "Is it against the law, rules, or the teachings of my religion? Is it harmful to me or to others? Would it disappoint my family or other important adults? Is it wrong to do? Would I be hurt or upset if someone did this to me?"

The questions clearly are designed to elicit a complete rejection of drug use. Is it against the law? Yes, drugs are against the law. Therefore, you must reject them. Is it harmful? Yes, they can be harmful. Reject them. Would it disappoint my family or other adults? Yes, reject. There's no way to make any other decision. "If the only decision that's the right decision is the decision to say no, you've effectively cut off the discussion again," observes Marsha Rosenbaum, director of the West Coast office of the Drug Policy Alliance and author of *Safety First: A Reality-Based Approach to Teens, Drugs, and Drug Education.*

Another program praised by the Department of Education is Project ALERT, which it calls "exemplary." A series of anti-drug and anti-tobacco lessons used in about a fifth of the nation's 15,000 school districts, Project ALERT boasts that it "helps students build skills that will last a lifetime," including "how to identify the sources of pressure to use substances," "how to match specific resistance techniques with social pressures," "how to counter pro-drug arguments," and "how to say 'no' several different ways."

Eliminate the psychobabble, and Project ALERT's message is almost indistinguishable from that of the 1980s anti-drug programs that teachers now roundly scorn: Peer pressure is bad. Drugs are bad. Just say no.

In a room plastered with posters titled "Pressures" and "Ways to Say No," I join a class of Los Angeles middle schoolers in November 2002 as it breaks into small groups to plod through an anti-drug lesson from Project ALERT. The adolescents have just finished watching a video about smoking cigarettes featuring former teenaged smokers who say things like, "Life is too short. I'm not eager to die."

Each of the four groups is assigned a different question to answer: How can you help people quit? What's good about quitting? How do people quit? What gets people to quit?

There is little discussion. The kids know what the teacher expects. How can you help people quit? Tell them smoking is dumb. Don't hang out with them anymore.

When asked if she knows anyone who smokes, one girl nods.

Do you think any of this helps?

"No," she says without hesitation.

Why not?

The girl barely lifts her eyes from the paper, where she is decorating the "Smoking is dumb" and "Don't hang out with them anymore" list with bright red hearts. She shrugs. "Some people just don't care," she says.

The students are asked why they think kids use drugs.

They respond in unison, "Peer pressure"—the answer they know is expected. When asked to explain what this means, the students conjure up images of older kids hassling younger ones. "Sometimes they're your friends, but sometimes they're crazy people that come up and ask if you want some," one boy says, drawing on concepts that prevailed during the Just Say No era but have little basis in real life.

One boy defines peer pressure as other students "trying to force you, trying to convince you to do it." When asked if he's ever experienced peer pressure, he shakes his head. He's waiting for a group of sinister strangers to thrust drugs in his face. Drug education apparently has not helped him realize that peer pressure is far subtler, like wearing the same clothes as your friends or sharing inside jokes. And the teachers, by continuing to portray peer pressure as a palpable evil, fail to protect their students from anything.

Everything Old Is New Again

Today's anti-drug programs claim to have replaced all the scare tactics of years past with good, solid information about the physiological effects of drug use. But these programs, which are based on the same flawed "scientific" information that adults have been using for years to keep kids off drugs, are a lot like anti-alcohol propaganda from the late 19th and early 20th centuries.

Back in the late 1800s, health lessons endorsed by the Woman's Christian Temperance Union (WCTU) and its Department of Scientific Instruction portrayed alcohol as a wicked poison that created an uncontrollable appetite for more: "Many persons who at first take only a little beer, cider, or wine, form a great desire for them….The appetite for alcoholic liquors usually grows rapidly, and men who use but little at first often become drunkards in a short time." This selection comes from *The House I Live In*, a schoolbook written in 1887 and heartily endorsed by the WCTU.

A century later, another popular textbook offers a similar perspective on drug use. This passage comes from *Making Life Choices* (1999), lauded by teachers for its scientific content: "Attachment to the drug becomes almost like a great love relationship with another person. The only sure way to escape drug addiction is never to experiment with taking the drugs that produce it."

In the popular classroom video *Marijuana Updates*, produced in 1997, teenagers and Leo Hayden, a former college football player turned drug counselor, describe how pot ruined their lives. They say the drug made them feel invincible, tired, hungry, and numb. Soon they were slacking off in school, shirking responsibilities, and turning to harder drugs for a better high. Their testimonials, which suggest that pot turns people into useless zombies eager to snort cocaine and shoot heroin, draw on two major themes in anti-marijuana propaganda: "amotivational syndrome" and the "gateway effect."

"[Drug eduators] make you feel as bad as they can if you do it," says one Los Angeles teenager. Still, he says, "almost every person I know has tried marijuana. Even good people."

A century ago, kids heard the same warnings about tobacco, another target of the so-called temperance movement. *Our Bodies and How We Live* (1904) warned that "the mind of the habitual user of tobacco is apt to lose its capacity for study or successful effort." According to the 1924 *Primer of Hygiene*, a smoker "forgets the importance of the work he has to do, and idles away his time instead of going earnestly to work to finish his task." *The Essentials of Health* (1892) worried that cigarettes would lead to harder stuff: "It is to be feared that if our young men continue the use of cigarettes we shall soon see, as a legitimate result, a large number of adults addicted to the opium habit."

The scientific studies allegedly proving the effectiveness of the new drug education programs aren't much more impressive than the tired rhetoric. Consider Life

Skills Training, a fast-growing program that reaches about 2 percent of the nation's 47 million schoolchildren and tops the list of "exemplary" programs. Generally touted as the future of drug education, Life Skills Training purports to cut tobacco, alcohol, and marijuana use by up to 75 percent; to reduce the use of multiple drugs by two-thirds; and to decrease the use of inhalants, narcotics, and hallucinogens. These claims aren't based on testimonials or case studies about 12-year-old Johnny turning his life around after a few Life Skills Training lessons. The program's supporters cite actual scientific studies, reported in journals published by the American Medical Association and American Psychological Association.

But the lead scientist on those evaluations, Cornell University epidemiologist Gilbert Botvin, is the creator of Life Skills Training and the one profiting from its success. Botvin also sits on the expert panel that deemed his prevention program "exemplary." He is not the only program developer sitting on the expert panel; two other panelists have participated in rating prevention programs they helped develop. All of their programs have received "exemplary" marks.

Such conflicts of interest aren't proof that the conclusions are flawed. But independent researchers such as Joel Brown at the Center for Educational Research and Development in Berkeley have found problems with the Life Skills Training studies. Brown charges that the evaluations often focused only on positive outcomes and omitted results indicating that teenagers who went through the prevention program were *more* likely to use drugs or alcohol than their peers.

You Gotta Believe

In a 2001 analysis published by the *Journal of Drug Education*, Brown noted that a six-year evaluation of Life Skills Training reported data only from students who had completed 60 percent or more of the curriculum, just two-thirds of the original 2,455-student sample. The students left out were the ones who missed many of the anti-drug lessons—probably students who skipped class a lot or were less motivated. Such students, other research suggests, would be especially prone to drug use. Carving them out of the picture inflated the program's apparent effectiveness, Brown's study shows.

Brown also found that when students completed anything less than 60 percent of the Life Skills Training curriculum, even 59 percent, their drug use was no lower, and in many cases higher, than that of students who did not participate in any lessons at all. Since the researchers don't give a good reason for using 60 percent as the cutoff point (only saying it was "a reasonably complete version of the intervention"), it seems they simply chose the point at which the outcomes turned positive.

Furthermore, Brown says, real students in real classrooms are unlikely ever to see 60 percent of the curriculum, because most teachers simply pick out lessons and squeeze them in whenever possible. The Life Skills Training research reinforces this caveat: Even under pristine conditions, with teachers getting constant training and monitoring, one-third of the students failed to reach the 60 percent mark. And those kids, Brown's research shows, were more likely to use drugs than the students who did not participate at all.

> What all of these programs continue to ignore is the most crucial piece in the drug prevention puzzle—the kids, and their stubbornly independent reactions to propaganda. They aren't fooled by "decision making" skills or "healthy choices."

The National Academy of Sciences found similar gaps in drug education research in its 2001 report *Informing America's Policy on Illegal Drugs: What We Don't Know Keeps Hurting Us.* Too many studies omit negative results, exclude students from the original sample, and inflate statistical evidence, the report concluded. But because the federal government only requires a prevention study to demonstrate a single positive outcome, programs backed by weak evidence stay in business.

Another problem with many of the new "science-based" prevention programs is that they continue to rely on statistics measuring student attitudes toward drugs. Project ALERT celebrates outcomes such as these: "Anti-drug beliefs were significantly enhanced," among them "intentions not to use within the next six months," "beliefs that one can successfully resist pro-drug pressures," and "beliefs that drug use is harmful and has negative consequences." But whether a student *intends* to abstain or *believes* he can resist drugs does not tell us whether he actually will do so.

DARE officials likewise tried to counter bad publicity by falling back on beliefs, trumpeting that 97 percent of teachers rated DARE as good to excellent, 93 percent of parents believed DARE teaches children to avoid drugs, and 86 percent of school principals believed students would be less likely to use drugs after DARE. With only beliefs to cite, DARE was left off the federal government's list of "exemplary" and "promising" prevention curricula in 2000. Many schools have dropped it from their anti-drug lineups or scaled it back to the point of irrelevance, a fact that DARE officials concede while refusing to release numbers on the decline.

Desperate to retain its dominance in the prevention market, DARE has embarked on a dramatic retooling of its lessons to keep up with the current emphasis on scientific research, decision-making skills, and resistance techniques. The Robert Wood Johnson Foundation has given DARE a $13.7 million grant to create a new middle school curriculum, which teachers began testing last fall. DARE officials said the new curriculum was drastically different.

"It's not just say no, it's not Nancy Reagan," says Charlie Parsons, executive director of DARE America. "We're teaching kids *how* to say no."

It remains to be seen how this revamped DARE curriculum is going to be any different from the old one—or, for that matter, how any of the new prevention programs are different from the old DARE. Many of the DARE tactics now scorned by educators are quite similar to those used in the new, supposedly revised programs. Project ALERT and Life Skills Training have "Ways to Say No" almost identical to the ones taught in DARE.

Drug Education as if Reality Matters

What all of these programs continue to ignore is the most crucial piece in the drug prevention puzzle—the kids, and their stubbornly independent reactions to propaganda. They aren't fooled by "decision making" skills or "healthy choices." They know what the teachers expect: Just say no.

"They make you feel as bad as they can if you do it," says one Los Angeles teenager. Still, he says, "almost every person I know has tried marijuana. Even good people."

At Mira Costa High School in Manhattan Beach, California, a 10th-grade summer health teacher, Guy Gardner, recognizes his difficult position. About one in four Manhattan Beach students are "current" (past-month) marijuana users, according to the district's own studies, which puts them near the national average. "A lot of them know more than I do," Gardner confesses. Yet he plays the game, rattling off a list of warnings—cocaine will rot out your nose, marijuana could kill you, there's no such thing as recreational drug use—even as most of his students know how unlikely or just plain wrong it all is.

In one lesson, Gardner asks students to name the first thing that comes to their minds when they hear the word *drugs*. "Don't give me answers I want to hear, give me your answers," he urges.

A couple of kids call out: Crime. Death. Stupid. Something that alters your mind and screws up your body.

But a few offer another point of view.

"I think it's bad, but people have the choice to do it, and if they do it, it's their problem," says one boy.

"If you really want to do it, you're going to do it," says another, even going so far as to advocate legalizing drugs. "We'd be so much more chill in the nation."

That may be, but saying so is untenable in the abstinence-only world of drug education. Gardner pulls back the debate. You can't legalize drugs, he tells the students, because they're harmful. "The ultimate message" of legalization, he says, "is it's OK to do drugs." And that, he implies, just isn't true.

In the end, meaningful drug education reform probably won't come from educators. It will have to come from those who have far more at stake when it comes to drug use by teenagers: their parents. They are the ones who see their kids stumble home with bloodshot eyes, who can't fall asleep when their kids are partying the night away, who know their kids are experimenting with drugs and want, above all, for them to be safe.

That's why drug experts such as *Safety First* author Marsha Rosenbaum are calling for a truly new approach to drug education, one that abandons the abstinence-only message and gives kids the unbiased, factual information they need to stay safe, even if they choose to experiment. Such information could include now-forbidden advice on real but avoidable hazards such as driving under the influence, having sex when you're high, mixing alcohol with other depressants, and overheating while using Ecstasy.

One possible model is Mothers Against Drunk Driving (MADD), which recognized that if it couldn't stop young people from drinking, it could at least stop them from getting behind the wheel while intoxicated. MADD's efforts, which made *designated driver* a household term, seem to have worked: Since 1982, according to the National Highway Traffic Safety Administration, the number of teenagers killed in drunk driving accidents has plunged 57 percent. MADD thus helped prove that we can make drug use safer without eliminating it entirely.

"There are kids who are not going to use drugs for religious reasons, because they're athletes, because they're focused on school, because they don't like the way they feel," Rosenbaum notes. "These kids don't need a program to tell them no. They're already not using. But for the kids who are amenable to the experience, it doesn't matter how many DARE programs they sit through; they're going to do it anyway ... If we can't prevent drug use, what we can prevent is drug abuse and drug problems. But we have to get real."

Renee Moilanen (rmoilanen@adelphia.net) is a freelance journalist studying drug policy at UCLA.

Dangerous Supplements Still At Large

If you can buy it at a clean, well-lighted store, if it's "all natural," it's not going to do you serious harm, right? That's what many Americans assume about dietary supplements. But while most supplements are probably fairly benign, CONSUMER REPORTS has identified a dozen that according to government warnings, adverse-event reports, and top experts are too dangerous to be on the market. Yet they are. We easily purchased all 12 in February in a few days of shopping online and in retail stores.

These unsafe supplements include Aristolochia, an herb conclusively linked to kidney failure and cancer in China, Europe, Japan, and the U.S.; yohimbe, a sexual stimulant linked to heart and respiratory problems; bitter orange, whose ingredients have effects similar to those of the banned weight-loss stimulant ephedra; and chaparral, comfrey, germander, and kava, all known or likely causes of liver failure. (For a complete list of the "dirty dozen," see the table: Twelve supplements you should avoid.)

U.S. consumers shelled out some $76 million in 2002 for just three of these supplements: androstenedione, kava, and yohimbe, the only ones for which sales figures were available, according to the Nutrition Business Journal, which tracks the supplement industry.

The potentially dangerous effects of most of these products have been known for more than a decade, and at least five of them are banned in Asia, Europe, or Canada. Yet until very recently, the U.S. Food and Drug Administration had not managed to remove a single dietary supplement from the market for safety reasons.

After seven years of trying, the agency announced a ban on the weight-loss aid ephedra in December 2003. And in March 2004 it warned 23 companies to stop marketing the body-building supplement androstenedione (andro).

Despite these actions against high-profile supplements, whose dangers were so well known that even industry trade groups had stopped defending them, the agency continues to be hamstrung by the 1994 Dietary Supplement Health and Education Act (DSHEA, pronounced de-*shay*). While drug manufacturers are required to prove that their products are safe before being marketed, DSHEA makes the FDA prove that supplements on the market are *unsafe* and denies the agency all but the sketchiest information about the safety record of most of them.

CR Quick Take

A CR investigation found that many dangerous supplements can easily be purchased in stores and online. Many of these supplements have been banned in other countries. Why can't the U.S. Food and Drug Administration ban these products now?
We found that regulatory barriers created by Congress, supplement industry pressure, and a lack of resources at the FDA have resulted in major risks for consumers.

- These widely available dietary supplements (see table) may cause cancer, severe kidney or liver damage, heart problems, or even death. They should be avoided by consumers.

- These supplements are sold under a profusion of names, making it difficult for consumers to know what they're purchasing.

- Most also appear in combination products marketed for a broad array of uses, such as asphrodisiacs, athletic-performance boosters, and treatments for anxiety, arthritis, menstrual problems, ulcers, and weight loss.

"The standards for demonstrating a supplement is hazardous are so high that it can take the FDA years to build a case," said Bruce Silverglade, legal director of the Center for Science in the Public Interest, a Washington, D.C., consumer advocacy group.

At the same time, the FDA's supplement division is understaffed and underfunded, with about 60 people and a budget of only $10 million to police a $19.4 billion-a-year industry. To regulate drugs, annual sales of which are 12 times the amount of supplement sales, the FDA has almost 43 times as much money and almost 48 times as many people.

"The law has never been fully funded," said William Hubbard, FDA associate commissioner for policy and planning. "There's never been the resources to do all the things the law would command us to do."

Twelve supplements you should avoid

The 12 supplements ingredients in this table have been linked to serious adverse events or, in the case of glandular supplements, to strong theoretical risks. They're all readily available on the Web, where our shoppers bought them both individually and in multi ingredient "combination products." We think it's wise to avoid all of them. But the strength of that warning varies with the strength of the evidence and the size of the risk. So we've divided the dirty dozen into three categories: definitely hazardous, very likely hazardous, and likely hazardous.

NAME (ALSO KNOWN AS)	DANGERS	REGULATORY ACTIONS
DEFINITELY HAZARDOUS *Documented organ failure and known carcinogenic properties*		
Aristolochic acid (*Aristolochia*, birthwort, snakeweed, sangree root, snagrel, serpentary, serpentaria; asarum candense, wild ginger)	Potent human carcinogen; kidney failure, sometimes requiring transplant; deaths reported.	FDA warning to consumers and industry and import alert, in April 2001. Banned in 7 European countries and Egypt, Japan, and Venezuela.
VERY LIKELY HAZARDOUS *Banned in other countries, FDA warning, or adverse effects in studies*		
Comfrey (*Symphytum officinale*, ass ear, black root, blackwort, bruisewort, consolidae radix, consound, gum plant, healing herb, knitback, knitbone, salsify, slippery root, symphytum radix, wallwort)	Abnormal liver function or damage, often irreversible; deaths reported.	FDA advised industry to remove from market in July 2001.
Androstenedione (*4-androstene-3, 17-dione*, andro, androstene)	Increased cancer risk, decrease in HDL cholesterol.	FDA warned 23 companies to stop manufacturing, marketing, and distributing in March 2004. Banned by athletic associations.
Chaparral (*Larrea divaricata*, creosote bush, greasewood, hediodilla, jarilla, larreastat)	Abnormal liver function or damage, often irreversible; deaths reported.	FDA warning to consumers in December 1992.
Germander (*Teucrium chamaedrys*, wall germander, wild germander)	Abnormal liver function or damage, often irreversible; deaths reported.	Banned in France and Germany.
Kava (*Piper methysticum*, ava, awa, gea, gi, intoxicating pepper, kao, kavain, kawa-pfeffer, kew, long pepper, malohu, maluk, meruk, milik, rauschpfeffer, sakau, tonga, wurzelstock, yagona, yangona)	Abnormal liver functin or damage, occasionally irreversible; deaths reported.	FDA warning to consumers in March 2002. Banned in Canada, Germany, Singapaore, South Africa, and Switzerland.
LIKELY HAZADOUS *Adverse-event reports or theoretical risks*		
Bitter orange (*Citrus aurantium*, green orange, kijitsu, neroli oil, Seville orange, shangzhou zhiqiao, sour orange, zhi oiao, zhi zhi)	High blood pressure; increased risk of heart arrythmias, heart attack, stroke.	None
Organ/glandular extracts (brain/adrenal/pituitary/placenta/other gland "substance" or "concentrate")	Theoretical risk of mad cow disease, particularly from brain extracts.	FDA banned high-risk bovine materials from older cows in foods and supplements in January 2004. (High-risk parts from cows under 30 months still permitted.) Banned in France and Switzerland.
Lobelia (*Lobelia inflata*, asthma weed, bladderpod, emetic herb, gagroot, lobelie, indian tobacco, pukeweed, vomit wort, wild tobacco)	Breathing difficulty, rapid heartbeat, low blood pressure, diarrhea, dizziness, tremors; possible deaths reported.	Banned in Bangladesh and Italy.
Pennyroyal oil (*Hedeoma pulegioides*, lurk-in-the-ditch, mosquito plant, piliolerial, pudding grass, pulegium, run-by-the-ground, squaw balm, squawmint, stinking balm, tickweed)	Liver and kidney failure, nerve damage, convulsions, abdominal tenderness, burning of the throat; deaths reported.	None
Scullcap (*Scutellaria lateriflora*, blue pimpernel, helmet flower, hoodwort, mad weed, mad-dog herb, quaker bonnet, scutelluria, skullcap)	Abnormal liver function or damage.	None
Yohimbe (*Pausinystalia yohimbe*, johimbi, yohimbehe, yohimbine)	Change in blood pressure, heart arrythmias, respiratory depression, heart attack; deaths reported.	None

Sources: Natural Medicines Comprehensive Database 2004 and Consumers Union's medical and research consultants.

The agency has learned that it must tread carefully when regulating supplements. The first time it tried to regulate the dangerous stimulant ephedra, in 1997, overwhelming opposition from Congress and industry forced it to back down.

As a result, the FDA is sometimes left practicing what Silverglade calls "regulation by press release"—issuing warnings about dangerous supplements and hoping that consumers and health practitioners read them.

There are signs of hope. The FDA has said that if the ban on ephedra holds up against likely legal challenges, it plans to go after other harmful supplements. Legislation has been introduced to strengthen the FDA's authority under DSHEA and give the agency more money to enforce the act.

But the supplement marketplace still holds hidden hazards for consumers, especially among products that aren't in the headlines. "Consumers are provided with more information about the composition and nutritional value of a loaf of bread than about the ingredients and potential hazards of botanical medicines," said Arthur Grollman, M.D., professor of pharmacological sciences at the State University of New York, Stony Brook, and a critic of DSHEA.

A QUESTION OF SAFETY

Supplement-industry advocates say the ephedra ban demonstrates that DSHEA gives the FDA enough power to protect consumers from unsafe products. "I don't think there's anything wrong except that FDA has only recently begun vigorous and active enforcement of the law," said Annette Dickinson, Ph.D., president of the Council for Responsible Nutrition, a major trade association for the supplement industry.

But critics of DSHEA think the ban illustrates the extremes to which FDA must go to outlaw a hazardous product.

When the agency initially tried to rein in ephedra use in 1997, after receiving hundreds of reports of adverse events, it sought not an outright ban but dosage restrictions and sterner warning labels. The industry mounted a furious counterattack, including the creation of a public-relations group called the Ephedra Education Council and a scientific review from a private consulting firm, commissioned by Dickinson's trade group, that concluded ephedra was safe. After the U.S. General Accounting Office said the FDA "did not establish a causal link" between taking ephedra and deaths or injuries, the agency was forced to drop its proposal.

The industry continued to vigorously market and defend ephedra. Metabolife International, a leading ephedra manufacturer, did not let the FDA know that it had received 14,684 complaints of adverse events associated with its ephedra product, Metabolife 356, in the previous five years, including 18 heart attacks, 26 strokes, 43 seizures, and 5 deaths. It took the pressure of congressional and Justice Department investigations to get the company to turn over the complaints in 2002. Then Steve Bechler, a pitcher for the Baltimore Orioles, died unexpectedly in 2003 while taking another ephedra supplement, Xenadrine RFA-1. With sales suffering from the bad publicity, manufacturers began to replace ephedra with other stimulants such as bitter orange, which mimics ephedra in chemical composition and function.

"All of a sudden Congress dropped objections to an ephedra ban and started demanding the FDA act," said Silverglade.

To amass the necessary scientific evidence that it hoped would satisfy the demanding standard set by DSHEA, the FDA took aggressive action: It commissioned an outside review from the RAND Corporation, analyzed adverse-event reports, and pored over every available shred of scientific evidence.

"We've gone the whole nine yards to collect and evaluate all the possible evidence," Mark McClellan, commissioner of the FDA, said in announcing the ban. "We will be doing our best to defend this in court, and if that's not sufficient, it may be time to re-examine the act."

DRUGS VS. SUPPLEMENTS

In an October 2002 nationwide Harris Poll of 1,010 adults, 59 percent of respondents said they believed that supplements must be approved by a government agency before they can be sold to the public. Sixty-eight percent said the government requires warning labels on supplements' potential side effects or dangers. Fifty-five percent said supplement manufacturers can't make safety claims without solid scientific support.

SUFFERED SIEZURE

Gretchen Fitzgerald, age 21, Fort Collins, Colo.

PROBLEM She took Xenadrine EFX "thermogenic" diet pills to boost her energy while studying for final exams, believing they were safe because they were labeled ephedra-free. After three weeks of taking the product she had a seizure. The neurologist consulted told her the bitter orange in the Xenadrine was the probable cause. Xenadrine's manufacturer did not return our phone calls. Since going off the Xenadrine, Fitzgerald has had no further problems.

They were wrong. None of those protections exist for supplements—only for prescription and over-the-counter medicines. Here are the major differences in the safety regulations:

Testing for hazards. Before approval, drugs must be proved effective, with an acceptable safety profile, by means of lab research and rigorous human clinical trials

KIDNEYS FAILED

**Beverly Hames, age 59,
Beaverton, Ore.**

PROBLEM Hames went to an acupuncturist in 1992 seeking a "safe, natural" treatment for an aching back. She got a selection of Chinese herbal products, at least five of which were later found to contain aristolochic acid. By mid-1994, she had symptoms of kidney failure, and in 1996 she underwent a kidney transplant. She must take anti-rejection drugs for life. The herbs' distributor said his Chinese suppliers had substituted Aristolochia for another herb without his knowledge.

involving a minimum of several thousand people, many millions of dollars, and several years.

In contrast, supplement manufacturers can introduce new products without any testing for safety and efficacy. The maker's only obligation is to send the FDA a copy of the language on the label (see Names & Claims).

"Products regulated by DSHEA were presumed to be safe because of their long history of use, often in other countries," said Jane E. Henney, M.D., commissioner of the FDA from 1998 to 2001. "As their use dramatically increased in this country after the passage of DSHEA, the presumption of safety may have been misplaced, particularly for products other than traditional vitamins and minerals. Some, like ephedra, act like drugs and thus have similar risks."

The only exceptions to this "presumption of safety" are supplement ingredients that weren't being sold in the U.S. when DSHEA took effect. Makers of such "new dietary ingredients" must show the FDA evidence of the products' safety before marketing them. The FDA invoked that rarely used provision in its action against androstenedione. After years of allowing andro to be marketed without restriction, the agency declared that it was "not aware" that the supplement was used before DSHEA, so it couldn't be sold without evidence of safety.

Disclosing the risks. Drug labels and package inserts must mention all possible adverse effects and interactions. But supplement makers don't have to put safety warnings on the labels, even for products with known serious hazards.

We bought a product called Relaxit whose label had no warning about the kava it contained, even though the American Herbal Products Association, an industry trade group, recommends a detailed, though voluntary warning label about potential liver toxicity on all kava products.

Ensuring product quality. Drugs must conform to "good manufacturing practices" that guarantee that their contents are pure and in the quantities stated on the label. While DSHEA gave the FDA authority to impose similar standards on supplements, it took until 2003 for the

agency to propose regulations—as yet not final—to implement that part of the law.

Contaminants, too, regularly turn up in supplements. In 1998 Richard Ko, Ph.D., of the California Department of Health Services reported that 32 percent of the Asian patent medicines he tested contained pharmaceuticals or heavy metals that weren't on the label. The FDA has seized supplements adulterated with prescription drugs, including, in 2002, an herbal "prostate health" supplement called PC SPES that turned out to contain a powerful prescription blood thinner, warfarin.

Reporting the problems. By law, drug companies are required to tell the FDA about any reports of product-related adverse events that they receive from any source. Almost every year, drugs are removed from the market based on safety risks that first surfaced in those reports.

In contrast, supplement makers don't have to report adverse events. Indeed, in the five years after DSHEA took effect, 1994 to 1999, fewer than 10 of the more than 2,500 reports that the FDA received came from manufacturers, according to a 2001 estimate from the inspector general of the U.S. Department of Health and Human Services. (Other sources of reports included consumers, health practitioners, and poison-control centers.) Overall, the FDA estimates that it learns of less than 1 percent of adverse events involving dietary supplements.

THE 'NATURAL' MYSTIQUE

Many makers market their supplements as "natural," exploiting assumptions that such products can't harm you. That's a dangerous assumption, said Lois Swirsky Gold, Ph.D., director of the Carcinogenic Potency Project at the University of California, Berkeley, and an expert on chemical carcinogens. "Natural is hemlock, natural is arsenic, natural is poisonous mushrooms," she said.

A cautionary example is aristolochic acid, which occurs naturally in species of Aristolochia vines that grow wild in many parts of the world. In addition to being a powerful kidney toxin, it is on the World Health Organization's list of human carcinogens. "It's one of the most potent chemicals of 1,400 in my Carcinogenic Potency Database," Gold said. "People have taken high doses similar to the doses that animals are given in tests, and they both get tumors very quickly."

The dangers of aristolochic acid have been known since at least 1993, when medical-journal articles began appearing about 105 patrons of a Belgian weight-loss clinic who had suffered kidney failure after consuming Chinese herbs adulterated with Aristolochia. At least 18 of the women also subsequently developed cancer near the kidney.

These findings prompted the FDA to issue a nationwide warning against Aristolochia in 2001 and to impose a ban on further imports of the herb. But in early 2004, more than two years after the import ban went into effect, CONSUMER REPORTS was able to purchase products online that were labeled as containing Aristolochia. In

names&claims

THE ART AND LAW OF SUPPLEMENT LABELS

- "New 21st century 'designer' D-Bol is so potent it turns genetically average guys into supernatural studs no one messes with!"

- Xenadrine EFX "provides the most effective approach to losing weight ever developed!"

- "Thousands of testimonials" credit chaparral "for tumor remission and complete cures. Other medical evidence indicates it is an anti-inflammatory and antimicrobial agent and a possible treatment for asthma."

Does the government really allow supplement companies to make extravagant promises like those, which we found on Web sites promoting products we purchased? The answer is murky at best.

Under the 1994 Dietary Supplement Health and Education Act, manufacturers can't claim that a product prevents or treats a disease or disorder. But they can say it affects the "structure and function" of the body— "supports healthy prostate function," for example—or shows a "link" to a disease or disorder, and allow consumers to draw their own, often erroneous, conclusions. The FDA can require that a manufacturer change a label that it decides is making an unauthorized claim.

DSHEA does say, confusingly, that supplement makers must be able to "substantiate" their claims. But it does not specify what that means, nor does it require that the evidence be shown to anybody, not even the FDA.

The Federal Trade Commission has the authority to punish companies whose ads are intentionally misleading. Unlike the FDA, it can force companies to give it documents substantiating suspect claims and order the products off the market if it decides that the substantiation isn't sufficient. But it can't move against a category of products, such as those containing ephedra, nor can it act against dangerous products that aren't advertising to the public.

Since DSHEA's passage, the FTC has brought more then 100 cases against supplement marketers for deceptive advertising. But "there are literally hundreds, perhaps thousands, of companies out there that probably deserve scrutiny," said Richard Cleland, assistant director of the FTC's division of advertising practices, "We don't have the resources to look at every one."

2003, Gold identified more than 100 products for sale on known or suspected to contain aristolochic acid.

Donna Andrade-Wheaton, a former aerobics instructor in Rhode Island, learned those facts too late to save her kidneys. After taking Chinese herbs containing Aristolochia for more than two years, she suffered severe kidney damage; her kidney tissues were found to contain aristolochic acid. In late 2002, at age 39, she underwent a kidney transplant.

Andrade-Wheaton is suing both the acupuncturist who gave her the herbs and several companies that manufactured them. The acupuncturist declined to discuss the case on the record, and the manufacturer did not return our phone calls.

There's another widespread and false assumption about natural supplements: that they're always pure, unprocessed products of the earth. Because DSHEA permits the marketing of concentrates and extracts, supplement makers can and do manipulate ingredients to increase the concentrations of pharmacologically active compounds.

That's especially true of the many weight-loss supplements designed for "thermogenic" stimulant effects-boosting calorie expenditure by revving the metabolic rate.

On one Internet shopping tour, for instance, we bought a product called Thermorexin—"the Hottest new Thermogenic on the market!" Its label says it contains, among its 22 ingredients, 30 milligrams of theophylline derived from a black tea extract and the stimulant bitter orange. Sold as Theo-Dur and other brands, theophylline is a prescription drug and an effective asthma treatment, but most doctors seldom prescribe it because it can cause seizures and irregular heartbeats at relatively low doses.

Larry Berube, president of Anafit, Thermorexin's manufacturer, based in Orlando, Fla., described how the product's combination of ingredients was developed: "Once we find out that the FDA says it's OK, we put them together in the lab, run our tests, and do our trials, and if it comes up good, we capsulate it, put it online and in the stores and sell it," he said.

Those tests involved asking fitness professionals to use the supplement, and measuring their heart rate and blood pressure, Berube said. The company doesn't use a control group, he said. Then "we go to the fitness discussion boards and let trainers and people know we have a new product and do they want to try it," he said. "And then they try it, and they report back." Berube said he has not heard of any bad reactions to Thermorexin.

WHAT YOU CAN DO

Sen. Richard Durbin, Democrat of Illinois, and Rep. Susan Davis, Democrat of California, have each intro-

KIDNEYS FAILED

**Donna Andrade-Wheaton, age 40,
Cranston, R.I.**

PROBLEM Andrade-Wheaton's acupuncturist prescribed more than a half dozen Chinese herbal supplements to treat health conditions, including endometriosis. At least one of the products listed Aristolochia as an ingredient, even after the FDA issued a nationwide Aristolochia safety warning in 2001. She underwent a kidney transplant in September 2002 and must take anti-rejection drugs for life.

duced legislation that for the first time would require supplement manufacturers to disclose reports they receive of "serious" adverse events. Durbin's bill also sets up a separate category for stimulants, which would have to receive FDA safety approval before being marketed, and reclassifies androstenedione and similar "steroid precursors" as controlled drugs. The Davis bill also strengthens the FDA's powers to investigate emerging supplement safety problems. Davis's bill exempts vitamins and minerals from its provisions. (Consumers Union, publisher of CONSUMER REPORTS, supports both bills.)

Though the bills are still in committee, the supplement industry has mobilized in opposition. On its Web site and in flyers handed out at supplement stores, the National Nutritional Foods Association, a supplement retailers' trade group, says the legislation "would significantly undermine many of the freedoms that American consumers of dietary supplements like you hold dear."

The industry is supporting a more limited bill introduced by Sen. Orrin Hatch, Republican of Utah, and Sen. Tom Harkin, Democrat of Iowa, that would give the FDA an extra $20 million this year, and more in subsequent years, to enforce DSHEA and would reclassify androstenedione and other steroid precursors as controlled drugs. Unlike the Durbin bill, however, this measure would exempt the steroid dehydroepiandrosterone, or DHEA, allowing it to continue to be marketed as an anti-aging product. Some $47 million worth was sold in 2002, according to the Nutrition Business Journal.

Until the law is substantially changed and the FDA is adequately funded, you cannot rely on the federal government to ensure that dietary supplements are safe and effective. Here are some steps you can take to minimize your risk from any supplements you decide to take:

Stay away from the dirty dozen. All carry risks that in our view are unacceptable (see table). In combination products, you need to read the detailed ingredient list in the tiny print on the back. Who could otherwise guess, for instance, that Gaia Herbs' PMS Day 14-28 capsules contain kava? (To the company's credit, the label includes a warning about liver toxicity.)

Do not take daily doses of vitamins and minerals that exceed the safe upper limits. While vitamins and minerals are by far the safest and best-studied of supplements, it's possible to overdose on some of them. For more information, see "Fortified Foods: Too Much of a Good Thing?," CONSUMER REPORTS, October 2003. Recommended allowances and safe upper limits can be found online at www.ific.org/publications/other/driupdateom.cfm.

Limit your intake of other supplements. Over the years, our medical and nutritional consultants have identified and tested a few products, other than standard multivitamins, with possible benefits and sufficiently low risks to recommend for general use: saw palmetto for benign enlarged prostate in men, glucosamine and chondroitin for arthritis, and fish-oil capsules (omega-3 fatty acids) for heart disease. (We plan to test additional supplements with potential benefits, such as probiotics.)

Tell your doctor about your supplements. "The Achilles' heel of unregulated supplements is the risk created by herb-prescription drug interactions," said Grollman, the pharmacologist at the State University of New York. "St. John's wort, used to treat depression, for instance, may reduce the effectiveness of prescription drugs used by millions of Americans for hypertension, AIDS, heart failure, asthma, and other chronic diseases."

Stay away from supplements for weight control. These products frequently contain several stimulants that have never been adequately tested separately, let alone in combinations. "I'd just as soon experiment with rats first rather than using the U.S. population as guinea pigs," said Bill Gurley, Ph.D., professor of pharmaceutical sciences at the University of Arkansas.

Do your own research. Health-foodstore clerks and marketers, alternative medicine practitioners, herbal company Web sites, and even physicians are not necessarily knowledgeable about the scientific evidence regarding dietary supplements. These two Web sites contain reliable information: the National Institutes of Health site at ods.od.nih.gov/databases/ibids.html and Memorial Sloan-Kettering Cancer Center's site at www.mskcc.org/mskcc/html/11570.cfm.

Watch for adverse events. Let your doctor know if you experience anything worrisome after starting a supplement. If your doctor concludes that the side effect may be related to the supplement, be sure to report it to the FDA, by calling 800-332-1088 or by visiting www.fda.gov/medwatch.

UNIT 6

Sexuality and Relationships

Unit Selections

Key Points to Consider

- Do you feel at risk of contracting AIDS or other STDs? If not, why not? If you do, what are you doing to reduce your risk?

- What is meant by a "love culture"?

- What would be the benefits of male contraceptives other than condoms?

- What are the physical benefits of lovemaking?

Student Website

www.mhcls.com/online

Internet References

Further information regarding these websites may be found in this book's preface or online.

Planned Parenthood
   http://www.plannedparenthood.org/
Sexuality Information and Education Council of the United States (SIECUS)
   http://www.siecus.org/

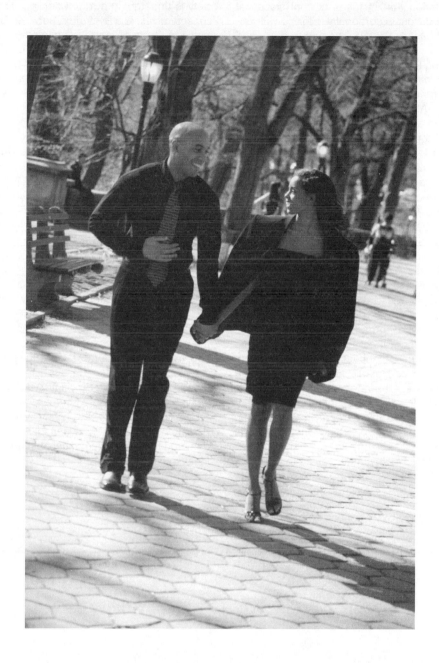

Sexuality is an important part of both self awareness and intimate relationships.

How important is physical attraction in establishing and maintaining intimate relationships? Researchers in the area of evolutionary psychology have proposed numerous theories that attempt to explain the mutual attraction that occurs between the sexes. The most controversial of these theories postulates that our perception of beauty or physical attractiveness is not subjective but rather a biological component hardwired into our brains. It is generally assumed that perceptions of beauty vary from era to era and culture to culture, but evidence is mounting that suggests people everywhere share a common sense of beauty that is based on physical symmetry.

While physical attraction is clearly an important issue when it comes to dating, how important is it in long-term loving relationships? For many Americans the answer may be very important, because we tend to be a "Love Culture," a culture that places a premium on passion in the selection of our mates. Is passion an essential ingredient in love, and can passion serve to sustain a long-term meaningful relationship? Since most people can't imagine marrying someone that they don't love, we must assume that most marriages are based on this feeling we call love. That being the case, why is it that so few marriages survive the rigors of day-to-day living? Perhaps the answer has more to do with our limited definition of love than love itself. "It's Just Mechanics" examines the issue of love as it relates to intimate relationships that last and identifies several key factors that relate to sex and aging including the use of Viagra and similar drugs. "Promiscuous Plague" examines the state of America's sexual health through a presentation that includes current statistical data and interviews with individuals personally involved with unintended pregnancies, STDs, HIV/AIDS, homosexuality, and abortion. A topic related to sexual health is that sex is good for health. Studies are showing that an active sex life may lead to a longer life, better ability to withstand pain, a healthy immune system, less heart disease and cancer, and lower rates of depression. In "Sexual Healing," Alice Park addresses all the health benefits associated with an active sex life.

An important topic of interest in the area of human sexuality is birth control. According to Dennis Barbour, president of the Association of Reproductive Health Professionals, the contraceptive choices that Americans have are safe and effective, but a method that is good for one woman may not work for another. Some of the factors that must be considered in making a contraceptive choice include the health of the individual, frequency of sexual activity, number of partners, future plans for having children, effectiveness rates, side effects, convenience, and cost. Another issue is that most birth control methods are designed for women; the one exception is the condom. In "Male Contraception: Search is On for Options," research on new male birth control choices is addressed.

Perhaps no topic in the area of human sexuality has garnered more publicity and public concern than the dangers associated with unprotected sex. Although the concept of "safe sex" is nothing new, the degree of open and public discussion regarding sexual behaviors is. With the emergence of AIDS as a disease of epidemic proportions and the rapid spreading of other sexually transmitted diseases (STDs), the surgeon general of the United States initiated an aggressive educational campaign based on the assumption that knowledge would change behavior. If STD rates among teens are any indication as to the effectiveness of this approach, then we must conclude that our educational efforts are failing. Conservatives believe that while education may play a role in curbing the spread of STDs, the root of the problem is promiscuity, and promiscuity rises when a society is undergoing a moral decline. The solution, according to conservatives, is a joint effort between parents and educators in which students are taught the importance of values such as respect, responsibility, and integrity. Liberals, on the other hand, think that preventing promiscuity is unrealistic, and instead the focus should be on establishing open and frank discussions between the sexes. Their premise is that we are all sexual beings, and the best way to combat STDs is to establish discussions between sexual partners so that condoms will be used correctly when couples engage in intercourse. While education undoubtedly has had a positive impact on slowing the spread of STDs, perhaps it was unrealistic to think that education alone was the solution, given the magnitude and the nature of the problem. Most experts agree that for education to succeed in changing personal behaviors the following conditions must be met: (1) The recipients of the information must first perceive themselves as vulnerable and, thus, be motivated to explore replacement behaviors, and (2) the replacement behaviors must satisfy the needs that were the basis of the problem behaviors. To date, most education programs have failed to meet these criteria. Given all the information that we now have on the dangers associated with AIDS and STDs, why is it that people do not perceive themselves at risk? It is not so much the denial of risks as it is the notion that when it comes to choosing sex partners most people think that they use good judgment. Unfortunately, most decisions regarding sexual behavior are based on subjective criteria that bear little or no relationship to one's actual risk. Even when individuals do view themselves as vulnerable to AIDS and STDs, there are currently only two viable options for reducing the risk of contracting these diseases. The first is the use of a condom and the second is sexual abstinence, neither of which is an ideal solution to the problem.

Sexual Healing

What feels good is good for you too. Making love can boost the heart, relieve pain and help keep you healthy

By Alice Park

The "sex glow." Carrie Bradshaw and her *Sex and the City* trio may be the champions of detecting it, getting it and keeping it, but you don't need a closetful of Prada to appreciate the rosy radiance that follows a pleasant sexual encounter. The fact is, sex leaves its mark, not just on the mind but on the body as well. Researchers have begun to explore its effects on almost every part of the body, from the brain to the heart to the immune system.

Studies are showing that arousal and an active sex life may lead to a longer life, better heart health, an improved ability to ward off pain, a more robust immune system and even protection against certain cancers, not to mention lower rates of depression.

But finding mechanisms for these benefits and proving cause and effect are no easy matter. "The associations are out there, so there has to be an explanation for it," says Dr. Ronald Glaser, director of the Institute of Behavioral Medicine Research at Ohio State University. Thanks to a better understanding of the biochemistry of arousal, as well as advances in imaging techniques, doctors are closing in on some possibilities. Their efforts are leading them to the hormone oxytocin, which may be the key lubricant for the machinery of sex. Known for controlling the muscles of the uterus during childbirth, oxytocin surges up to five times as high as its normal blood level during orgasm. Studies in animals have also revealed oxytocin's softer side. It is responsible for helping individuals forge strong emotional bonds, earning its moniker as the cuddle hormone. Released in the brain, oxytocin works in the blood, where it travels to tissues as distant as the uterus, as well as along nerve fibers, where it regulates body temperature, blood pressure, wound healing and even relief from pain.

While it is unlikely that oxytocin alone is responsible for sex's wide-ranging effects on the body, researchers hope that by tracking the hormone they can expose the network of body systems affected by sexual activity and identify other biochemical players along the way. Here's what they have learned so far:

THE HEART OF THE MATTER

The strongest case that can be made for the benefits of sex come from studies of aerobic fitness. The act of intercourse burns about 200 calories, the equivalent of running vigorously for 30 minutes. During orgasm, both heart rate and blood pressure typically double, all under the influence of oxytocin. It would be logical to conclude that sex, like other aerobic workouts, can protect against heart disease, but studies in support of this link have yet to be done. "Can we make the claim that having sex is equal to walking a mile or bicycling? We don't know," says Robert Friar, a biologist at Michigan's Ferris State University. "The data don't really exist."

At least not yet. A study conducted in Wales in the 1980s showed that men who had sex twice a week or more often experienced half as many heart attacks after 10 years as men who had intercourse less than once a month. The trial, however, did not include a parallel group of randomly chosen control subjects, the scientific gold standard. So it's unclear whether frequent intercourse was responsible for the lower rate of heart attacks or whether, for example, the men who were sexually active were healthier or less prone to heart disease to begin with.

More recent research has focused on the hormones dehydroepiandrostone (DHEA) and testosterone, both important for libido. They have been linked to reducing the risk of heart disease as well as protecting the heart muscle after an attack. That may explain why doctors maintain that sex after a heart attack is relatively safe.

How Your Body Benefits

Sexual activity affects you from head to toe. Here's what doctors have learned about its positive effects on health:

Heart Disease
Lovemaking is good aerobic exercise that improves the circulation and works the heart. Sexually active people tend to suffer from fewer heart attacks, possibly owing to their better fitness

Weight
Intercourse can burn around 200 calories, not bad for a few minutes' work and far more entertaining than a 15-minute churn on a treadmill at the gym

Pain
Endorphins released during orgasm can dull the chronic pain of backaches and arthritis as well as migraines

Depression
Sexually active people appear to be less vulnerable to depression and suicide, perhaps because they are more comfortable with their sexuality. Researchers are also looking at the brain chemicals involved

Anxiety
Hormones released during arousal can calm anxiety, ease fear and break down inhibitions

Immunity
Frequent intercourse may boost levels of key immune cells that help fight off colds and other infections

Cancer
Early studies hint that oxytocin and the hormone DHEA, both released during orgasm, may prevent breast-cancer cells from developing into tumors

Longevity
Frequent orgasm has been linked to longer life; this may have something to do with sex's beneficial effects on the heart and immune system

PAIN CONTROL

In the 1970s Dr. Beverly Whipple of Rutgers University identified the female G spot, the vaginal on-switch for female arousal, and stumbled upon one of oxytocin's more potent effects: its ability to dull pain. Whipple showed that gentle pressure on the G spot raised pain thresholds by 40% and that during orgasm women could tolerate up to 110% more pain. But she could not explain the link until the advent of functional magnetic resonance imaging (fMRI). Using fMRI to view the brains of easily orgasmic women as they climaxed, either with visual stimuli or by self-stimulation, Whipple found that the body's pain-killing center in the midbrain is activated during peak arousal. Signals from this part of the brain instruct the body to release endorphins and corticosteroids, which can temporarily numb the raw nerve endings responsible for everything from menstrual cramps to arthritis and migraine for several minutes. Activating this region also reduces anxiety and has a calming effect.

THE HEALING POWER OF SEX

A trial involving more than 100 college students in 1999 found that the levels of immunoglobulin, a microbe-fighting antibody, in students who engaged in intercourse once or twice a week were 30% higher than in those who were abstinent. Curiously, those who had sex more than twice a week had the same levels as those who were celibate. Could there be an optimal rate of sexual frequency for keeping the body's defenses strong?

Researchers in Sweden are meanwhile exploring how sex affects another immunological function: the healing of wounds. Here again, oxytocin may lead the way. Using injections of oxytocin as a surrogate for arousal, Swedish investigators have found that sores on the backs of lab rats heal twice as fast under the influence of the hormone as without it.

To find out whether the hormone has the same healing effect in people, Ohio State's Glaser and his wife Janice Kiecolt-Glaser, a psychologist at the same institution, are enrolling married couples in an unorthodox study in which each spouse's arm is blistered and then covered with a serum-collecting device. Over a 24-hour observation period, the couples discuss positive aspects of their marriage and mates as well as points of contention, such as finances or in-laws. The Glasers will analyze how levels of oxytocin change during these discussions, along with rates of healing.

A LONG, HAPPY LIFE?

It's well known that married folk tend to live longer and suffer less depression than singles do. But is this because of more frequent sex, simple companionship or some benign aspect of personality that lends itself to marriage? Teasing apart such matters is difficult, but sex itself appears to be factor. A study of 3,500 Scottish men, for example, found a link between frequent intercourse and greater longevity. A much smaller study of elderly men found that those who masturbated appeared to experience less depression than those who did not. In addition, frequent sexual activity has been tied to lower risk of breast cancer in women and prostate cancer in men, a relationship that is still not fully understood but may involve some interaction between oxytocin and the sex hormones estrogen and testosterone and their roles in cell signaling and cell division. "Scientifically, it's an exciting time that will lead to a lot of rethinking and reconceptualizing of human sexuality," says Dr. John Bancroft, director of the Kinsey Institute. As the answers come in, the human race may begin to appreciate that the "sex glow" stays with them a lot longer than they realized.

Male contraception: Search is on for options

When women enter your family planning clinic, you have a wide array of contraceptive options to offer them. But when men ask about prevention methods, you have three choices: hand them condoms, advise abstinence, or counsel on vasectomy.

While 2002 saw the introduction of the contraceptive patch and vaginal ring for women, no contraceptive method emerged on the commercial marketplace for men. However, researchers report that investigation of male methods is enjoying a resurgence in interest, as hormonal approaches may have acquired the critical mass needed to make the transition from academic research to pharmaceutical development.[1]

To expedite development of new approaches to regulating fertility, the Bethesda-based National Institutes of Health has awarded a five-year, $9.5 million grant to the Seattle-based University of Washington to establish an interdisciplinary Male Contraception Research Center. The center will be part of the Cooperative Contraceptive Research Centers Program, funded by the Contraception and Reproductive Health (CRH) Branch of the National Institute of Child Health and Human Development.

In addition, the CRH has issued a request for applications that are focused on novel approaches to male fertility regulation, and it has issued a request for proposal for clinical trial expertise in male contraception, says **Diana Blithe**, PhD, CRH scientific officer.

Defining the challenge

Why has it been so difficult to develop a viable male contraceptive? Consider the challenging physiological task of controlling the male reproductive system. While a woman produces one egg a month, a man produces hundreds of millions of sperm each day. Women are fertile only until menopause; men continue to produce sperm throughout their adult lives.[2]

Current research approaches in male contraception primarily are focusing on two mechanisms of action. One approach is aimed at suppressing the production of sperm, by hormonal or nonhormonal means, while the second avenue seeks to inhibit the fertilizing ability of sperm.[2]

Researchers have looked at administering doses of testosterone to achieve blood concentrations that are significantly higher than normal. This causes the male pituitary gland to slow the release of two hormones—follicle stimulating hormone (FSH) and luteinizing hormone (LH)—that produce the signals necessary for sperm development. FSH and LH act in a feedback loop to maintain normal concentrations of testosterone.[3]

Scientists also have looked at progestins to block testosterone production in the testes, which hinders sperm formation. Since this approach results in a drop in testosterone concentrations in the blood, researchers have administered low doses of testosterone in conjunction with the progestins.[3]

Results of two recent investigations indicate such approaches may be effective. One study, which looked at the use of testosterone decanoate injections and etonogestrel implants, suggests that spermatogenic suppression is achieved.[4] In the other study, investigators compared levonorgestrel implants and testosterone transdermal patch to testosterone patch alone on the suppression of spermatogenesis.[5] The scientists expanded their research to include use of a combination of oral levonorgestrel and testosterone patch, as well as use of levonorgestrel implants and testosterone enanthate injection. Results indicate that the implant/injection option was the most efficient in suppressing spermatogenesis to a level acceptable for contraceptive efficacy.[5]

New androgen eyed

The New York City-based Population Council is examining several research options in male contraception using its trademarked synthetic androgen, MENT (7 alpha-methyl-19-nortestosterone). While the synthetic steroid resembles testosterone, MENT does not enlarge the prostate, a drawback that occurs when testosterone is given exogenously. The Population Council is researching a MENT implant, transdermal gel, and patch formulation for contraception purposes.

Dose-ranging studies are under way in Germany, Chile, and the United States, using MENT alone and MENT associated with other agents to achieve a complete suppression of sperm production in male volunteers, states **Regine Sitruk-Ware**, MD, the council's executive director of contraceptive development. When the appropriate dose is determined, researchers will begin a study with couples volunteering to test the method for contraception. This step will not be possible before scientists are certain of achieving 100% suppression of sperm production, she notes.

A large-scale contraceptive efficacy and safety study would not start before mid-2004; it would include 300 couples followed for one year, and it also would document recovery of fertility in a further year of follow-up, says Sitruk-Ware.

"If the results are successful, we would then have to document efficacy and safety in 1,200 couples followed over one year of therapy," she states. "Given these requirements, the method would be approved and available for general use most likely in year 2008 or 2009."

References

1. Anderson RA, Baird DT. Male contraception. *Endocr Rev* 2002; 23: 735–762.
2. Best K. Experimental male methods inhibit sperm. *Network* 1998; 18: 16–19, 31.
3. Christensen D. Male choice. The search for new contraceptives for men. *Science News* 2000; 158: 222.
4. Anderson RA, Zhu H, Cheng L., et al. Investigation of a novel preparation of testosterone decanoate in men: Pharmacokinetics and spermatogenic suppression with etonogestrel implants. *Contraception* 2002; 66: 357–364.
5. Gonzalo IT, Swerdloff RS, Nelson AL, et al. Levonorgestrel implants (Norplant II) for male contraception clinical trials: Combination with transdermal and injectable testosterone. *Clin Endocrinol Metab* 2002; 87: 3,562–3,572.

From *Contraceptive Technology Update*, February 2003, pp. 18-20. © 2003 by American Health Consultants.

It's just mechanics

Viagra is just the start: we'll soon have pills that make you feel deep love and video games that give vibrations. Ziauddin Sardar on the masturbatory society

ZIAUDDIN SARDAR

Is your sex life normal? The question was raised recently on the *Oprah Winfrey Show*. Tell us, the show asked its 20 million viewers, what turns you on, what turns you off, and what makes good sex.

The problem with such questions is that there are no "normal" answers. The normal is problematic because our ideas about sex have changed fundamentally. What constitutes normal is constantly refurbished. Its boundaries shift rapidly, and continue to shift. So what was abnormal yesterday—say, pornography—becomes normal today. And what is shunned today (say paedophilia) may just as easily become normal tomorrow.

One huge jump was provided by Viagra. In less than six years since the impotence pill came on the market, Viagra and its competitors, Levitra and Cialis, have transformed sexual norms and practices. As Meika Loe argues in *The Rise of Viagra* (New York University Press), it has redefined the concept of normal and changed the language of sex.

From the beginning, this was a treatment branded and marketed as normal. Impotence was called "erectile dysfunction", or simply ED—a common condition, as the football legend Pele assured us in TV ads, but not normal. Moreover, it did not arise from psychological causes or physical damage; rather, it was a simple medical condition rectified by a pill. Suddenly, drug company surveys discovered that more than half the US adult male population suffered from ED; figures for Europe were not far behind.

So if you can't get it up because you're pissed, stressed out, simply not in the mood or no longer find your partner attractive, you are actually suffering from a disease. And like all diseases, it must be cured. The cure is to swallow a pill and have sex no matter what, any where, any time, whenever. This has now become the norm.

Viagra is another step in stripping sex of all its complexity. Sex has been reduced to a simple question: for men, "how big?"; for women, "how long?". Combine these conundrums with other features of a market economy, such as availability on demand, choice, flexibility to mix'n'match, and we have new definitions not just of sex and love but of what it means to be human.

Today, to be normal, humans have sex right up to their last breath. It's the way to go. Sex is no longer the indulgence of the young. Nowadays, it is people over 50 who are having the most sex. With demographic shifts, high divorce rates and early retirement, the erstwhile golden generation of Sixties swingers who let it all hang out are now the "silver singles" (as they are called in America). The preoccupations of their youth have been sustained through their later years by medical enhancements. The wet dreams of 60-year-olds, who turned on to chemical enhancement in the Sixties, are a manifest example of future normality for us all.

What Viagra actually treats is loss of male power. In a confusing, depersonalising world busy reassigning status, regendering the social order, manipulating the ever-increasing demands of a commodified existence, sexual potency is the last bastion. Men, who have lost status and power almost everywhere, from workplace to home, must repair to the bedroom. Only there can they find the redemption of their true nature.

However, in an age of sexual equality, men cannot be left alone with their predicament. The other half of humanity, too, finds it is not exempt from malfunction. Just a few months ago, the disease "female sexual dysfunction" hit the headlines. But female sexuality being what it is, women probably need something more than a pill. Simple enhanced blood flow, as laboratory tests have shown, is not good enough. So a female Viagra won't do the job as well as a vibrator or a dildo—soon to be widely and cheaply available from a Boots near you. A vibrator outperforms even a man on Viagra.

More serious aids to female performance are in the pipeline. In the next few years, patches and drugs to enhance vaginal lubrication and sensitivity will become available. A US surgeon has already patented a pacemaker-sized device which, implanted under the skin, triggers an orgasm. Last month, clinical trials for the device were approved by the US Food and Drug Administration. Within a decade, it will be normal for every woman to have a perpetual orgasm whenever she wants it, wherever she needs it.

Love, too, will be available on demand. Recent research on love suggests that it consists of three basic biochemical elements. First, testosterone—which produces lust. Second, a group of amphetamine-like chemicals (dopamine, noradrenaline and phenylethylamine) produces feelings of euphoria that lead to infatuation. Third, if a relationship survives the first two rushes, a new biochemical response emerges, based on oxytocin, vasopressin and endorphins. This produces feelings of intimacy, trust and affection. Pharmaceutical companies are currently working on this third phase. So a "love pill" that modulates your subtler emotions and takes you straight to deep feelings of intimacy, trust and affection is just over the horizon. Science will fulfil the fairy tale. It will come up with a genuine love potion.

> **Science will fulfil the fairy tale. It will come up with a genuine love potion, modulating your subtler emotions**

The sexual liberation of every woman and man approaches its apotheosis: availability on demand with peak performance, assured gratification and enduring emotion. But much more has been let out of the bottle. The physical and psychological barriers to sex, identified as the ultimate metaphor for all the ills of humanity, had to be overcome. The consequence is that most sexual taboos have evaporated. No matter how dark your thoughts, how unethical your desires, how absurd your fetish, everything is normal. Your desire to dress up as a stuffed toy, your dreams of having sex with obese or dead people, your obsession with plastic or rubber, your fixation with asphyxiation—all that is sexually driven is OK.

Pornography's status as a taboo is rapidly disappearing. It has become part of the mainstream of western culture. Ancient Egyptians, Greeks and Romans had their erotica as esoterica on scrolls, pottery and frescos. Hindus have their erotic sculptures on temples. But in western culture pornography in unparalleled quantities and forms is communicated in every mass medium. Never before in history has there been so much pornography to be had by so many in such numerous ways.

Everyone is now just a click away from explicit, hardcore material. It is impossible to miss pornography on the internet because it seeks you out persistently, unannounced, at every opportunity. It is there on Channels 4 and 5, Sky and innumerable digital channels every night.

On MTV's reality show *The Real World*, you can witness bisexual group sex. Explicit sex, including shots of erect penises, can be viewed on Sky's revisionist western drama *Deadwood*. Michael Winterbottom's *9 Songs*, which will go on general release shortly, offers a stream of close-ups of intercourse, fellatio, ejaculation and cunnilingus. The French art-house director Catherine Breillat has pioneered the transfer of porn stars into mainstream cinema. Her new film, *Anatomy of Hell*, is as graphic as it is bizarre. And if that doesn't satisfy you, you can go to a new breed of "pornaoke bars", just opened in Edinburgh, where you can groan and grind karaoke-style to porno tapes.

When pornography becomes normal, where will we go next?

There are only two taboos left: sex with children, and incest. Attempts to "normalise" paedophilia have begun. A thesis by Richard Yuill, awarded a PhD by Glasgow University in December 2004, suggests that sex between adults and minors is a good and positive thing. Yuill's research, based on interviews with paedophiles and their victims, "challenges the assumption" that paedophiles are inherently abusive. It is only a matter of time before other academics start arguing that incest, too, is decent and wholesome. Graphic art films and television documentaries will follow. The organisations campaigning for the rights of paedophiles will have their case for "normality" made for them.

They may then be able to take their place among the bewildering array of sexual orientations already being normalised. Once upon a time, there were heterosexuals and the love that dared not speak its name. Gay men and lesbians have long since lost their reticence. Then bisexuals, transsexuals and the "kinky" found their identity. Now we have intersexuals and the polyamorous. A few months ago, *New Scientist* announced the discovery, in breathless prose, of asexuals. These folk don't like to have sex—horror of horrors—with *anybody*. There are even orientations within orientations. So we have such self-definition as non-op transsexual, TG butch, femme queen, gender-queer, cross-dresser, third gender, drag king or queen and transboy. In one recent episode of Channel 5's *CSI: crime scene investigation*, a murder victim was said to be part of a community of "plushies", people who enjoy sex while dressed up as stuffed animals.

It is now normal to have your breasts removed or added to, have new genitals constructed, or sprinkle a dash of hormones for the appropriate, desired effect. Things are about to become even more complex. Within a decade or so, you will be able to modify your body almost totally, as you wish. You will be able to turn off all physical signs of gender, switch off the hormones and get rid of all secondary sexual characteristics. Then you can add on the bits you wish and "sculpt" your body in any shape you like. When gene therapy becomes common, things will be even easier. Already, there are people who are experimenting with this; and a "body-mod" subculture is thriving on the internet.

The shifting of the boundaries of what is normal and our obsession with sex have not improved our sex lives

What you can't do in reality will soon be available in simulation. The emerging technology of haptics, or the telecommunication of sensation using a computer interface, will enable you to live your most horrific dreams in virtual reality. Haptic technologies simulate physical sensation of real objects and feed them to the user. The first generation of haptic technology can be experienced in certain video games for the Sony PlayStation where the joystick is used to simulate vibrations. The next generation, on its way from Rutgers University, will simulate pressure, texture and heat. Combine this with state-of-the-art graphics and some innovative software and you have a complete pornographic universe. As Eric Garland points out in the December 2004 issue of the American magazine *The Futurist*, among its first uses could be "pornography involving children and featuring violence". But what's the harm, as it is only a digitised child?

Am I the only person to wonder if the constant shifting of the boundaries of the normal, while increasing our obsession with sex, has really improved our sex lives? On the contrary, I would argue, it has led to a decline in real sex. Genuine intimacy cannot be generated through a pill. Neither can sincere, unconditional love be simulated. When sex is reduced to mechanics and endurance, there is little to differentiate it from plumbing and maintenance. When gender becomes meaningless, sex becomes empty. When sexual choice becomes an end in itself, then the end is destined to be tragic.

Sex used to be intercourse because it was part of a context, a loving relationship. When sex is just sex, without any context, what good does it do you? That is the crux of the problem. It becomes the ultimate narcissism, the sole gratification of self-love.

Welcome to the masturbatory society.

Ziauddin Sardar is editor of Futures, *the monthly journal of policy, planning and futures studies*

Promiscuous Plague

Sexually transmitted diseases (STDs) are the single greatest health threat affecting our youth. A girl is four times more likely to contract an STD than she is to become pregnant, and a young mother has had an average of 2.3 STDs.

KAREN TESTERMAN

We are facing a plague of massive proportions, a plague made more sinister because it attacks not only adults but our youth. What is this crisis? It is a pandemic of sexually transmitted diseases (STDs) that is encouraged by a message of "safe sex" and an adult population that acts as if self-control and traditional morality are outdated and without value.

Society focuses on out-of-wedlock and teen births. Meanwhile STDs tear through our youth and adult population at alarming and deadly rates. They are "not your father's" STDs, which were few and easily cured with penicillin (see sidebar).

In the 1960s, syphilis and gonorrhea were the two most prevalent STDs; today, there are more than 20 and some have as many as 80-100 strains. Despite the fitting publicity that the deadly epidemic of human immunodeficiency virus/acquired immune disorder syndrome (HIV/AIDS) commands, according to research at the University of New Mexico, human papilloma virus (HPV), not HIV, is the most common STD transmitted today.

What is the magnitude of the problem? According to recent testimony before the House Committee on Energy and Commerce, "Three to four million STDs are contracted yearly by 15- to 19-year-olds, and another five to six million STDs are contracted annually by 20- to 24-year-olds."

Perhaps the most tragic aspect of this plague is the role adults play in it. Failures by grown-ups are the primary cause of the pandemic among our youth. Adults are failing our children by promoting a fatal message about sex: both in education and in actions. Youth are allowed to believe that there is such a thing as safe sex outside of marriage and that any sexual practice is acceptable as long as the participants are smiling.

Marketing sex

Billboards, TV, magazines, movies, and catalogs promote the message that sex is the way to be cool, to fit in, to solve life's challenges. Today, the initial onset of sexual activity is occurring at younger ages, while couples delay the decision to marry or prefer cohabitation. Dr. Meg Meeker, a pediatrician and author of *Epidemic: How Teen Sex Is Killing Our Kids*, reports that half of all students in the ninth through twelfth grades have had sexual intercourse. Additionally, the average age for the onset of puberty in girls has dropped from 12 to 10.

There are physical and emotional consequences of engaging in sexual activity outside of marriage. Unwed childbearing costs American taxpayers $29 billion a year in social services and lost tax revenue, and results in delinquency and poverty among teenage parents. These teens will enter adulthood disadvantaged and will convey this disadvantage to their children.

In 1960, 15 percent of teen births in the United States were out-of-wedlock. More recently, despite the reduction in teen pregnancy, the out-of-wedlock birthrate was 78 percent among teens, according to the National Center for Health Statistics (2000).

Meanwhile, a primary indicator of poverty in our nation is single-parent households among 15- to 19-year-olds. Ninety percent of these young people will never attend college. Eighty percent of women who choose to parent while they are teens will live at the poverty level for 10 years or more.

Linda Waite, professor of urban sociology at the University of Chi-

Not So Free Sex

(!) There are physical and emotional consequences of engaging in sexual activity outside of marriage.

(!) Unwed childbearing costs American taxpayers $29 billion a year in social services, lost tax revenue, and the consequences of delinquency and poverty among the teenage parents.

(!) In 1960, 15 percent of teen births in the United States were out-of-wedlock.

(!) More recently, despite the reduction in teen pregnancy, the out-of-wedlock birthrate was 78 percent.

(!) Adolescents raised by single parents or stepfamilies are more likely to engage in sexual intercourse and to be sexually active at an earlier age.

(!) Most sexually active, infected youth do not know they have a disease.

cago, and Maggie Gallagher, affiliate scholar at the Institute for American Values, have found that children born to unmarried mothers are more likely to die in infancy. Boys raised in single-parent homes are twice as likely to commit a crime that leads to incarceration by their early thirties.

Adolescents raised by single parents or stepfamilies are more likely to engage in sexual intercourse and to be sexually active at an earlier age, according to Dawn M. Upchurch, professor at the UCLA School of Public Health. None of this takes into account the impact of post-abortive trauma or the emotional trauma of making tough decisions to allow adoption so that the child will have better opportunities.

A girl is four times more likely to contract an STD than she is to become pregnant. Today, a young mother has had on average 2.3 STDs. Syphilis, gonorrhea, herpes, chlamydia, hepatitis A and B, HIV, and HPV are the most common. Many of the viral STDs have multiple strains.

Sexual Russian roulette

A leading risk factor is the number of sexual partners. Vital health statistics directly link this factor to the early onset of sexual activity. Consider the infected teen who has sex with 6 people, each of whom has 6 partners. According to Dr. Meeker, this means that 36 people have been exposed to disease.

Marcel T. Saghir, coauthor of *Male and Female Homosexuality: A Comprehensive Investigation*, cites the magnification of this problem in the homosexual community, even among those who define themselves as monogamous. The average such relationship among homosexual males lasts less than three years. Despite attempts to portray their choice for living as normal and healthy, homosexuals are in the highest risk group for several of the most serious STDs.

Evidence from the National Cancer Institute that smoking shortens a person's life by 7-10 years led to a multibillion-dollar lawsuit by state governments. However, despite numerous studies that reveal homosexual relationships can reduce male or female lives by 10-30 years, tolerance and political correctness reign.

As even homosexual supporters and the media admit, the increasing pressure to accept homosexual practices as mainstream is dramatically affecting our society. According to the *New York Blade News Reports*, gay men are in the highest-risk group for several of the most serious diseases, including STDs.

Instability and promiscuity are characteristic of homosexual relationships. Even the Gay Lesbian Medical Association agrees with mainstream reports that, despite decades of intensive efforts to educate, HIV/AIDS continues to increase among the homosexual community.

According to another homosexual newspaper, the *Washington Blade*, HPV is "almost universal" among homosexuals. HPV, often asymptomatic, is believed to be the caus-

ative vector of cervical cancer in women. It can also lead to anal cancer in men.

Add to this the confusion about what constitutes sexual activity. Is it just penile penetration of the vagina? Does oral sex count? Is heavy petting to be included? What about practices of homosexuals? Conventional wisdom seems to promote the idea that these questions are irrelevant, as a condom can prevent the passing of bodily fluids, and thus STDs.

Beyond bodily fluids

Sadly, this misconception leads to even more danger, as the passing of body fluids is not the only way to contract these diseases. Even a properly used and defect-free latex condom will not completely protect against all STDs. Any genital contact can cause an infection. Genital warts are the common name for HPV. The most common and contagious of STDs, HPV is passed by skin-to-skin contact. It is the leading cause of cervical cancer and in its cancerous form does not exhibit any symptoms.

Alas, most of our sexually active, infected youth do not know they have a disease. Some viruses can lie dormant in the body for up to 30 years before symptoms develop. Ninety percent of those infected with chlamydia exhibit no symptoms and receive no treatment.

According to abstinence speaker Pam Stenzel, the statistics of this disaster are staggering, especially among our youth. Every day in America, 12,000 teenagers contract a sexually transmitted disease.

The American Medical Association recommends that sexually active girls be tested for chlamydia every six months. Why just girls? Aren't boys infected as well? Yes, men carry the infection, but as is often the case, girls endure most of the consequences. Stenzel points out that the female reproductive system is open; scar tissue builds up on the cervix, fallopian tubes, and ovaries as a result of pelvic inflammatory disease (PID) from the chlamydia infection.

STDs: Yesterday and Today

The basic types of organisms responsible for STDs are bacteria, parasites, and viruses. Bacterial diseases are treatable with antibiotics such as penicillin, but the organism often develops a resistance to the antibiotic, complicating treatment. Most parasitic diseases are treatable, but viruses often remain in the host for life. Many produce symptoms with a secondary impact to the host—a reduced immune system, stress, or another infection. There are no known cures for viruses, and many hosts infected with them exhibit no symptoms.

In 1960 there were 5 primary STDs: gonorrhea, syphilis, granuloma inguinale, chancroid, and lymphogranuloma venereum. Today there are over 20. Unless otherwise noted, the following figures refer to the United States.

Herpes simplex virus (HSV) Types I and II—Genital herpes results from viral infection transmitted through intimate contact with the moist mucous lining of the genitals. Once in the body it remains, and there is no cure. A rash or ulcerations may be exhibited. Genital herpes can be transmitted without the host experiencing symptoms. Only 80 percent of those infected will test positive for the virus.

Human papilloma virus (HPV)—HPV is the most commonly transmitted STD. There are between 80 and 100 strains of the virus. Some cause genital warts, but the strains that cause cervical cancer and were recently linked to anal cancer do not produce symptoms in the host. HPV is spread through skin-to-skin contact.

Gonorrhea—A bacterial infection, gonorrhea is one of the oldest STDs. Estimates are that over 1 million women are infected with gonorrhea-causing bacteria, which infect the vagina, cervix, urethra, throat, and rectum. The disease is treatable.

Syphilis—A chronic disease, syphilis is caused by a bacterial spirochete that bores into the mucous membranes of the mouth or genitals. It is treatable but in the secondary stage is highly contagious, with a rash on the hands that can be transmitted through casual contact.

Chlamydia—A bacterial infection, first reported in 1984, chlamydia affects an estimated 3-5 million women annually. It infects the cervix, urethra, throat, and rectum. While treatable, it is highly destructive to the fallopian tubes and can cause infertility or ectopic pregnancies.

Human herpes virus 8 (HHV8)—HHV8 is a virus associated with Kaposi's sarcoma, an unusual skin tumor usually found in HIV-infected men. While the virus has been found in the semen of HIV-infected men, its impact is yet to be determined.

Trichomoniasis—Caused by *Trichomonas vaginalis*, a sexually transmitted parasite, trichomoniasis affects approximately 5 million people annually.

HIV/AIDS—Acquired immune deficiency syndrome is caused by the human immunodeficiency virus. An HIV infection weakens the body's immune system and increases the body's vulnerability to many infections as well as the development of certain cancers. AIDS is one of the most frightening of the STDs because it is the most uniformly fatal of the group.

Hepatitis A, B, C*, D*—These viruses cause inflammation of the liver and can lead to cirrhosis, liver failure, and liver cancer. The B virus form is transmitted through sexual intimacy in about 30 percent of the cases. The C form is spread mainly through blood contact, although it has been spread through semen.

Chancroid—One of the older bacterial STDs, chancroid is usually diagnosed through a culture of the ulcer. It must be distinguished from syphilis or herpes. All partners should be treated whether or not the ulcer was present at the time of exposure.

Lymphogranuloma venereum— Caused by a type of chlamydia, this disease affects the genitals, anus, or rectum. Another strain of the bacteria affects the urethra and can coexist with the former. Both are treatable with an oral antibiotic.

Donovanosis (granuloma inguinale)—A chronic bacterial infection of the genitals that is found in tropical areas, donovanosis can cause severe complications if left untreated.

Molluscum contagiosum—A common noncancerous skin growth, molluscum is caused by a viral infection in the top layers of the skin. The growths are similar to warts but are caused by a different virus. The virus and growths are easily spread by skin contact.

Ureaplasma urealyticum—A bacterial infection, generally asymptomatic in nature, ureaplasma is sexually transmitted between partners. The bacteria can survive undetected in the reproductive tract for many years, until a patient is specifically tested for the infection. Although generally asymptomatic, ureaplasma can lead to fertility problems including tubal disease, recurrent miscarriages, decreased sperm motility and count.

Shigellosis* and salmonellosis*—These bacterial infections cause diarrhea and are spread through contamination from the stool or soiled fingers of one person to the mouth of another. These are STDs common among men having sex with men.

Cytomegalovirus*—An asymptomatic disease, cytomegalovirus is caused by a virus that usually remains dormant in the body for life. Severe impairment of the immune system by medication or disease reactivates it. Infectious CMV may be shed in the bodily fluids of any infected person and thus may be found in urine, saliva, blood, tears, semen, and breast milk.

Giardiasis*—A diarrheal illness, giardiasis is caused by a one-celled, microscopic parasite that lives in the intestines of people and animals and is passed in the stool. The parasite is protected by an outer shell that allows it to survive outside the body for long periods. Giardiasis is more common at present among homosexuals, as it may be spread through oral-anal sexual contact.

Amoebiasis*—Caused by a one-celled parasite, amoebiasis is most commonly found in Mexico, South America, India, and South and West Africa. The parasite is harbored in the human intestinal tract and is passed along by contamination of food and water or by anal or anal/oral sex.

Bacterial vaginosis*—The condition is caused by excessive bacteria that may normally be present in the vagina. It is not clear whether it is sexually transmitted, but it is associated with other sexually transmitted diseases. Bacterial vaginosis is more common in women with multiple sexual partners, and it often develops soon after intercourse with a new partner. The disorder is relatively common among women with female partners, where the condition may be triggered by shared objects used in sexual acts.

*Sexual transmission occurs but is not the primary mode of transmission.

With a single chlamydia infection, there is a 25 percent chance of sterility. With a second infection there is a 50 percent chance of sterility. If there is a third infection, it is almost certain that the girl will be sterile—all due to PID.

This is why, some people reason, we should promote a dual message and sell teens on abstinence with "safe sex" as a backup. The dual message approach says that abstinence is best, but if you choose to engage in genital contact, use some

form of contraception, usually condoms. This comprehensive message indicates that our youth are no more than bundles of uncontrollable hormones—that they are no more than mere animals. Many public school sexuality education programs in-

Homosexuality and Health

Little is heard today about the devastating health effects of homosexual promiscuity. A panoply of diseases—not only the well-publicized AIDS but lesser-known scourges such as hepatitis A, B, and C; herpes; cytomegalovirus; gay bowel syndrome; amoebiasis; anal warts and anal cancer; shigellosis; chlamydia; gonorrhea; and syphilis-serve to truncate the average gays life expectancy to roughly 50 years. And these pestilences not only shorten lives but sharply erode quality of life.

Behavioral disorders and mental illnesses also are far more prevalent among homosexuals than their heterosexual counterparts. High rates of alcoholism, drug addiction, "spousal" abuse, depression, and suicide all militate against living to old age.

Gay sex is of particular concern because among homosexuals, promiscuity is more the rule than the exception. For example, the December 1989 *Archives of Internal Medicine* refers to a Los Angeles report's finding that gay males averaged over 20 sex partners annually Some studies show that those in supposedly "steady" relationships are even more promiscuous, engaging in dozens of trysts a year outside the relationship.

A 1998 study that appeared in *Psychological Reports* used four databases to investigate the life spans of gays versus heterosexuals. It concluded that the homosexual lifestyle sliced 20 to 30 years from practitioners' life expectancy. Supporting this was a 1994 obituary investigation, which determined that the median age of death for gay males was 42 and for lesbians 49. It ran in the *Omega Journal of Death and Dying*.

Medical statistics show the gay community to be virtually awash in pathogens:

- Over 50 percent of all homosexual men are carriers of the human papilloma virus, which produces anal warts and can often lead to anal cancer, according to Stephen Goldstone, assistant clinical professor of surgery at Mount Sinai Medical Center, speaking at a 1999 Gay Men's Health Summit in Boulder, Colorado.
- Male homosexuals are about 1,000 times more likely to acquire AIDS than the general population (National Center for Infectious Diseases, 1992).
- A survey of more than 2,300 gays in New York and three other cities found that 37 percent of the men and 14 percent of the women reported having a non-HIV sexually transmitted infection (*Washington Blade*, October 9, 1998). Ten years earlier, male homosexuals (less than 1 percent of the population) accounted for 50 percent of U.S. syphilis cases (*Atlantic Monthly*, January 1988).
- Hepatitis B is about five times more prevalent among homosexuals than among heterosexual men, according to the National Health and Nutrition Examination Surveys, 1976-1994 (*American Journal of Public Health*).
- A young gay man has about a 50 percent chance of acquiring the AIDS virus by middle age, and the incidence of gonorrhea rose 74 percent among homosexuals from 1993-1996 (*New York Times*, November 23, 1997).
- Behavioral and mental disorders are likewise widespread in the gay community. Among the evidence is the following:
- A 1992 Boston study found that of 262 gay male subjects, 49 percent used drugs with sex, 9 percent weekly; 57 percent used alcohol with sex, 9 percent weekly (*AIDS*).
- Forty-six percent of homosexual and bisexual youths in a 1997 study of Massachusetts high-school students had attempted suicide in the preceding year (*Newsweek*).
- Forty percent of male homosexual subjects had a history of major depressive disorder (*Archives of General Psychiatry*, February 1991; *Comprehensive Psychiatry*, May/June 1993).

—*The Editor*

struct youth in the proper use of condoms and contraception. The information given is that condoms significantly reduce the chance of STD infection.

In reality, even if a condom is used 100 percent of the time, a sexually active young person is at risk to contract STDs including gonorrhea, chlamydia, and trichomoniasis. Even when used, a condom fails to prevent pregnancy 12 percent of the time, according to the Maryland Center for Mental and Child Health. Despite faithful use of the condom, the person who engages in genital contact is not immune from contract-

ing an STD that spreads through skin-to-skin contact.

It is time that adults clean up their act and encourage youth to aspire to achieve the goal of being responsible, thinking people. Young people need adults who will trust them enough to give them the information they need to make good choices.

Knowledge is power

Young people need to know that sex without boundaries is deadly. There are consequences when engaging in genital contact outside the bonds of marriage. Young people need to know that both parties

should wait until they make a lifelong commitment to one another in marriage to have sex. Within marriage, they have a better chance to be healthier, to attain a higher level of education, to be financially secure, to be happier and enjoy sex more, but only if that sex is with their marital partner.

The only way to protect against STDs that can have lifelong, physically and emotionally painful consequences is to abstain from genital contact outside of marriage. According to the University of Chicago research in *Sex in America*, researchers report that when a marriage is intact, the couple almost never have sex outside their marital relationship.

Promiscuous sexual practices, whether heterosexual or homosexual, are highly costly to Americans. The health of present and future generations is in jeopardy. Simply avoiding pregnancy or homosexual behavior is not enough. This attitude completely ignores the possibility and consequences of exposure to STDs. Add to this the disease of substance abuse and emotional trauma due to abortion, depression, anxiety, and subsequent problems, and it is clear that one should avoid promiscuity at all costs.

Despite the rhetoric, everyone is not doing it. Over 50 percent of our youth are not engaging in genital contact with one another. Given the information, our young people are capable of making informed decisions. Once we realize this, we can give them (and society) a future without this plague.

The promiscuous plague has many facets. Messages in the media, peer pressure, alcohol, and drugs all influence teen sexual behavior. The biggest influences, of course, are parents. The actions of young people reflect what adults transmit. This is done through how adults behave and what is communicated as acceptable. By allowing the media to undermine morality, the plague is fostered. By engaging in dangerous sexual practices, the plague is encouraged.

More important, by abdicating parental responsibility, the plague is promoted. A recent survey of teens conducted by L.B. Whitbeck, professor of sociology at the University of Nebraska, found that parents have the strongest effect on a teen's decision whether to have sex. Parents influence the attitude of their teens by their own marital status, their attitudes, the amount of supervision they provide, and how involved they are with their children.

Ultimately, the most effective inoculation against this plague is effective parenting. Certainly parenting would be made easier if the entertainment media reduced their hard sell of "anything goes" sex and schools truly taught nonmarital abstinence and credited our youth with the ability to use good sense. If given the opportunity, teens can and will make good choices. Our next generation needs to know it is okay to say no!

Young people need to know that sex without boundaries is deadly.

Karen Testerman is executive director of Cornerstone Policy Research, a family policy think tank located in Concord, New Hampshire. She has taught anatomy and physiology at the secondary-school level and sits on the New Hampshire Abstinence Task Force.

UNIT 7

Preventing and Fighting Disease

Unit Selections

Key Points to Consider

- What role might inflammation play in the risk of cardiovascular disease?

- What is the relationship between obesity and diabetes (Type 2)?

- What lifestyle changes could you make that would reduce your risk of developing cardiovascular disease, cancer, diabetes, and AIDS?

- Assuming that you live long enough, which chronic disease do you think you are most likely to contract, based on your family history and lifestyle?

- What are some steps individuals can take to reduce their risk of contracting cancer? What life changes could you make to reduce your risk of cancer?

- Why is discovering the origin of AIDS an important goal for researchers?

Student Website

www.mhcls.com/online

Internet References

Further information regarding these websites may be found in this book's preface or online.

American Cancer Society
http://www.cancer.org

American Heart Association
http://www.amhrt.org

National Institute of Allergy and Infectious Diseases (NIAID)
http://www.niaid.gov

Cardiovascular disease and cancer are the leading killers in this country. This is not altogether surprising given that the American population is growing increasingly older and one's risk of developing both of these diseases is directly proportional to one's age. Another major risk factor, which has received considerable attention over the past 30 years, is one's genetic predisposition or family history. Historically the significance of this risk factor has been emphasized as a basis for encouraging at-risk individuals to make prudent lifestyle choices, but this may be about to change as recent advances in genetic research, including mapping the human genome, may significantly improve the efficacy of both diagnostic and therapeutic procedures.

Just as cutting-edge genetic research is transforming the practice of medicine, startling new research findings in the health profession are transforming our views concerning adult health. This new research suggests that the primary determinants of our health as adults are the environmental conditions we experienced during life in the womb. According to Dr. Peter Nathanielsz of Cornell University, conditions during gestation, ranging from hormones that flow from the mother to how well the placenta delivers nutrients to the tiny limbs and organs, program how our liver, heart, kidneys, and especially our brains function as adults. While it is too early to draw any firm conclusions regarding the significance of the "life in the womb factor," it appears that this avenue of research may yield important clues as to how we may best prevent or forestall chronic illness.

Of all the diseases in America, coronary heart disease is this nation's number one killer. Frequently, the first and only symptom of this disease is a sudden heart attack. Epidemiological studies have revealed a number of risk factors that increase one's likelihood of developing the disease. These include hypertension, a high serum cholesterol level, diabetes, cigarette smoking, obesity, a sedentary lifestyle, a family history of heart disease, age, sex, race, and stress. In addition to these well-established risk factors, scientists think they may have discovered several additional risk factors. These include the following: low birth weight, cytomegalovirus, *Chlamydia pneumoniae*, porphyromonasgingivalis, and c-reactive protein (CRP). CRP is a measure of inflammation somewhere in the body. In theory, a high CRP reading may be a good indicator of an impending heart attack. The article, "The Battle Within" addresses research related to yet another possible link to heart disease. Is the search for stroke and cardiovascular risk factors over? Probably not, but as more risk factors are discovered our ability to accurately assess one's risk of developing cardiovascular disease improves.

One of the most startling and ominous health stories was the recent announcement by the Centers for Disease Control and Prevention (CDC) that the incidence of Type 2 adult onset diabetes increased significantly over the past 15 years. This sudden rise appears to cross all races and age groups, with the sharpest increase occurring among people aged 30 to 39 (about 70 percent). Health experts at the CDC believe that this startling rise in diabetes among 30- to 39-year-olds is linked to the rise in obesity observed among young adults (obesity rates rose from 12 to 20 percent nationally during this same time period). Experts at the CDC believe that there is a time lag of about 10-15 years between the deposition of body fat and the manifestation of Type 2 diabetes. This time lag could explain why individuals in their 30s are experiencing the greatest increase in developing Type 2 diabetes today. Current estimates suggest that 16 million Americans have diabetes; it kills approximately 180,000 Americans each year. Many experts now believe that our couch-potato culture is fueling the rising rates of both obesity and diabetes. Given what we know about the relationship between obesity and Type 2 diabetes, the only practical solution is for Americans to watch their total calories and exercise regularly. "Diabesity, a Crisis in an Expanding Country" examines the rapid rise in the incidence of Type 2 diabetes among our youth and young adults and suggests that the term "adult onset diabetes" may be a misnomer given the growing number of young adults and teens with this form of diabetes.

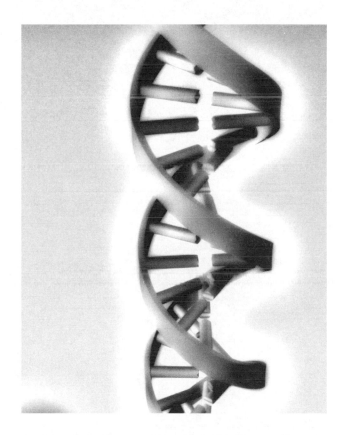

Cardiovascular disease is America's number one killer, but cancer takes top billing in terms of the "fear factor." This fear of cancer stems from an awareness of the degenerative and disfiguring nature of the disease. Today, cancer specialists are employing a variety of complex agents and technologies, such as monoclonal antibodies, interferon, and immunotherapy, in their attempt to fight the disease. Progress has been slow, however, and the results, while promising, suggest that a cure may be several years away. A very disturbing aspect of this country's battle against cancer is the fact that millions of dollars are spent each year trying to advance the treatment of cancer, while funding for the technologies used to detect cancer in its early stages is quite limited. A reallocation of funds would seem appropriate, given the medical community's position that early detection and treatment are the key elements in the successful management of cancer. Until such time that we have more effective methods for detecting cancer in the early stages, our best hope for managing cancer is to prevent it through our lifestyle choices. "Why We're Losing the War on Cancer and How to Win" takes an extensive look at the major forms of cancer in the United States and provides useful suggestions on the steps one can take to lower one's risk. While many questions remain unanswered regarding both cardiovascular disease and cancer, scientists are closing in on important clues.

It has now been over 20 years since the CDC first became aware of HIV/AIDS, and over that period of time more than 58 million people worldwide have been infected with the HIV virus and 22 million have died of AIDS. Despite medical advances in the war against AIDS, there is no cure in sight and a vaccination may be several years away. The complications associated with AIDS are not only medical, but include complex financial, political, and social issues. With medical advances in the treatment of AIDS, complacency grew, and many people abandoned the philosophy of safe sex. Today many medical experts are worried that unless we remain vigilant in our fight against this disease we will find ourselves back where we were in the early days in terms of infection rates. "The Puzzling Origins of AIDS" examines the disease, its origins, and the importance of finding the source of the disease and its transmission to help prevent future viral pandemics.

'Diabesity,' a Crisis in an Expanding Country

By JANE E. BRODY

I can't understand why we still don't have a national initiative to control what is fast emerging as the most serious and costly health problem in America: excess weight. Are our schools, our parents, our national leaders blind to what is happening—a health crisis that looms even larger than our former and current smoking habits?

Just look at the numbers, so graphically described in an eye-opening new book, "Diabesity: The Obesity-Diabetes Epidemic That Threatens America—and What We Must Do to Stop It" (Bantam), by Dr. Francine R. Kaufman, a pediatric endocrinologist, the director of the diabetes clinic at Children's Hospital Los Angeles and a past president of the American Diabetes Association.

In just over a decade, she noted, the prevalence of diabetes nearly doubled in the American adult population: to 8.7 percent in 2002, from 4.9 percent in 1990. Furthermore, an estimated one-third of Americans with Type 2 diabetes don't even know they have it because the disease is hard to spot until it causes a medical crisis.

An estimated 18.2 million Americans now have diabetes, 90 percent of them the environmentally influenced type that used to be called adult-onset diabetes. But adults are no longer the only victims—a trend that prompted an official change in name in 1997 to Type 2 diabetes.

More and more children are developing this health-robbing disease or its precursor, prediabetes. Counting children and adults together, some 41 million Americans have a higher-than-normal blood sugar level that typically precedes the development of full-blown diabetes.

'Then Everything Changed'

And what is the reason for this runaway epidemic? Being overweight or obese, especially with the accumulation of large amounts of body fat around the abdomen. In Dr. Kaufman's first 15 years as a pediatric endocrinologist, 1978 to 1993, she wrote, "I never saw a young patient with Type 2 diabetes. But then everything changed."

Teenagers now come into her clinic weighing 200, 300, even nearly 400 pounds with blood sugar levels that are off the charts. But, she adds, we cannot simply blame this problem on gluttony and laziness and "assume that the sole solution is individual change."

The major causes, Dr. Kaufman says, are "an economic structure that makes it cheaper to eat fries than fruit" and a food industry and mass media that lure children to eat the wrong foods and too much of them. "We have defined progress in terms of the quantity rather than the quality of our food," she wrote.

Her views are supported by a 15-year study published in January in The Lancet. A team headed by Dr. Mark A. Pereira of the University of Minnesota analyzed the eating habits of 3,031 young adults and found that weight gain and the development of prediabetes were directly related to unhealthful fast food.

Taking other factors into consideration, consuming fast food two or more times a week resulted, on average, in an extra weight gain of 10 pounds and doubled the risk of prediabetes over the 15-year period.

Other important factors in the diabesity epidemic, Dr. Kaufman explained, are the failure of schools to set good examples by providing only healthful fare, a loss of required physical activity in schools and the inability of many children these days to walk or bike safely to school or to play outside later.

Genes play a role as well. Some people are more prone to developing Type 2 diabetes than others. The risk is 1.6 times as great for blacks as for whites of similar age. It is 1.5 times as great for Hispanic-Americans, and 2 times as great for Mexican-Americans and Native Americans.

Unless we change our eating and exercise habits and pay greater attention to this disease, more than one-third of whites, two-fifths of blacks and half of Hispanic people in this country will develop diabetes.

It is also obvious from the disastrous patient histories recounted in Dr. Kaufman's book that the nation's medical structure is a factor as well. Many people do not have readily accessible medical care, and still many others have no coverage for preventive medicine. As a result, millions fall between the cracks until they are felled by heart attacks or strokes.

A Devastating Disease

There is a tendency in some older people to think of diabetes as "just a little sugar," a common family problem. They fail to take it seriously and make the connection between it and the costly, crippling and often fatal diseases that can ensue.

Diabetes, with its consequences of heart attack, stroke, kidney failure, amputations and blindness, among others, already ranks No. 1 in direct health care costs, consuming $1 of every $7 spent on health care.

Nor is this epidemic confined to American borders. Internationally, "we are witnessing an epidemic that is the scourge of the 21st century," Dr. Kaufman wrote.

Unlike some other killer diseases, Type 2 diabetes issues an easily detected wake-up call: the accumulation of excess weight, especially around the abdomen. When the average fasting level of blood sugar (glucose) rises above 100 milligrams per deciliter, diabetes is looming.

Abdominal fat is highly active. The chemical output of its cells increases blood levels of hormones like estrogen, providing the link between obesity and breast cancer, and de-creases androgens, which can cause a decline in libido. As the cells in abdominal fat expand, they also release chemicals that increase fat accumulation, ensuring their own existence.

The result is an increasing cellular resistance to the effects of the hormone insulin, which enables cells to burn blood sugar for energy. As blood sugar rises with increasing insulin resistance, the pancreas puts out more and more insulin (promoting further fat storage) until this gland is exhausted. Then when your fasting blood sugar level reaches 126 milligrams, you have diabetes.

Two recent clinical trials showed that Type 2 diabetes could be prevented by changes in diet and exercise. The Diabetes Prevention Program Research Group involving 3,234 overweight adults showed that "intensive lifestyle intervention" was more effective than a drug that increases insulin sensitivity in preventing diabetes over three years.

The intervention, lasting 24 weeks, trains people to choose low-calorie, low-fat diets; increase activity; and change their habits. Likewise, the randomized, controlled Finnish Diabetes Prevention Study of 522 obese patients showed that introducing a moderate exercise program of at least 150 minutes a week and weight loss of at least 5 percent reduced the incidence of diabetes by 58 percent.

Many changes are needed to combat this epidemic, starting with schools and parents. Perhaps the quickest changes can be made in the workplace, where people can be encouraged to use stairs instead of elevators; vending machines can be removed or dispense only healthful snacks; and cafeterias can offer attractive healthful fare. Lunchrooms equipped with refrigerators and microwaves will allow workers to bring healthful meals to work.

Dr. Kaufman tells of a challenge to get fit and lose weight by Caesars Entertainment in which 4,600 workers who completed the program lost a total of 45,000 pounds in 90 days. Others could follow this example.

the battle within

OUR ANTI-INFLAMMATION DIET

Michael Downey

What do paper cuts, spicy foods, stubbed toes and intense workouts at the gym have to do with your odds of getting colon cancer, drifting into Alzheimer's or succumbing to a heart attack? A lot more than you might think.

The more scientists learn about these and other serious diseases, the more they are being linked with the long-term effects of inflammation on the body.

The inflammation-disease connection has become a hot research topic. And it's about to explode.

Vital Nuisance

Inflammation is a vital immune response to infection, injury or irritation. It is the basis of humanity's earliest survival.

It's what causes the redness in that paper cut—the result of extra blood walling off the area and rushing macrophages, histamine and other bacteria-fighting immune factors to the wound.

The same inflammatory process is what makes your throat burn when you decide to impress your friends by chugging the extra-spicy suicide sauce—blood vessels leak fluid, proteins and cells to repair or remove damaged tissues. And fever is yet another form of that inflammatory burning.

Inflammation sparks the swelling in that stubbed toe—caused by fluid released into the banged-up cells to speed healing and cushion that toe against further injury.

It also causes that tenderness you feel after hours at the gym—because your immune system rushes fluids to the torn muscles to protect and re-

pair them, compressing sensitive nerve endings in the process.

Inflammation isolates foreign invaders and rushes our strongest natural infection-fighters to the site deemed under attack. It cleans away debris from destroyed tissue; slows bleeding; starts clotting; and—if tissues cannot be restored—produces scar tissue. Without this sophisticated immune response, our species would have died out long ago.

But it's a double-edged sword. In addition to its telltale redness, heat, swelling or pain, inflammation can cause serious dysfunction.

Problems begin when—for one reason or another—the inflammatory process becomes chronic, persisting long after it's needed.

Heart disease researchers were the first to notice that inflammation can play a role in cardiovascular disease.

Heart Mystery

Not long ago, doctors viewed heart disease as a plumbing problem. Cholesterol levels in the blood get too high, and, over the years, fatty deposits clog the pipes and cut off the blood supply.

There's just one problem with that explanation: Sometimes, it's dead wrong.

Defensive Nutrition

- oily fish and fish oil supplements
- olive, walnut or flaxseed oil
- walnuts, flaxseeds and soy foods
- fruits and vegetables
- red wine
- antioxidant supplements
- garlic, ginger and turmeric (enreumin)
- sunflower seeds, eggs, herring, nuts or zinc tablets
- pineapple or bromelain supplements
- S-adenosyl-methionine (SAMe)

Half of all heart attacks occur in people with normal cholesterol levels and normal blood pressure. Something causes relatively minor deposits to burst, triggering massive clots that block the blood supply.

That something has turned out to be inflammation.

C-reactive protein (CRP)—a blood measure of inflammation—shoots up during an acute illness or infection. But CRP is also somewhat elevated among otherwise healthy people. And studies show that those with the highest CRP levels have three times the heart attack risk as those with the lowest levels. The inflammatory response, possibly reacting to cholesterol that has seeped into the lining of the artery, makes even normal fatty deposits unstable.

There are several causes of heart disease: smoking, high blood pressure and, yes, cholesterol. But we must now add inflammation to that list.

Runaway Reaction

Heart disease is just the tip of the inflammation iceberg. Studies over the past couple of years have suggested that higher CRP levels raise the risk of diabetes. It's too early to say whether lowering inflammation will keep diabetes from developing. But before insulin was isolated at the University of Toronto in the 1920s, doctors found that blood sugar levels could be decreased by using salicylates, a group of aspirin-like compounds known to reduce inflammation.

In the 1860s, German pathologist Rudolph Virchow speculated that cancerous tumors start at the site of chronic inflammation—basically, a wound that never heals. Then, in the middle of the 20th century, we came to understand the role of genetic mutations in cancerous tissue. Today, researchers are investigating the possibility that mutations and inflammation work together to turn normal cells into deadly tumors. Reducing chronic inflammation may yet become a prescription for keeping cancer at bay.

Researchers have found that people who take anti-inflammation medications—for arthritis, for example—succumb to Alzheimer's disease later in life than those who don't. Plaque and tangles accumulate in the brains of Alzheimer's patients. Perhaps the immune system mistakenly sees these abnormalities as damaged tissue that should be eliminated. Early information suggests that low-dose aspirin and fish oil capsules—both known to reduce inflammation—lower the risk of Alzheimer's.

The cause of asthma is still unknown, but some suspect the inflammatory attack. The treatments that help relieve asthma work by reducing the inflammation involved.

Sometimes, for reasons that are not clear, perfectly healthy cells trigger the body's immune system. The inflammatory response is launched against normal cells in the joints, nerves, connective tissue or any part of the body. These autoimmune disorders include rheumatoid arthritis, multiple sclerosis, lupus, vitiligo, psoriasis and other versions of a body at war with itself. Even Crohn's disease and cystic fibrosis are associated with inflammation.

Some level of inflammatory immune reaction is usually present in our bodies, whether we're aware of it or not. And if inflammation really is the biological engine that drives many of our most feared illnesses, it suggests a new and possibly much simpler way of warding off disease. Instead of different treatments for all of these disorders, simply turning down the degree of our inflammatory attack might be a partial prevention for all of them.

Dampening the Fires

Many attributes of a Western lifestyle—such as a diet high in sugars and saturated fats, accompanied by little or no exercise—make it much easier for the body to become inflamed.

Losing weight helps because fat cells produce cytokines, which crank up inflammation. Thirty minutes a day of moderate exercise dampens the fire as well. Flossing your teeth combats gum disease, another source of chronic inflammation. And, of course, you should avoid excess alcohol intake and smoking.

Despite the injury they can do to the stomach, anti-inflammatory drugs such as aspirin and ibuprofen are often prescribed for treatment of inflammatory diseases, but they're not appropriate for prevention. Fish oil capsules have been shown to produce the same reduction in inflammatory cytokines.

Inflammation-promoting prostaglandins are made from the trans fats found in partially hydrogenated oils. So avoid margarines and vegetable shortenings that are made with them.

Getting a good supply of omega-3 fatty acids—and a minimum of omega-6 fats—is key to an immune system that's not overreactive. Opt for oily fish such as salmon, sardines, herring and mackerel; and on days that you don't have fish, take a fish oil supplement, eat walnuts, freshly ground flaxseeds or flaxseed oil and soy foods. Steer away from safflower, sunflower, corn and sesame oils, as well as polyunsaturated vegetable oils. Use walnut, flaxseed or extra virgin olive oils instead.

Fruits and vegetables are full of antioxidants that disable free radicals and minimize inflammation. All are good, but you should focus your diet on those that produce the highest antioxidant activity: blueberries and kiwi. Consider antioxidant supplements such as resveratrol, grape seed extract, quercetin, pycnogenol or citrus bioflavonoids, as well as beta-carotene and vitamins, C and E. And drink red wine in small quantities.

Garlic, ginger and turmeric are natural anti-inflammatory agents. Include them in your diet.

Zinc controls inflammation while promoting healing. It is found in sunflower seeds, eggs, nuts, wheat germ, herring and zinc supplements.

S-adenosyl-methionine (SAMe), alpha lipoic acid and coenzyme Q10 act as inflammation fighters. Also, bromelain—found in pineapple and supplements—may reduce inflammation.

So if you want to stop inflammation, get off that couch and head out to pick up oily fish, fresh produce, garlic and supplements. And try not to stub your toe on the way.

WHY WE'RE LOSING THE WAR ON CANCER

[AND HOW TO WIN IT]

Avastin, Erbitux, Gleevec … The new wonder drugs might make you think we're finally beating this dreaded scourge. We're not. Here's how to turn the fight around.

BY CLIFTON LEAF

It's strange to think that I can still remember the smell after all this time. The year was 1978, not long after my 15th birthday, and I'd sneaked into my brother's bedroom. There, on a wall of shelves that stretched to the ceiling, were the heaviest books we had in our house—24 volumes of the *Encyclopedia Britannica*. The maroon spines were coated in a film of dust, I remember. The pages smelled as if a musty old pillow had been covered in mint.

I carefully pulled out the volume marked HALICARNASSUS TO IMMINGHAM and turned to the entry for Hodgkin's disease. It took forever to read the half-dozen paragraphs, the weighty book spread open on my lap like a Bible. There was talk of a mysterious "lymphatic system," of "granulomas" and "gamma rays," as though this disease—the one the doctor had just told me I had—was something out of science fiction. But the last line I understood all too well: Seventy five percent of the people who got it would die within five years.

As it turns out, I did not die from Hodgkin's, though the cancer had already spread from my neck to my lungs and spleen. I lost my spleen to surgery and most of my hair to chemotherapy and radiation. But I was lucky enough to get into a clinical trial at the National Cancer Institute that was testing a new combination therapy— four toxic chemicals, together called MOPP, plus those invisible gamma rays, which flowed from an enormous cobalt 60 machine three stories below ground. The nurses who stuck needles in my arm were so kind I fell in love with them. The brilliant doctor who tattooed the borders of an imaginary box on my chest, then zapped me with radiation for four weeks, had warm pudgy hands and a comic look of inspiration, as though he'd thought of something funny just before entering the exam room. The American taxpayer even footed the bill.

Most of all, of course, I was lucky to survive. So it makes the question I am about to ask sound particularly ungrateful: Why have we made so little progress in the War on Cancer?

The question may come as a shock to anyone who has witnessed a loved one survive the dread disease— or marveled at Lance Armstrong powering to his fifth Tour de France victory after beating back testicular cancer, or received a fundraising letter saying that a cure is within our grasp. Most recently, with media reports celebrating such revolutionary cancer medicines as Gleevec, Herceptin, Iressa, Erbitux, and the just approved Avastin, the cure has seemed closer than ever.

PUBLIC ENEMY NO. 1

Doctors have dramatically reduced deaths from heart disease. But cancer is as lethal as ever and may soon overtake it as the biggest killer of Americans.

But it's not. Hope and optimism, so essential to this fight, have masked some very real systemic problems that have made this complex, elusive, relentless foe even harder to defeat. The result is that while there have been substantial achievements since the crusade began with the National Cancer Act in 1971, we are far from winning the war. So far away, in fact, that it looks like losing.

Just count the bodies on the battlefield. In 2004, cancer will claim some 563,700 of your family, friends, coworkers, and countrymen. More Americans will die of cancer in the next 14 months than have perished in every war the nation has ever fought … *combined.* Even as research and treatment efforts have intensified over the past three decades and funding has

125

soared dramatically, the annual death toll has risen 73%—over one and a half times as fast as the growth of the U.S. population.

> ## Optimism is essential, but the percentage of Americans dying from cancer is still what it was in 1970 ... and in 1950.

Within the next decade, cancer is likely to replace heart disease as the leading cause of U.S. deaths, according to forecasts by the NCI and the Centers for Disease Control and Prevention. It is already the biggest killer of those under 75. Among those ages 45 to 64, cancer is responsible for more deaths than the next three causes (heart disease, accidents, and stroke) put together. It is also the leading disease killer of children, thirty-somethings—and everyone in between.

Researchers point out that people live a lot longer than they used to, and since cancer becomes more prevalent with age, it's unfair to look just at the raw numbers when assessing progress. So when they calculate the mortality rate, they adjust it to compare cancer fatalities by age group over time. But even using this analysis (in which the proportion of elderly is dialed back to what it was during the Nixon administration), the percentage of Americans dying from cancer is about the same as in 1970 ... and in *1950*. The figures are all the more jarring when compared with those for heart disease and stroke—other ailments that strike mostly older Americans. Age-adjusted death rates for those diseases have been slashed by an extraordinary 59% and 69%, respectively, during the same half-century.

Researchers also say more people are surviving longer with cancer than ever. Yet here, too, the complete picture is more disappointing. Survival gains for the more common forms of cancer are measured in additional *months* of life, not years. The few dramatic increases in cure rates and patient longevity have come in a handful of less common malignancies—including Hodgkin's, some leukemias, carcinomas of the thyroid and testes, and most childhood cancers. (It's worth noting that many of these successes came in the early days of the War on Cancer.) Thirty-three years ago, fully half of cancer patients survived five years or more after diagnosis. The figure has crept up to about 63% today.

Yet very little of this modest gain is the result of exciting new compounds discovered by the NCI labs or the big cancer research centers—where nearly all the public's money goes. Instead, simple behavioral changes such as quitting smoking have helped lower the incidence of deadly lung cancer. More important, with the help of breast self-exams and mammography, PSA tests for prostate cancer, and other testing, we're catching more tumors earlier. Ruth Etzioni, a biostatistician at Seattle's Fred Hutchinson Cancer Research Center, points out that when

you break down the Big Four cancers (lung, colon and rectal, breast, and prostate) by stage—that is, how far the malignant cells have spread—long-term survival for advanced cancer has barely budged since the 1970s.

And the new cases keep coming. Even with a dip in the mid-1990s, the incidence rate has skyrocketed since the War on Cancer began. This year an additional 1.4 million Americans will have that most frightening of conversations with their doctor. One in two men and one in three women will get the disease during their lifetime. As a veteran Dana-Farber researcher sums up, "It is as if one World Trade Center tower were collapsing on our society every single day."

So why aren't we winning *this* decades-old war on terror—and what can we do now to turn it around?

That was the question I asked dozens of researchers, physicians, and epidemiologists at leading cancer hospitals around the country; pharmacologists, biologists, and geneticists at drug companies and research centers; officials at the FDA, NCI, and NIH; fundraisers, activists, and patients. During three months of interviews in Houston, Boston, New York, San Francisco, Washington, D.C., and other cancer hubs, I met many of the smartest and most deeply committed people I've ever known. The great majority, it should be said, were optimistic about the progress we're making, believing that the grim statistics belie the wealth of knowledge we've gained—knowledge, they say, that will someday lead to viable treatments for the 100-plus diseases we group as cancer. Most felt, despite their often profound misgivings about the way research is done, that we're on the right path.

Yet virtually all these experts offered testimony that, when taken together, describes a dysfunctional "cancer culture"—a groupthink that pushes tens of thousands of physicians and scientists toward the goal of finding the tiniest improvements in treatment rather than genuine breakthroughs; that fosters isolated (and redundant) problem solving instead of cooperation; and rewards academic achievement and publication over all else.

At each step along the way from basic science to patient bedside, investigators rely on models that are consistently lousy at predicting success—to the point where hundreds of cancer drugs are thrust into the pipeline, and many are approved by the FDA, even though their proven "activity" has little to do with curing cancer.

"It's like a Greek tragedy," observes Andy Grove, the chairman of Intel and a prostate-cancer survivor, who for years has tried to shake this cultural mindset as a member of several cancer advisory groups. "Everybody plays his individual part to perfection, everybody does what's right by his own life, and the total just doesn't work."

Tragedy, unfortunately, is the perfect word for it. Heroic figures battling forces greater than themselves. Needless death and destruction. But unlike Greek tragedy, where the Fates predetermine the outcome, the nation's cancer crusade didn't have to play out this way. And it doesn't have to stay this way.

"A VERY TOUGH SET OF PROBLEMS"

NUCLEAR FISSION WAS A MERE eight months old when the Panzers rolled into Poland in September 1939, beginning the Second World War. Niels Bohr had announced the discovery at a conference on theoretical physics at George Washington University. Three years later the crash program to build an atomic device from a uranium isotope began in earnest. And within three years of that— Aug. 6, 1945—a bomb named Little Boy exploded over Hiroshima.

NASA came into existence on Oct. 1, 1958. Eleven years later, two men were dancing on the moon. Sequencing the entire human genome took just 18 years from the time the idea was born at a small gathering of scientists in Santa Cruz, Calif. Go back as far as Watson and Crick, to the discovery of the structure of DNA, and the feat was still achieved in a mere half-century.

Cancer researchers hate such comparisons. Good science, say many, can't be managed. (Well, sure, maybe easy stuff like nuclear physics, rocket science, and genetics—but not cancer.)

And to be sure, cancer *is* a challenge like no other. The reason is that this killer has a truly uncanny ability to change its identity. "The hallmark of a cancer cell is its genetic instability," says Isaiah "Josh" Fidler, professor and chair of the department of cancer biology at Houston's M.D. Anderson Cancer Center. The cell's DNA is not fixed the way a normal cell's is. A normal cell passes on pristine copies of its three-billion-letter code to every next-generation cell. But when a cancer cell divides, it may pass along to its daughters an altered copy of its DNA instructions—and even the slightest change can have giant effects on cell behavior. The consequence, says Fidler, is that while cancer is thought to begin with a single cell that has mutated, the tumors eventually formed are made up of countless cellular cousins, with a variety of quirky traits, living side by side. "That heterogeneity of tumors is the major, major obstacle to easy therapy," he says.

Harold Varmus, president of Memorial Sloan-Kettering Cancer Center in New York City, agrees. "I just think this is a very tough set of problems," says Varmus, who has seen those problems from more angles than just about anybody. He shared a Nobel Prize for discovering the first oncogene (a normal gene that when mutated can cause cancer) in 1976. That crucial finding, five years into the War on Cancer, helped establish that cancers are caused by mutated genes. Later Varmus served as NIH director under Bill Clinton, presiding over a period of huge funding increases. "Time always looks shorter in retrospect," he says. "I think, hey, in 30 years mankind went from being almost completely ignorant about how cancer arises to being pretty damn knowledgeable."

Yet all that knowledge has come at a price. And there's a strong argument to be made that maybe that price has been too high.

President Nixon devoted exactly 100 words of his 1971 State of the Union speech to proposing "an intensive campaign to find a cure for cancer." The word "war" was never mentioned in the text, yet one would flare up in the months that followed—a lobbying war over how much centralized control the proposed na-

---

CANCER'S BIG FOUR KILLERS

In 1971, when the war on cancer began, 50% of people diagnosed with the disease went on to live at least five years. Today, 33 years and some $200 billion later, the five-year survival rate is 63%, a modest 13-point gain. But a look behind the numbers for the four biggest killers—lung, colon and rectal, breast, and prostate cancer—reveals that progress isn't being made where you might think it is. With the help of early detection and treatment, more patients are living longer. Once a cancer has spread, however, chances of survival are scarcely better now than they were three decades ago.

---

tional cancer authority would exert. Between the speech and the signing of the National Cancer Act that December, there was a "battle line between 'creative research' and 'structured research'" as a news report headlined it. A massive alliance of virtually all the medical societies, the medical schools, the then—Big Three cancer hospitals (Memorial Sloan-Kettering, M.D. Anderson, and Roswell Park in Buffalo) said yes to federal money but wanted very little direction and only loose coordination from Uncle Sam.

On the other side was Sidney Farber, the Boston physician known as the godfather of cancer research. He wanted public backing for a massive, coordinated assault. "We cannot wait for full understanding; the 325,000 patients with cancer who are going to die this year cannot wait; nor is it necessary, in order to make great progress in the cure of cancer, for us to have the full solution of all the problems of basic research," Farber testified in congressional hearings that fall. "The history of medicine is replete with examples of cures obtained years, decades, and even centuries before the mechanism of action was understood for these cures—from vaccination, to digitalis, to aspirin."

Farber lost.

Today the cancer effort is utterly fragmented—so much so that it's nearly impossible to track down where the money to pay for all this research is coming from. But let's try anyway.

We begin with the NCI budget. Set by Congress, this year's outlay for fighting cancer is $4.74 billion. Critics have complained that is a mere 3.3% over last year's budget, but Uncle Sam gives prodigiously in other ways too—a fact few seem to realize. The NIH, technically the NCI's parent, will provide an additional $909 million this year for cancer research through the National Institute of Environmental Health Sciences and other little-noticed grant mechanisms. The Department of Veterans Affairs will likely spend just over the $457 million it spent in 2003 for research and prevention programs. The CDC will chip in around $314 million for outreach and education. Even the Pentagon pays for cancer research—offering $249 million this year for nearly 500 peer-reviewed grants to study breast, prostate, and ovarian cancer.

Now throw state treasuries into the mix—governors signed 89 cancer-related appropriations from 1997 to 2003—plus the fundraising muscle of cancer charities, cancer centers, and research hospitals, which together will raise some $2 billion this

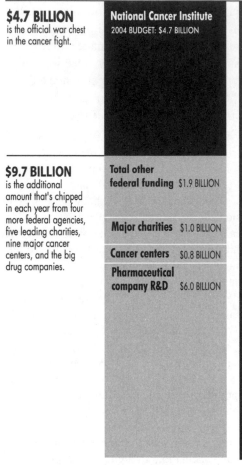

FUNDING APLENTY

The National Cancer Institute isn't the half of it. Major bucks for cancer R&D come from many sources—some you'd never expect (like the Pentagon).

$4.7 BILLION
is the official war chest in the cancer fight.

National Cancer Institute
2004 BUDGET: $4.7 BILLION

$9.7 BILLION
is the additional amount that's chipped in each year from four more federal agencies, five leading charities, nine major cancer centers, and the big drug companies.

Total other federal funding $1.9 BILLION

Major charities $1.0 BILLION

Cancer centers $0.8 BILLION

Pharmaceutical company R&D $6.0 BILLION

Annual cancer funding:
$14.4 BILLION

FORTUNE CHART/SOURCES: Totals derive from data for the most recent year available. Other federal funding includes cancer spending by NIH (except NCI) and the VA (excluding treatment), CDC, and Pentagon. Data on charities and cancer centers are from federal tax forms; state figures are not included. Pharma total is from Tufts Centers for the Study of Drug Development and *Fortune* estimates.

year from generous donors, based on recent tax forms. And finally, that huge spender Big Pharma. The Tufts Center for the Study of Drug Development estimates that drug companies will devote about $7.4 billion, or roughly a quarter of their annual R&D spending, to products for cancer and metabolic and endocrine diseases.

When you add it all up, Americans have spent, through taxes, donations, and private R&D, close to $200 billion, in inflation-adjusted dollars, since 1971. What has that national investment netted so far?

Without question, the money has bought us an enormous amount of knowledge, just as Varmus says. Researchers have mapped the human cell's intricate inner circuitry in extraordinary detail, identifying dozens of molecular chains of communication, or "signaling pathways," among various proteins, phosphates, and lipids made by the body. In short, scientists now know (or think they know) nearly all the biochemical steps that a healthy cell uses to multiply, to shut down its growth, and to sense internal damage and die at the right time—as well as many of the genes that encode for these processes. What's more, by extension, they know how these same gene-induced mechanisms go haywire in a cancer cell.

According to PubMed, the NCI's online database, the cancer research community has published 1.56 million papers—that's right: 1.56 million!—largely on this circuitry and its related genes in hundreds of journals over the years. Many of the findings are shared at the 100-plus international congresses, symposiums, and conventions held each year.

Yet somehow, along the way, something important has gotten lost. The search for knowledge has become an end unto itself rather than the means to an end. And the research has become increasingly narrow, so much so that physician-scientists who want to think systemically about cancer or the organism as a whole—or who might have completely new approaches—often can't get funding.

Take, for instance, the NCI's chief funding mechanism, something called an RO1 grant. The grants are generous, averaging $338,000 apiece in 2003. And they are one of the easiest sweepstakes to win: One in three applications is accepted. But the money goes almost entirely to researchers who focus on very specific genetic or molecular mechanisms within the cancer cell or other tissue. The narrower the research niche, it sometimes seems, the greater the rewards the researcher is likely to attain. "The incentives are not aligned with the goals," says Leonard Zwelling, vice president for research administration at M.D. Anderson, voicing the feeling of many. "If the goal is to cure cancer, you don't incentivize people to have little publications."

Jean-Pierre Issa, a colleague of Zwelling's who studies leukemias, is equally frustrated by the community's mindset. Still, he admits, the system's lure is powerful. "You get a paper where you change one gene ever so slightly and you have a drastic effect of cancer in the mouse, and that paper gets published in *Science* or *Nature*, and in your best journals. That makes your reputation. Then you start getting grants based on that," he says. "Open any major journal and 80% of it is mice or drosophila [fruit flies] or nematodes [worms]. When do you get human studies in there?"

Indeed, the cancer community has published an extraordinary 150,855 experimental studies on mice, according to a search of the PubMed database. Guess how many of them have led to treatments for cancer? Very, very few. In fact, if you want to understand where the War on Cancer has gone wrong, the mouse is a pretty good place to start.

THE MODELS OF CANCER STINK

OUTSIDE ERIC LANDER'S OFFICE is a narrow, six-foot-high poster. It is an org chart of sorts, a taxonomy, with black lines connecting animal species. The poster's lessons feel almost biblical—it shows, for example, that the zebrafish has much in common with the chicken; that hedgehog and shrew are practically kissing cousins; and that while a human might look more like a macaque than a platypus or a mouse, it ain't that big of a leap, really.

The connection, of course, is DNA. Our genomes share much of the same wondrous code of life. And therein lie both the temptation and the frustration inherent in cancer research today. Certain mutated genes cause cells to proliferate uncontrollably, to spread to new tissues where they don't belong, and to refuse to end their lives when they should. That's cancer. So research, as we've said, now revolves around finding first, the molecular mechanisms to which these mutated genes give rise, and second, drugs that can stop them.

The strategy sounds obvious—and nobody makes it sound more so than Lander, the charismatic founding director of the Whitehead Institute's Center for Genome Research in Cambridge, Mass., and a leader of the Human Genome Project. The "Prince of Nucleotides," as FORTUNE once called him, sketches the biological route to cancer cures as if he were directing you to the nearest Starbucks: "There are only, pick a number, say, 30,000 genes. They do only a finite number of things. There are only a finite number of mechanisms that cancers have. It's a large number; when I say finite, I don't mean to trivialize it. There may be 100 mechanisms that cancers are using, but 100 is only 100."

So, he continues, we need to orchestrate an attack that isolates these mechanisms by knocking out cancer-promoting genes one by one in mice, then test drugs that kill the mutant cells. "These are doable experiments," he says. "Cancers by virtue of having mutations also acquire Achilles' heels. Rational cancer therapies are about finding the Achilles' heel associated with each new mutation in a cancer."

The principle is, in all likelihood, dead on. The process itself, on the other hand, has one heck of an Achilles' heel. And that takes us back to the six-foot poster showing the taxonomy of genomes. A mouse gene may be very similar to a human gene, but the rest of the mouse is very different.

The fact that so many cancer researchers seem to forget or ignore this observation when working with "mouse models" in the lab clearly irks Robert Weinberg. A professor of biology at MIT and winner of the National Medal of Science for his discovery of both the first human oncogene and the first tumor-suppressor gene, Weinberg is as no-nonsense as Lander is avuncular. Small and mustachioed, with Hobbit-like fingers, he plops into a brown leather La-Z-Boy that is somehow wedged into the middle of his cramped office, and launches into a lecture:

"One of the most frequently used experimental models of human cancer is to take human cancer cells that are grown in a petri dish, put them in a mouse—in an immunocompromised mouse—allow them to form a tumor, and then expose the resulting xenograft to different kinds of drugs that might be useful in treating people. These are called preclinical models," Weinberg explains. "And it's been well known for more than a decade, maybe two decades, that many of these preclinical human cancer models have very little predictive power in terms of how actual human beings—actual human tumors inside patients—will respond." Despite the genetic and organ-system similarities

between a nude mouse and a man in a hospital gown, he says, the two species have key differences in physiology, tissue architecture, metabolic rate, immune system function, molecular signaling, you name it. So the tumors that arise in each, with the same flip of a genetic switch, are vastly different.

Says Weinberg: "A fundamental problem which remains to be solved in the whole cancer research effort, in terms of therapies, is that the preclinical models of human cancer, in large part, *stink*."

A few miles away, Bruce Chabner also finds the models lacking. A professor of medicine at Harvard and clinical director at the Massachusetts General Hospital Cancer Center, he explains that for a variety of biological reasons the "instant tumors" that researchers cause in mice simply can't mimic human cancer's most critical and maddening trait, its quick-changing DNA. That characteristic, as we've said, leads to staggering complexity in the most deadly tumors.

"If you find a compound that cures hypertension in a mouse, it's going to work in people. We don't know how toxic it will be, but it will probably work," says Chabner, who for many years ran the cancer-treatment division at the NCI. So researchers routinely try the same approach with cancer, "knocking out" (neutralizing) this gene or knocking in that one in a mouse and causing a tumor to appear. "Then they say, 'I've got a model for lung cancer!' Well, it ain't a model for lung cancer, because lung cancer in humans has a hundred mutations," he says. "It looks like the most complicated thing you've ever seen, genetically."

Homer Pearce, who once ran cancer research and clinical investigation at Eli Lilly and is now research fellow at the drug company, agrees that mouse models are "woefully inadequate" for determining whether a drug will work in humans. "If you look at the millions and millions and millions of mice that have been cured, and you compare that to the relative success, or lack thereof, that we've achieved in the treatment of metastatic disease clinically," he says, "you realize that there just has to be something wrong with those models."

Vishva Dixit, a vice president for research in molecular oncology at Genentech in South San Francisco, is even more horrified that "99% of investigators in industry and in academia use xenografts." Why is the mouse model so heavily used? Simple. "It is very convenient, easily manipulated," Dixit explains. "You can assess tumor size just by looking at it."

> **"People obsessed with cures, cures, cures are being— I hate to use the word—selfish by ignoring what could be done in terms of prevention.**

Although drug companies clearly recognize the problem, they haven't fixed it. And they'd better, says Weinberg, "if for no other reason than [that] hundreds of millions of dollars are being wasted every year by drug companies using these models."

Even more depressing is the very real possibility that reliance on this flawed model has caused researchers to pass over drugs that *would* work in humans. After all, if so many promising drugs that clobbered mouse cancers failed in man, the reverse is also likely: More than a few of the hundreds of thousands of compounds discarded over the past 20 years might have been truly effective agents. Roy Herbst, who divides his time between bench and bedside at M.D. Anderson and who has run big trials on Iressa and other targeted therapies for lung cancer, is sure that happens often. "It's something that bothers me a lot," he says. "We probably lose a lot of things that either don't have activity on their own, or we haven't tried in the right setting, or you don't identify the right target."

If everyone understands there's a problem, why isn't anything being done? Two reasons, says Weinberg. First, there's no other model with which to replace that poor mouse. Second, he says, "is that the FDA has created inertia because it continues to recognize these [models] as the gold standard for predicting the utility of drugs."

"WE HAVE A SHORTAGE OF GOOD IDEAS"

IT IS ONE OF THE MANY chicken-and-egg questions bedeviling the cancer culture. Which came first: the FDA's imperfect standards for judging drugs or the pharmaceutical companies' imperfect models for testing them?

The riddle is applicable not just to early drug development, in which flawed animal models fool bench scientists into thinking their new compounds will wallop tumors in humans. It comes up, with far more important ramifications, in the last stage of human testing, when the FDA is looking for signs that a new drug is actually helping the patients who are taking it. In this case, the faulty model is called tumor regression.

It is exciting to see a tumor shrink in mouse or man and know that a drug is doing that. A shrinking tumor is intuitively a good thing. So it is no surprise that it's one of the key endpoints, or goals, in most clinical trials. That's in no small part because it is a *measurable* goal: We can see it happening. (When you read the word "response" in a newspaper story about some exciting new cancer drug, tumor shrinkage is what it's talking about.)

But like the mouse, tumor regression by itself is actually a lousy predictor for the progression of disease. Oncologists can often shrink a tumor with chemo and radiotherapy. That sometimes makes the cancer easier to remove surgically. If not, it still may buy a little time. However, if the doctors don't get every rotten cell, the sad truth is that the regression is not likely to improve the person's chances of survival.

That's because when most malignant solid tumors are diagnosed, they are typically quite large already—the size of a grape, perhaps, with more than a billion cells in the tumor mass. By the time it's discovered, there is a strong chance that some of those cells have already broken off from the initial tumor and are on their way to another part of the body. This is called metastasis.

Most of those cells will not take root in another tissue or organ: A metastasizing cell has a very uphill battle to survive once it enters the violent churn of the bloodstream. But the process has begun— and with a billion cells dividing like there's no tomorrow, an ever-growing number of metastases will try to make the journey. Inevitably, some will succeed.

In the end, it is not localized tumors that kill people with cancer; it is the process of metastasis—an incredible *90% of the time*. Aggressive cells spread to the bones, liver, lungs, brain, or other vital areas, wreaking havoc.

So you'd think that cancer researchers would have been bearing down on this insidious phenomenon for years, intently studying the intricate mechanisms of invasion. Hardly. According to a FORTUNE examination of NCI grants going back to 1972, less than 0.5% of study proposals focused primarily on metastasis—trying to understand, for instance, its role in a specific cancer (e.g., breast, prostate) or just the process itself. Of nearly 8,900 NCI grant proposals awarded last year, 92% didn't even *mention* the word metastasis.

One accomplished researcher sent an elegant proposal into the NCI two years ago to study the epigenetics (changes in normal gene function) of metastases vs. primary tumors. It's now in its third resubmission, he says. "I mean, there is nothing known about that. But somehow I can't interest people in funding this!"

M.D. Anderson's Josh Fidler suggests that metastasis is getting short shrift simply because "it's tough. Okay? And individuals are not rewarded for doing tough things." Grant reviewers, he adds, "are more comfortable with the focused. Here's an antibody I will use, and here's blah-blah-blah-blah, and then I get the money."

Metastasis, on the other hand, is a big idea—an organism-wide phenomenon that may involve dozens of processes. It's hard to do replicable experiments when there are that many variables. But that's the kind of research we *need*. Instead, says Weinberg, researchers opt for more straightforward experiments that generate plenty of reproducible results. Unfortunately, he says, "the accumulation of data gives people the illusion they've done something meaningful."

That drive to accumulate data also goes to the heart of the regulatory process for drug development. The FDA's mandate is to make sure that a drug is safe and that it works before allowing its sale to the public. Thus, the regulators need to see hard data showing that a drug has had some effect in testing. However, it's hard to see "activity" in preventing something from happening in the first place. There are probably good biomarkers—proteins, perhaps, circulating in the body—that can tell us that cancer cells have begun the process of spreading to other tissues. As of yet, though, we don't know what they are.

So pharma companies, quite naturally, don't concentrate on solving the problem of metastasis (the thing that kills people); they focus on devising drugs that shrink tumors (the things that don't).

Dozens of these drugs get approved anyway. At the same time, many don't—and the FDA is invariably blamed for holding up the War on Cancer. The fault, however, is less the umpire's than the players'. That's because many tumor-shrinking drugs simply don't perform much better than the standard treatments. Or as Rick Pazdur, director of oncology drugs for the FDA, puts it, "It's efficacy, stupid! One of the major problems that we have is dealing with this meager degree of efficacy." When it's clear that something is working, the agency is generally quick to give it priority review and/or accelerated approval, two mechanisms that speed up the regulatory process for compounds aimed at life-threatening diseases. "We have a shortage of good ideas that are likely to work," agrees Bruce Johnson, a Dana-Farber oncologist who runs lung-cancer research for institutions affiliated with the Harvard Medical School, a huge partnership that includes Massachusetts General Hospital, Brigham and Women's Cancer Center, and others.

That is also the devastating conclusion of a major study published last August in the *British Medical Journal*. Two Italian pharmacologists pored over the results of trials of 12 new anti-cancer drugs that had been approved for the European market from 1995 to 2000, and compared them with standard treatments for their respective diseases. The researchers could find no substantial advantages—no improved survival, no better quality of life, no added safety—with any of the new agents. All of them, though, were several times more expensive than the old drugs. In one case, the price was 350 times higher.

WHY THE NEW DRUGS DISAPPOINT

FLAWED MODELS FOR DRUG development. Obsession with tumor shrinkage. Focus on individual cellular mechanisms to the near exclusion of what's happening in the organism as a whole. All these failures come to a head in the clinical trial—a rigidly controlled, three-phase system for testing new drugs and other medical procedures in humans. The process remains the only way to get from research to drug approval—and yet it is hard to find *anyone* in the cancer community who isn't maddeningly frustrated by it.

In February 2003 a blue-ribbon panel of cancer-center directors concluded that clinical trials are "long, arduous," and burdened with regulation; without major change and better resources, the panel concluded, the "system is likely to remain inefficient, unresponsive, and unduly expensive."

All that patients know is that the process has little to offer them. Witness the fact that a stunning 97% of adults with cancer don't bother to participate.

There are two major problems with clinical trials. The first is that their duration and cost mean that drug companies—which sponsor the vast majority of such trials—have an overwhelming incentive to test compounds that are likely to win FDA approval. After all, they are public companies by and large, with shareholders demanding a return on investment. So the companies focus not on breakthrough treatments but on incremental improvements to existing classes of drugs. The process does not encourage risk taking or entrepreneurial approaches to drug discovery. It does not encourage brave new thinking. Not when a drug typically takes 12 to 14 years to develop. And not with $802 million—that's the oft-cited cost of developing a drug—on the line.

What's more, the system essentially forces companies to test the most promising new compounds on the sickest patients—where it is easier to see some activity (like shrinking tumors) but almost impossible to cure people. At that point the disease has typically spread too far and the tumors have become too ridden with genetic mutations. Thus drugs that might have worked well in earlier-stage patients often never get the chance to prove it. (As you'll see, that may be a huge factor in the disappointing response so far of one class of promising new drugs.)

The second problem is even bigger: Clinical trials are focused on the wrong goal—on doing "proper" science rather than saving lives. It is not that they provide bad care—patients in trials are treated especially well. But the trials' very reason for being is to test a hypothesis: Is treatment X better than treatment Y? And sometimes—too often, sadly—the information generated by this tortuously long process doesn't much matter. If you've spent ten-plus years to discover that a new drug shrinks a tumor by an average of 10% more than the existing standard of care, how many people have you really helped?

Take two drugs approved in February for cancer of the colon and rectum: Erbitux and Avastin. In each case it took many months just to enroll the necessary number of patients in clinical trials. Participating doctors then had to administer the drugs according to often arduous preset protocols, collecting reams of data along the way. (ImClone's well-known troubles with the FDA occurred because it had not set up its trials properly.)

And here's what clinicians learned after years of testing. When Avastin was added to the standard chemotherapy regimen, the combination managed to extend the lives of some 400 patients with terminal colorectal cancer by a median 4.7 months. (A previous trial of the drug on breast cancer patients failed.) Oncologists consider the gain substantial, considering that those in advanced stages of the disease typically live less than 16 months.

And Erbitux? Although it did indeed shrink tumors, *it has not been shown to prolong patients' lives at all*. Some certainly have fared well on the drug, but survival on average for the groups studied didn't change. Still, Erbitux was approved for use primarily in "third line" therapy, after every other accepted treatment has failed. A weekly dose costs $2,400.

Remember, it took several years and the participation of thousands of patients in three stages of testing, tons of data, and huge expense to find out what the clinicians and researchers already knew in the earliest stage of human testing: Neither drug will save more than a handful of the 57,000 people who will die of colorectal cancer this year.

> **"If you look at the millions of mice that have been cured of cancer, and compare it to humans, you realize there just has to be something wrong with those models."**

You could say the same for AstraZeneca's Iressa, another in the new class of biological wonder drugs—compounds specifically "targeted" to disrupt the molecular signals in a cancer cell. Not a single controlled trial has shown Iressa to have a major patient benefit such as the easing of symptoms or improved survival—a fact that the company's upbeat press releases admit as if it were legal boilerplate. Even so, the FDA okayed the pill last year for last-ditch use against a type of lung cancer, citing the fact that it had shrunk tumors in 10% of patients studied.

"Very smart people, with a lot of money, have done trials of over 10,000 patients around the world—testing these new molecular targeted drugs," says Dana-Farber's Bruce Johnson. "AstraZeneca tested Iressa. Isis Pharmaceuticals and Eli Lilly tested a compound called Isis 3521. Several different companies ended up investing tens of millions of dollars, and all came up with a big goose egg."

The one targeted drug that clearly isn't a goose egg is Novartis's Gleevec, which has been shown to save lives as well as stifle tumors. The drug has a dramatic effect on an uncommon kind of leukemia called CML and an even more rare stomach cancer named GIST. Early reports say it also seems to work, in varying degrees, in up to three other cancers. Gleevec's success has been held out as the "proof of principle" that the strategy we've followed in the War on Cancer all these years has been right.

But not even Gleevec is what it seems. CML is not a complicated cancer: In it, a single gene mutation causes a critical signaling mechanism to go awry; Gleevec ingeniously interrupts that deadly signal. Most common cancers have perhaps as many as five to ten different things going wrong. Second, even "simple" cancers get smarter: The malignant cells long exposed to the drug (which must be taken forever) mutate their way around the molecular signal that Gleevec blocks, building drug resistance.

No wonder cancer is so much more vexing than heart disease. "You don't get multiple swings," says Bob Cohen, senior director for commercial diagnostics at Genentech. Use a drug that does not destroy the tumor completely and "the heterogeneity will evolve from the [surviving] cells and say, 'I don't give a rat's ass! You can't screw me up with this stuff.' Suddenly you're squaring and cubing the complexity. That's where we are." And that's why the only chance is to attack the disease earlier—and on multiple fronts.

Three drugs, four drugs, five drugs in combination. Cocktails of experimental compounds, of course, were what doctors used to control HIV, whose rapidly mutating virus was once thought to be a death sentence. Virtually every clinician and scientist interviewed for this story believes a similar approach is needed with the new generation of anticancer drugs. But once again, institutional forces within the cancer world make it nearly impossible.

Combining unapproved drugs in clinical trials brings up a slew of legal and regulatory issues that cause pharma companies to squirm. While many drug-company oncologists are as committed to the public's well-being as government or cancer-center researchers, they have less flexibility to take chances on an idea. Ultimately, they need FDA approval for their investigational compounds. If two or three unapproved drugs are tested in concert, it's even harder to figure out what's working

> **"It's like a Greek tragedy," says Intel's Andy Grove. "Everybody plays his part, everybody does what's right by his own life, and the total just doesn't work."**

MIRACLE CURES THAT WEREN'T

Decades of breakthroughs have raised hopes again and again for people with cancer—but have failed to deliver on expectations.

Radiation therapy Soon after Wilhelm Roentgen's discovery of X-rays in 1895, some doctors predicted that the high-energy waves from exotic "cyclotrons" could be used to kill most cancerous tumors. A century-plus later, targeted radiation is a critical weapon in the oncologist's arsenal but not the magic bullet many thought.

Interferon In 1980, the world was afrenzy about the big "IF"—an immune-system booster produced by the body in tiny quantities—as word spread that this natural virus fighter could also shrink tumors. Though still in use in some cancer therapies, IF has not fulfilled its early promise.

Interleukin-2 Like Interferon, this protein helps activate the body's immune system. And like IF, IL-2 was once thought to be the "cancer breakthrough" we were waiting for (see FORTUNE's 1985 cover, lower right). But after years of testing and tweaking, the therapy has led to only scattered remissions in patients.

Endostatin After a flurry of early hype, this first of many compounds designed to fight tumor angiogenesis failed dramatically in human tests. The jury is still out on its next-generation kin.

Gleevec The little yellow pill from Novartis has wondrous effect in a few rare cancers involving simple mutations, although the disease can grow resistant to this "targeted" biological drug.

and what isn't, and whether one drug is responsible for side-effects or the combination. "It becomes much more challenging in the context of managing the databases, interpreting the results, and owning the data," adds Lilly's Pearce.

Over dinner at Ouisie's Table in Houston, M.D. Anderson's Len Zwelling, who oversees regulatory compliance for the center's 800-plus clinical trials, and his wife, Genie Kleinerman, who is chief of pediatrics there, have no trouble venting about the legal barriers that seem to be growing out of control. It takes no more than ten minutes for Kleinerman to rattle off three stories about trying to bring together different drug companies in clinical trials for kids with cancer. In the first attempt, the trial took so long that the biotech startup with the promising agent went out of business. In the second the lawyers haggled over liability concerns until both companies pulled out. The third, however, was the worst. There were two drugs that together seemed to jolt the immune system into doing a better job of targeting malignant cells of osteosarcoma, a bone cancer that occurs in children. "Working with the lawyers, it was just impossible," she says, "because each side wanted to own the *rights* to the combination!"

CHANGING THE WAY WE THINK ABOUT CANCER

STRANGE AS IT MAY SEEM, much of our failure in fighting cancer—and more important, much of the potential for finally winning this fight—has to do with a definition. Some 2,400 years ago the Greek physician Hippocrates described cancer as a disease that spread out and grabbed on to another part of the body like "the arms of a crab," as he elegantly put it. Similarly, medical textbooks today say cancer begins when the cells of an expanding tumor push through the thin protein "basement" membrane that separates them from another tissue. It's a fancy way of saying that to be cancer, a malignant cell has to invade another part of the body.

Michael Sporn, a professor of pharmacology and medicine at Dartmouth Medical School, has two words for this: "Absolute nonsense!" He goes on: "We've been stuck with this definition of what cancer is from 1890. It's what I was taught in medical school: 'It's not cancer until there's invasion.' That's like saying the barn isn't on fire until there are bright red flames coming out of the roof."

In fact, cancer begins much earlier than that. And therein lies the best strategy to contain it, believes Sporn, who was recently named an Eminent Scholar by the NCI. Let's aggressively find those embers that have been smoldering in many of us for years—and douse them before they become a full-fledged blaze. Prevent cancer from ever entering that deadly stage of malignancy in the first place.

Sporn, who spent more than three decades at the NCI, has been struggling for many years to get fellow researchers to start thinking about cancer not as a state of being (that is, an invasive group of fast-growing cells) but as a *process*, called carcinogenesis. Cancer, as Sporn tells it, is a multistage disease that goes through various cell transformations and sometimes long periods of latency in its progression.

Thus, the trick is to intervene earlier in that process—especially at key points when lesions occur (known to doctors as dysplasias, hyperplasias, and other precancerous cell phases). To do that, the medical community has to break away from the notion that people in an early stage of carcinogenesis are "healthy" and therefore shouldn't be treated. People are not healthy if they're on a path toward cancer.

If this seems radical and far-fetched, consider: We've prevented millions of heart attacks and strokes by using the very same strategy. Sporn likes to point out that heart disease doesn't start with the heart attack; it starts way earlier with the elevated blood cholesterol and lipids that cause arterial plaque. So we treat those. Stroke doesn't start with the blood clot in the brain. It starts with hypertension. So we treat it with both lifestyle

changes and drugs. "Cardiovascular disease, of course, is nowhere near as complex as cancer is," he says, "but the principle is the same." Adds Sporn: "All these people who are obsessed with cures, cures, cures, and the miraculous cure which is still eluding us, they're being—I hate to use this word, but if you want to look at it pragmatically—they're being selfish by ignoring what could be done in terms of prevention."

The amazing thing about this theory—other than how obvious it is—is that we can start applying it *right now*. Precancerous cell changes mark the progression to many types of solid-tumor cancers; many such changes are relatively easy to find and remove, and others are potentially reversible with current drugs and other treatments.

A perfect example is the Pap smear, which detects premalignant changes in the cells of the cervix. That simple procedure, followed by the surgical removal of any lesions, has dropped the incidence and death rates from cervical cancer by 78% and 79%, respectively, since the practice began in the 1950s. In countries where Pap smears aren't done, cervical cancer is a leading killer of women.

Same goes for colon cancer. Not every adenomatous polyp in the colon (a lesion in the organ's lining) goes on to become malignant and invasive. But colon cancers have to go through this abnormal step on their way to becoming deadly. The list of other dysplasia-like conditions goes on and on, from Barrett's esophagus (a precursor to cancer there) to hyperkeratosis (head and neck cancers). Obviously, doctors are already doing this kind of testing with some cancers, but they need to do it much, much more.

Some complain that the telltale biomarkers of carcinogenesis, while getting more predictive, still are far from definitive, and that we should wait until we know more. (Sound familiar?) Researchers in heart disease, meanwhile, have taken an opposite tack and been far more successful. Neither high cholesterol nor hypertension guarantees future cardiovascular disease, but they're treated anyway.

A few cancer researchers have made great strides in finding more early warning signs—looking for protein "signatures" in blood, urine, or even skin swabs that can identify precancerous conditions and very early cancers that are likely to progress. For instance, Lance Liotta, chief of pathology at the NCI, has demonstrated that ovarian cancer can be detected by a high-tech blood test—one that identifies a unique "cluster pattern" of some 70 different proteins in a woman's blood. "We've discovered a previously unknown ocean of markers," he says. And it's potentially a mammoth lifesaver. With current drugs, early-stage ovarian cancer is more than 90% curable; late stage is 75% deadly. Early results on a protein test for pancreatic cancer are promising as well, says Liotta.

Yes, the strategy has costs. Some say wholesale testing of biomarkers and early lesions—many of which won't go on to become invasive cancers—would result in a huge burden for the health-care system and lead to a wave of potentially dangerous surgeries to remove things that might never become lethal anyway. But surely the costs of not acting are much greater.

Indeed, it is an encouraging sign that Andy von Eschenbach, director of the NCI, and Elias Zerhouni, who leads the NIH, are both believers in this strategy. "What our investment in biomedical research has led us to is understanding cancer as a disease process and the various steps and stages along that pathway—from being very susceptible to it, to the point where you get it, and ultimately suffer and die from it," says von Eschenbach, a former urologist who has survived prostate and a pair of skin cancers. So, he says, he wants to lead the NCI on a "mission to prevent the process from occurring in the first place or detect the occurrence of cancer early enough to eliminate it with less morbidity."

HOW TO WIN THE WAR

THERE HAS BEEN TALK like this before. But the money to fund the assault never came. And several cancer experts interviewed for this story worry that the new rhetoric from the NCI, while encouraging, has yet to move beyond lip service.

For the nation finally to turn the tide in this brutal war, the cancer community must embrace a coordinated assault on this disease. Doctors and scientists now have enough knowledge to do what Sydney Farber hoped they might do 33 years ago: to work as an army, not as individuals fighting on their own.

The NCI can begin this transformation right away by drastically changing the way it funds research. It can undo the culture created by the RO1s (the grants that launched a million me-too mouse experiments) by shifting the balance of financing to favor cooperative projects focused on the big picture. The cancer agency already has such funding in place, for endeavors called SPOREs (short for specialized programs of research excellence). These bring together researchers from different disciplines to solve aspects of the cancer puzzle. Even so, funding for individual study awards accounts for a full quarter of the agency's budget and is more than 12 times the money spent on SPORE grants. The agency needs to stop being an automatic teller machine for basic science and instead use the taxpayers' money to marshall a broad assault on this elusive killer—from figuring out how to stop metastasis in its tracks to coming up with testing models that better mimic human response.

At the same time, the NCI should commit itself to finding biomarkers that are predictive of cancer development and that, with a simple blood or urine test (like PSA) or an improved molecular imaging technique (PET and CT scans), can give patients a chance to preempt or control the disease. For that matter, as a nation we could prevent tens of thousands of cancers—and 30% of all cancer deaths, according to the NCI—by getting people to stop smoking. This all-too-obvious observation was made by every researcher I interviewed.

Alas, this is not a million-dollar commitment. It's a billion-dollar one. But the nation is already investing billions in research, and that doesn't even include the $64 billion a year we spend on treatment. To make the resource shift easier, Congress should move the entire federal war chest for cancer into one bureaucracy, not five. Cancer research should be managed by the NCI, not the VA and Pentagon.

Just as important, the cancer leadership, the FDA, and lawmakers need to transform drug testing and approval into a process that delivers information on what's working and what's not to the patients far faster. If the best hope to treat most cancer lies in using combinations of drugs, we're going to have to remove legal constraints and give drug companies incentives to test investigational compounds together in shorter trials. Those should be funded by the NCI—in a process that's distinct from individual drug approval. One bonus for the companies: If joint activity showed marked improvement in survival, the FDA process could be jump-started.

"It's going to require a community conversation to facilitate this change," says Eli Lilly's Homer Pearce. "I think everyone believes that at the end of the day, cancer is going to be treated with multiple targeted agents—maybe in combination with traditional chemotherapy drugs, maybe not. Because that's where the biology is leading us, it's a future that we have to embrace—though it will definitely require different models of cooperation."

When clinical trials begin to offer patients more than incremental improvements over existing drug treatments, people with cancer will rush into the studies. And when participation rates go up, it will accelerate the process so that we can test more combinations faster and cheaper.

> "Metastasis is a big idea. It's hard to do replicable experiments with so many variables. But it's the kind of reseach we need."

To see which drugs truly have promise, however, we need to do one thing more: test them on people in less advanced stages of disease. The reason, once again, comes back to cancer's genetic instability— a progression that not only ravages the body but also riddles tumors with mutations. When cancer patients are in the end stage of the disease, drugs that might have a potent effect on newer cancers fail to show much progress at all. Our current crop of rules, however, pushes drug companies into this can't-win situation, where the only way out is incremental improvements to existing therapies. Drugs that might well help some cancer patients are now getting tossed by the wayside because they don't help people whom they couldn't have helped in any case. This has to stop.

Witness what has happened with the new class of drugs developed to fight the process called angiogenesis ("angio" refers to blood vessels, and "genesis" to new growth)—compounds designed to block the development of capillaries that supply oxygen and nutrients to tumors. Avastin is the best known, but there are some 40 anti-angiogenesis drugs in clinical trials.

This, by the way, is one of those big ideas that the cancer culture didn't take seriously, and would barely fund, for decades. The concept was pioneered 43 years ago by Judah Folkman, now a surgeon at Children's Hospital Boston. While studying artificial blood in a Navy lab, he was struck by a simple and seemingly obvious idea: Every cell needs oxygen to grow, including cancer cells. Since oxygen in the body comes from blood, fast-growing tumors couldn't develop without access to blood vessels.

Folkman later figured out that tumors actually recruited new blood vessels by sending out a protein signal. If you could turn off that growth signal, he reasoned, you could starve the tumors and keep them tiny. The surgeon submitted a paper on his experiments to various medical journals, but the article was rejected time and again. That is, until an editor at the *New England Journal of Medicine* heard Folkman give a lecture and offered to publish it in the *Journal*'s Beth Israel Hospital Seminars in 1971—ironically, the year the War on Cancer began.

After decades of resistance, the cancer culture has finally come around to Folkman's thinking—as the reception greeting Avastin makes clear. Still, the biggest promise of anti-angiogenesis drugs will be realized only when doctors can use them to treat earlier-stage patients. That's because the drugs designed to choke the tumor's blood supply often take a far longer time to work than traditional toxic chemo—time that people with advanced disease and fast-growing cancers may not have. Doctors also need the freedom to administer such drugs in combination. Tumors recruit blood vessels through several signaling mechanisms, researchers believe, so the best approach is to apply several drugs, cutting off all routes.

Who knows? A new paradigm in treatment may emerge from Folkman's 40-year-old idea. Yet to make this simple and seemingly obvious shift, the entire cancer culture must change—from the rules governing drug approval to tort law and intellectual property rights. Science now has the knowledge and the tools; we need to act.

THE GOOD DOCTOR

IN THE WEEKS SINCE I finished my reporting and began writing this story, one image has stuck with me: a drawerful of letters. The letters belong to Eric Winer, a 47-year-old physician at Dana-Farber. He and I had been talking for close to an hour when he showed me the drawer.

It was late on a Friday evening, and Winer, still in the clinic, was describing the progress we were making in this war, his reedy voice cracking higher every so often. He was telling me of his optimism. That's when he mentioned the drawer: "That enthusiasm is very much tempered by the fact that we have 40,000 women dying of breast cancer every year. Um, and you know, I've got a file full of letters that are almost entirely from family members of my patients who died...."

I asked to see it, and then asked again, and there it was, in the bottom drawer of his filing cabinet—two overstuffed folders of mostly handwritten notes. Once the letters go in, Winer confessed, he never looks at them again. "I don't go back," he said sheepishly. "My excuse initially was that if anyone wanted to say I was a bad doctor, I'd hold on to these things that people said about me. And I could prove that I wasn't."

If the walls of his office are any indication, there is no way Winer is a bad doctor. They are covered with loving mementos from patients. There is a picture of Tolstoy from a woman whose breast tumors were initially shrunk by Herceptin, but who died within five years. (Winer had once mentioned to her to that he had majored in Russian history at Yale.) There's a photo of the Grand Canyon taken by a young nurse who was determined to take a trip out West with her 10-year-old son before she died. The daughter of another patient even cornered Lance Armstrong and begged him to sign a neon-yellow jersey for Winer, who is an avid cyclist. It is the most prominent thing in his office.

No, it isn't just the patients in this War on Cancer who need renewed hope. It is the foot soldiers as well.

The Puzzling Origins of
AIDS

*Although no one explanation has been universally accepted,
four rival theories provide some important lessons*

Jim Moore

Shortly after the 1983 discovery of the human immunodeficiency virus (HIV), the pathogen responsible for AIDS, investigators became aware of a strangely similar immune deficiency disease afflicting Asian monkeys (macaques) held in captivity in various U.S. research labs. Soon, virologists identified the culprit: a simian immunodeficiency virus (SIV) that is found naturally in a West African monkey species, the sooty mangabey (*Cercocebus atys*), but is harmless to that host. This virus, denoted SIVsm, is genetically similar to a weakly contagious form of the AIDS virus that is largely restricted to parts of West Africa, HIV-2, and thus is considered its likely precursor. More recent work has shown that the closest relative of the primary human immunodeficiency virus (HIV-1) is another simian immunodeficiency virus, one carried by chimpanzees (SIVcpz).

After comparing the SIVs in chimpanzees and sooty mangabeys with HIV-1 and HIV-2 strains, investiga-

tors concluded that there must have been multiple transmission "events" from simians to humans—at least seven for HIV-2 (some of which are known from only a single person who lives near mangabeys carrying a uniquely similar SIV) and three for HIV-1, the virus now infecting some 40 million people worldwide.

How did SIVcpz and SIVsm cross over into humans and become pathogenic? Given the lack of historical references to AIDS-like disease in Africa prior to the mid-20th century, as well as its absence previously in the New World (which imported some 10 million African slaves during the 16th through 19th centuries), that transfer appears to have happened relatively recently—exactly when is a point of considerable debate. And why did two distinct simian viruses with which humans have apparently coexisted for centuries, or even millennia, suddenly pass into humans multiple times within a few decades?

The answers to these questions have been slow in coming, despite the considerable efforts of molecular biologists to understand the nature and evolution of primate immunodeficiency viruses. I am not one of those molecular biologists; rather, I became a player in the field of AIDS-origin research through my interest in chimpanzee socioecology. Although I am partial to a theory I helped to fashion for why AIDS emerged when it did, with time it might become clear that a competing idea better accounts for genesis of the epidemic. Or perhaps the answer will prove to lie with some complex combination of factors that no single explanation presently encompasses. Whatever the case, the solution almost certainly will come from one or more of four competing theories.

Theory 1: Tainted Polio Vaccine

The first theory is the most controversial. In a 1992 article in the magazine *Rolling Stone*, journalist Tom

Curtis suggested that HIV could have resulted from the use in Africa of an experimental oral polio vaccine (OPV), one contaminated by a then-unknown SIV carried most probably (Curtis supposed) by African green monkeys. Green-monkey kidney cells were widely used as a substrate to grow viruses for research and vaccine production. And one of the first major trials of an experimental oral polio virus vaccine took place from 1957 to 1960 in what are now the Democratic Republic of the Congo, Burundi and Rwanda, seemingly the "hearth" of the global AIDS epidemic. When interviewed by Curtis, Hilary Koprowski, the polio-vaccine pioneer who mounted that massive campaign, could not recall or find documentary evidence as to whether his group had used kidney cells from green monkeys or Asian macaques (which do not naturally carry an SIV). If culture media contained SIV (a possibility, given that the techniques available during that era were unable to guard against unknown viruses that did not cause overt symptoms in their monkey hosts), more than 900,000 people might have received it with their medicine, laying the basis for the current epidemic.

Curtis credited this theory to Blaine Elswood, a Californian AIDS activist. Interestingly, the idea that the administration of a contaminated oral polio vaccine might have been involved in the genesis of AIDS was suggested independently by two others at about the same time. The first to do so was Louis Pascal, who like Elswood is not a scientist. After years of rejections, Pascal, a New Yorker, finally managed in 1991 to get the University of Wollongong in Australia to publish a paper describing his ideas. Not surprisingly, few noticed it. Attorney Walter Kyle also published a broadly similar theory in *The Lancet*, a British medical journal, in 1992. Since then, writer Edward Hooper, author of the controversial 1999 book *The River*, has become the contaminated-vaccine theory's most ardent supporter. Hooper, noting a passing mention by Curtis of a chimpanzee colony run by Koprowski's team, suggested that kidneys from these chimpanzees—not from green monkeys—may have been the original source of the virus.

Multiple localized strains of HIV have now been discovered, and mass vaccination appears unlikely to account for all of them. But the early distribution of the major pandemic strain, HIV-1 group M (for "main"), seems to fit reasonably well with the location of Koprowski's campaigns, and the OPV theory now is applied primarily to this strain.

Contamination of OPV is the only one of the four current theories that is readily falsifiable: Finding the HIV-1 group M virus in a tissue sample that predated the suspect vaccine would eliminate this possibility. So far that has not happened. Still, many investigators give the theory little weight for other reasons, which has led to the widespread belief that the theory has been definitively disproved. In 2001, for example, *Science* magazine published a piece titled "Disputed AIDS Theory Dies its Final Death," and *Nature* ran one under the heading "Polio Vaccines Exonerated." Earlier this year *Nature* also published "Origin of AIDS: Contaminated Polio Vaccine Theory Refuted"—a surprising title given that this theory ostensibly died three years ago.

The recent findings of various molecular biologists have indeed failed to provide support for the OPV theory. For example, in 2000 a few existing samples of the vaccine from Koprowski's home institution (the Wistar Institute in Philadelphia) were tested and found negative for both chimpanzee DNA and SIV. However, this result did not rule out the possibility, previously suggested by Hooper, that local amplification of the live-virus vaccine in Africa (to create more doses) could have introduced the SIV. The key issue is thus whether chimpanzee kidneys were used as a culture medium at any stage of Koprowski's vaccine program. There is eyewitness testimony on both sides of this question, and failure to find SIVcpz in a handful of samples of the live vaccine strain of the type used in Africa does not prove the virus was absent in (putative) locally produced batches.

A second reason to question the OPV theory also came to light in 2000, with a report in *Science* by Bette T. Korber (of Los Alamos National Laboratory) and colleagues. They used molecular differences among HIV-1 group M subtypes to estimate the date of their last common ancestor. The conclusion: 1931 (with 95 percent confidence limits giving the range 1915 to 1941), preceding OPV administration by decades. However, the calculation of such common ancestor dates can be thrown off by genetic recombination among subtypes ("viral sex"), which can make such dates come out too early, and there is increasing evidence that such recombination may be common with HIV. So maybe this date is not right. On the other hand, independent analyses using different methods have supported the date, and an analogous study of HIV-2 came up with an origin for the main group between 1940 and 1945.

Another objection to the OPV theory concerns the subspecies of chimpanzee kept near Kisangani (formerly Stanleyville) at a facility called Camp Lindi, which Koprowski and colleagues maintain was used for safety-testing their vaccine, but which Hooper suspects was the source of chimpanzee tissues used to produce vaccine locally. The SIVcpz strain that is most similar to HIV-1 has so far only been identified in a subspecies of chimpanzee native to west-central Africa, *Pan troglodytes troglodytes*. A second, less similar strain has been identified only in Pan troglodytestes schweinfurthii, the subspecies found in east-central Africa—where Camp Lindi was located. The nearest known populations of *P. t. troglodytes* are more than 500 kilometers from Koprowski's chimp colony. So, this argument goes, the locally obtained captive chimps would not have been carrying the SIVcpz strain thought to have given rise to HIV-1.

One difficulty with this argument is that distance is not always measured in kilometers, particularly in Central Africa: Kisangani lies at the upstream end of the navigable portion of the Congo River, which borders the range of P. *t. troglodytes* for hundreds of kilometers, and river trade has been substantial since the colonial scramble for Africa in the late 19th century. If it became known that Americans were paying good money for young apes in Kisangani, it would be almost surprising if some hunters had not made the trip upriver. Another problem is the difficulty of proving the absence of something based on only a few samples, which requires some significant assumptions about the epidemiology of SIVcpz in the wild.

In short, although the majority of the biological evidence published in the last few years suggests that the OPV hypothesis is wrong, headlines reporting the death of this theory remain premature.

Theory 2: Cut Hunter

The main competing theory posits that SIV is occasionally transmitted to hunters via blood-to-blood contact with an infected primate. According to this view, the virus is usually cleared in its human host, but at least several times during the 20th century it survived and became established as HIV. It is not hard to imagine hunters suffering cuts or being injured by a wounded mangabey or chimpanzee, and some form of natural transfer between species presumably accounts for the widespread distribution of SIVs in African primates. Hence, one has the "cut hunter" or "natural transfer" theory, which is probably the most accepted idea today. According to that view, the timing of the widespread emergences of HIV-l and HlV-2 in the middle part of the 20th century is attributed to urbanization and regional commerce, which create conditions ideal for spreading a sexually transmitted disease.

Unlike the case with OPV, there is no easy way to disprove this theory—even a smoking gun linking oral polio vaccines to HIV-1 group M would leave multiple other HIV strains unaccounted for, and "modernization" is a diffuse enough explanation to cover any of them. Nor is the cut-hunter theory particularly limited in time. After all, many Africans began moving to colonial capitals and ports in the 19th century. A hypothesis that does not account for the timing of the AIDS epidemic and that is not falsifiable is of limited use. Still, the thinness of the theory does not make it wrong.

Theory 3: Contaminated Needles

The next proposal, a refinement of the cut-hunter theory, comes from Preston A. Marx, a virologist who holds positions at Tulane University and at the Aaron Diamond AIDS Research Center. In 1995 he noted (to Hooper) that a big change in medical practice took place in the 1950s with the worldwide introduction of disposable plastic syringes, making guaranteed sterile use possible and dropping the cost of syringe production by almost two orders of magnitude. The result was that the medical use of injections went up astronomically. Because doses can be measured and there is no possibility of patients losing or selling the medicine, injections became a popular way for doctors in the developing world to administer medicines, including vitamins, analgesics and other common drugs.

The problem is that trivial costs are still large to someone living outside the cash economy, and plastic syringes *cannot* be sterilized by boiling: they melt. According to this scenario, the widespread availability of disposable syringes increased the acceptance of injections to treat a variety of diseases, but the syringes were not so available (or cheap) as to permit users actually to dispose of them. The result was that unsterilized syringes were used again and again, spreading viruses, including those that eventually became HIV.

Marx suggests that people's immune systems would normally be able to overcome an SIV they acquired, say while butchering a monkey, within a week or two of infection. He further posits that the transition from SIV to HIV demands a series of mutations, with the probability of all the required mutations occurring being a function of viral population size. Thus, Marx contends, some way must be found to permit the SIV to remain at high levels in people for long enough that such spontaneous mutations might take place. He suggests that the required mechanism is "serial passaging" of virus through unsterile needles. That is, a cut hunter might get an injection while he is still harboring large numbers of viral particles in his bloodstream; that same needle would then be used to infect another person, who might soon receive a second injection, and so forth. High viral population levels can thus be maintained in a series of different people getting shots. With each transfer via contaminated needle, the virus finds itself in a fresh host, with an opportunity to proliferate before the infected person can mount an immune response. Chance mutations can thus accumulate, and eventually the SIV adapts, becoming HIV.

Theory 4: *Heart of Darkness*

Together with two undergraduate students, I am responsible for another variant to the cut-hunter theory, so perhaps I should explain how I became engaged in this field of inquiry. In late 1998 I became involved in an e-mail discussion about the conservation implications of the identification of central African chimpanzees as the source of HIV-1, a result that Beatrice H. Hahn of the University of Alabama at Birmingham and her colleagues had just published. At about the same time, a colleague urged me to read *King Leopold's Ghost*, Adam Hochschild's history of the Belgian Congo, and I was independently contacted by two students, Amit Chitnis and Diana Rawls, who were interested in doing something involving the intersection of biological anthropology and medicine. Then came the catalyst: an article in *Discover* magazine that mentioned the idea that the origin of AIDS might have had something to do with the chaos that followed colonial withdrawal from central Africa. The notion was that the colonial authorities had kept things under control, but when they left, "there was a free-for-all" that provided the conditions for the establishment of a new disease.

King Leopold's Ghost had more impact on me than any other book I have read. I had vaguely heard that Belgian rule was harsh, but I had not realized that more Africans probably died as a result of colonial practices in French Equatorial Africa and neighboring Belgian Congo between 1880 and the onset of World War II than had been taken from Africa as slaves during the preceding 400 years. "Probably," because no record was kept of the dead. The first censuses, taken in the 1920s, estimated that the population of the two colonies was then about 15 million. Census-takers recorded that wherever they asked, local people (colonial and native) reported that about twice as many had lived there two or three decades before, indicating that some 15 million had died. Losing 50 percent of the population exceeds even the 35-percent fatality rate of the Black Death in Europe.

It seems Joseph Conrad's *Heart of Darkness* was as much fact as fiction, and the horror described in that famous novel reflected official policies in the Congo as much as individual insanity. What appeared to many as colonial "control" of the region in the late 19th and early 20th centuries brought chaos to the lives of the Africans who lived and died under it. Chitnis, Rawls and I set out to see what disease-promoting factors might have existed prior to the withdrawal of colonial powers around 1960.

Candidates were not difficult to find, at least during the years prior to

World War I. Forced labor camps of thousands had poor sanitation, poor diet and exhausting labor demands. It is hard to imagine better conditions for the establishment of an immune-deficiency disease. Where imagination fails, let history serve. To care for the health of the laborers, well-meaning but undersupplied doctors routinely inoculated workers against smallpox and dysentery, and they treated sleeping sickness with serial injections. The problem is, the multiple injections given to arriving gangs of tens or hundreds were administered with only a handful of syringes. The importance of sterile technique was known but not regularly practiced: Transfer of pathogens would have been inevitable. And to appease the laborers, in some of the camps sex workers were officially encouraged.

And that was just the situation in the camps. Major efforts were made to eradicate smallpox and sleeping sickness elsewhere in the region (these diseases cut into productivity). The shortage of syringes was acute. One 1916 sleeping-sickness control expedition treated 89,000 people in Ubangi Shari (now Central African Republic) using just six syringes. And before the introduction of dried smallpox vaccine in about 1914, the only way to transport vaccine to the interior was by serially inoculating people, traveling during the eight-day interval required for the new carrier to develop pustules from which the next inoculation could be derived. There are records of at least 14,000 people receiving vaccine in this way. The method had been abandoned in Europe some 20 years before, because syphilis was all-too-often transmitted accidentally in the process.

Such circumstances easily could have promoted the evolution of HIV from SIVcpz. Imagine, for example, the following scenario:

A fisherman flees his small village to escape a colonial patrol demanding its rubber quota; as he runs, he grabs one of the unfamiliar shotguns recently arrived in the area. While hiding for sev-

eral days, he shoots a chimpanzee and, unfamiliar with the process of butchering it, is infected with SIVcpz. On return to the village he finds his family massacred and the village disbanded. He wanders for miles, dodging patrols, until arriving at a distant village. The next day he is seized by a railroad press gang and marched for days to the labor site, where he (along with several hundred others) receives several injections for reasons he does not understand. During his months working on the railroad, he has little to eat and is continually stressed, susceptible to any infection. He finds some solace in one of the camp prostitutes (themselves imported by those in charge), but eventually dies of an undiagnosed wasting— the fate of hundreds in that camp alone. Disease, starvation, abuse—no record is kept, none of the authorities knows, and those few doctors who care are overwhelmed.

We wrote up a short article laying out reasons to at least examine colonial-era practices seriously in regard to how they may have contributed to the origin and spread of HIV. It probably would have been ignored but for another coincidence: Our paper appeared in the journal *AIDS Research and Human Retroviruses* almost simultaneously with the report of Korber and her colleagues in *Science* placing the beginnings of HIV-1 Group M in the early decades of the 20th century. If this dating is correct, the colonial-policy theory offers an explanation. Note, however, that a version of the basic cut-hunter theory that does not rely on urbanization (or sets a much lower threshold for the critical level of city life) could also explain the genesis and initial spread of HIV during this period.

Neither of these scenarios neatly accounts for the decades between the postulated origin of HIV in the early part of the 20th century and the widespread emergence of AIDS in Africa, which did not take place until the early 1980s. But maybe that long delay is only an artifact of our perceptions: Starting with a single case and assuming a doubling in frequency every few years, one would need decades to pass for the prevalence to build appreciably; would colonial doctors have noticed an initially rare immune disease? Nor do these theories readily explain details of the spatial pattern in the early cases of HIV infection and AIDS, which indeed show a suggestive overlap with the sites of oral polio vaccination. But is that correspondence just a function of the distribution of population and doctors? As with all of the current ideas, one can suggest various explanations to account for intriguing observations or troubling discrepancies. For the moment, the fit between theory and observation remains loose enough that no one view has proved absolutely compelling.

Battling Theories

Arguments over rival theories of the origin of AIDS have raged viciously at times—far beyond the norms of most scientific debates. Indeed, both sides in the OPV controversy have in the recent scientific literature gone so far as to accuse their opponents of lying and manipulating evidence. I only became aware of the explosive nature of the debate after my students and I unwittingly wandered into this minefield.

Some of the participants in this controversy appear unwilling even to entertain the possibility of being wrong. Given the precarious status of each of the current theories, it seems more reasonable to try to keep an open mind until better evidence emerges and, in the meantime, to consider the literature on each of these origin stories as representing a highly refined simulation scenario. Insofar as there is any material benefit to come from understanding the origin of HIV in terms of cautionary tales, each model can and should be considered plausible—and worrisome. After all, unsterile needles *do* transmit diseases, contaminated polio vaccine *did* spread a simian virus (one called SV40) to millions of people, doctors *do* sometimes conduct risky research, colonial policies *did* have major health consequences,

and contact with wild animals *can* introduce pathogens into humans.

An obvious general lesson can be drawn from all four theories: For some very puzzling reason, the origin of HIV was not fundamentally natural, given that humans apparently failed to acquire an immunodeficiency virus from simians during thousands of years of exposure. Instead, the emergence of HIV involved social change in one form or another: the abuses carried out at the hand of an invading foreign power; abrupt urbanization overwhelming the ability of medical and political authorities to manage the process; the undersupervised transfer of medical technology and half-measures in development programs; doctors taking liberties in distributing medicines without adequate precautions. It is worth noting that three of the four theories postulate an origin for AIDS that involves the inadvertent results of medical efforts, with what were then state-of-the-art health programs and technologies carrying with them unforeseen dangers.

Whether understanding the origin of HIV and AIDS is useful for evaluating risks associated with present-day concerns (say, the consumption of wildlife that might be the natural reservoir for emerging diseases like SARS, or evaluating the likelihood that the transplantation of animal organs into people will unleash a dangerous new virus) is a matter of opinion. My own view is that a firmer grasp of what happened in the past—and what might easily have happened had circumstances been slightly different—helps society to understand these dangers and to minimize the risk of sparking the next global scourge.

Bibliography

Apetrei, C., D. L. Robertson and P. A. Marx. 2004. The history of SIVs and AIDS: Epidemiology, phylogeny and biology of isolates from naturally SIV infected non-human primates (NHP) in Africa. *Frontiers in Bioscience* 9:225-254.

Chitnis, A., D. Rawls and J. Moore. 2000. Origin of HIV-1 in colonial French Equatorial Africa? *AIDS Research and Human Retroviruses* 16:5-8.

Cohen, J. 2001. Disputed AIDS theory dies its final death. *Science* 292:615.

Curtis, T. 1992. The Origin of AIDS. *Rolling Stone* issue 626 (19 March): 54-59+.

Dicko, M., A.-Q. O. Oni, S. Ganivet, S. Kone, L. Pierre and B. Jacquet. 2000. Safety of immunization injections in Africa: Not simply a problem of logistics. *Bulletin of the World Health Organization* 78:163-169.

Hochschild, A. 1998. *King Leopold's Ghost: A Story of Greed, Terror, and Heroism in Colonial Africa.* New York, Boston: Houghton Mifflin.

Hooper, E. 2000. *The River: A Journey to the Source of HIV and AIDS.* Boston: Back Bay Books.

Hooper, E. 2003. Dephlogistication, imperial display, apes, angels, and the return of Monsieur Émile Zola: New developments in the origins of AIDS controversy, including some observations about ways in which the scientific establishment may seek to limit open debate and flow of information on "difficult" issues. *Atti dei Convegni Lincei* 187:27-230.

Korber, B., M. Muldoon, J. Theiler, F. Gao, R. Gupta, A. Lapedes. B. H. Hahn, S. Wolinsky and T Bhattacharya. 2000. Timing the ancestor of the HIV-1 pandemic strains. *Science* 288:1789-1796.

Kyle, W. S. 1992. Simian retroviruses, polio vaccine, and origin of AIDS. *The Lancet* 339:600-601.

Lemey, P., O. G. Pybus, B. Wang, N. K. Saksena, M. Salemi and A.-.M. Vandamme. 2003. Tracing the origin and history of the HIV-2 epidemic. *Proceedings of the National Academy of Sciences of the U.S.A.* 100:6588-6592.

Peeters, M., V. Courgnaud, B. Abela, P. Auzel, X. Pourrut, F. Bibollet-Ruche, S. Loul, F. Liegeois, C. Butel, D. Koulagna, E. Mpoudi- Ngole, G. M. Shaw, B. H. Hahn and E. Delaporte. 2002. Risk to human health from a plethora of simian immunodeficiency viruses in primate bushmeat. *Emerging Infectious Diseases* 8:451-457.

Peterson, D. 2003. *Eating Apes.* Berkeley: University of California Press.

Reeler, A. V. 1990. Injections: A fatal attraction? *Social Science & Medicine* 31:1119-1125.

Salemi, M., K. Strimmer, W. W. Hall, M. Duffy, E. Delaporte, S. Mboup, M. Peeters and A.- M. Vandamme. 2001. Dating the common ancestor of SIVcpz and HIV-1 group M and the origin of HIV-1 subtypes using a new method to uncover clock-like molecular evolution. *The FASEB Journal* 15:276-278.

Weiss, R. A. 2001. Polio vaccines exonerated. *Nature* 410:1035-1036.

Worobey, M., M. L. Santiago, B. F. Keele, J.-B. N. Ndjango, J. B. Joy, B. L. Labama, B. D. Dhed'a, A. Rambaut, P. M. Sharp, G. M. Shaw, B. H. Hahn. 2004. Contaminated polio vaccine theory refuted. *Nature* 428:820.

Jim Moore received his doctorate in biological anthropology from Harvard in 1985, where he studied demography and sociality in primates. Since then he has been on the faculty of the University of California, San Diego, where his research focuses on primate behavioral ecology. Address: Anthropology Department, University of California, San Diego, La Jolla, CA 92093. Internet: jj-moore@ucsd.edu

From *American Scientist*, November/December 2004, pp. 540, 542-547. Copyright © 2004 by American Scientist, magazine of Sigma Xi, The Scientific Research Society. Reprinted by permission.

UNIT 8

Health Care and the Health Care System

Unit Selections

Key Points to Consider

- Is health care just another commodity? Should it be treated differently from other consumer services?

- Is quality health care a right or a privilege? Defend your answer.

- What can you as an individual do to help reduce health care costs? Give specific actions that can be taken.

- What steps can you take to reduce your risk of injury during hospitalization?

- What can be done to reduce unnecessary medical treatment?

- How should health care be rationed?

Student Website
www.mhcls.com/online

Internet References
Further information regarding these websites may be found in this book's preface or online.

American Medical Association (AMA)
   http://www.ama-assn.org
MedScape: The Online Resource for Better Patient Care
   http://www.medscape.com

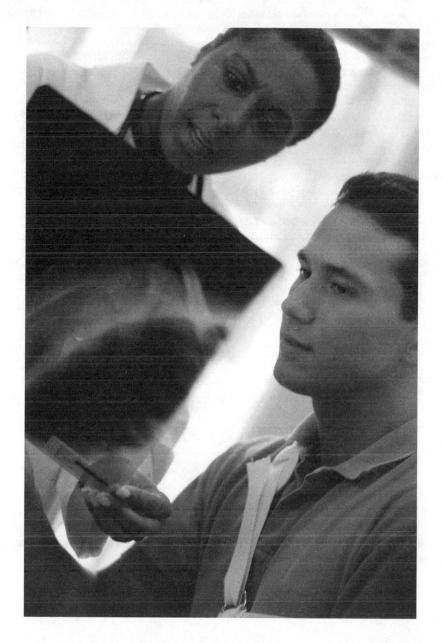

Americans are healthier today than at any time in this nation's history. Americans suffer more illness today than at any time in this nation's history. Which statement is true? They both are, depending on the statistics you quote. According to longevity statistics, Americans are living longer today and, therefore, must be healthier. Still other statistics indicate that Americans today report twice as many acute illnesses as did our ancestors 60 years ago. They also report that their pain lasts longer. Unfortunately, this combination of living longer and feeling sicker places additional demands on a health care system that, according to experts, is already in a state of crisis. In "Putting a Value on Health," Don Peck believes that the way to stop rising health care costs is to admit there already is a rationing system and try to better manage it.

Despite the clamor regarding the problems with our health care system, if you can afford health care, the American system is one of the best in the world. However, being the best does not mean that it is without its problems. Each year, more than half a million Americans are injured or die due to preventable mistakes made by medical care professionals. In addition, countless unnecessary tests are preformed that not only add to the expense of health care but also may actually place the patient at risk. Reports such as these fuel the fire of public skepticism regarding the quality of health care that Americans receive. While these aspects of our health care system indicate a system in need of repair, they represent just the tip of the iceberg. The article "Stay Safe in the Hospital" presents several key points that patients should consider to protect themselves from the hazards of hospitalization. A related issue is the high number of medical facilities and hospitals not utilizing technology. While we live in a technically advanced society, many hospitals have been reluctant to embrace modern systems that could positively impact health care. Many health centers are still writing prescriptions by hand and keeping paper records. Both of these practices can lead to medication errors and other errors.

While avoiding hospital blunders has been made easier, paying for services continues to be a challenge as medical costs continue to rise. Why have health care costs risen so high? The answer to this question is multifaceted and includes such factors as physicians' fees, hospital costs, insurance costs, pharmaceutical costs, and health fraud. It could be argued that while these factors operate within any health care system, the lack of a meaningful form of outcomes assessment has permitted and encouraged waste and inefficiency within our system. Ironically, one of the major factors driving up the cost of health care is our rapidly expanding aging population—tangible evidence of an improving health care delivery system. This is obviously one factor that we hope will continue to rise. Another significant factor that is often overlooked is the constantly expanding boundaries of health care. It is somewhat ironic that as our success in treating various disorders has expanded, so has the domain of health care, and often into areas where health care previously had little or no involvement. According to Shannon Brownlee, in the article, "The Overtreated American," health care costs continue to escalate due to unnecessary treatment, tests, and office visits.

Traditionally, Americans have felt that the state of their health was largely determined by the quality of the health care available to them. This attitude has fostered an unhealthy dependence upon the health care system and contributed to the skyrocketing costs. It should be obvious by now that while there is no simple solution to our health care problems, we would all be a lot better off if we accepted more personal responsibility for our health. While this shift would help ease the financial burden of health care, it might necessitate more responsible coverage of medical news to educate and enlighten the public on personal health issues.

THE OVERTREATED AMERICAN

*One of our biggest health-care problems is that there's just
too much health care. Cutting down on the excess could save
enough to cover everyone who is now uninsured*

BY SHANNON BROWNLEE

Americans enjoy the most sophisticated medical care that money can buy—and one of the most vexing health-care-delivery systems. We spend about $1.2 trillion each year, two to four times per capita what other developed nations spend, yet we can't find a way to provide health insurance for 41 million citizens. After a brief respite in the 1990s when HMOs held down expenses by squeezing profits from doctors and hospitals, medical costs are once again soaring by 10 to 12 percent a year. Yet reforms proposed by Congress and the White House are only nibbling around the edges of the problem.

Such political timidity is understandable, given the experience of would-be reformers of the past. Any attempt to expand coverage for the uninsured while holding down costs inevitably raises fear in the minds of voters that the only way to accomplish these seemingly opposing goals is by restricting access to expensive, life-saving medical treatment. Sure, we feel bad about the 18,000 or so of our fellow citizens who die prematurely each year because they lack health insurance, and about the seniors who are forced to choose between buying food and buying medicine. But Americans want nothing to do with a system like England's, which, for example, is reluctant to provide dialysis to the elderly, and most of us who are now covered by either Medicare or private insurance have little stomach for health-care reform that contains even a whiff of rationing.

Behind this fear lies an implicit assumption that more health care means better health. But what if that assumption is wrong? In fact, what if more medicine can sometimes be bad not just for our pocketbooks but also for our health?

An increasing body of evidence points to precisely that conclusion. "There is a certain level of care that helps you live as long and as well as possible," says John Wennberg, the director of the Center for Evaluative Clinical Sciences at Dartmouth Medical School. "Then there's excess care, which not only doesn't help you live longer but may shorten your life or make it worse. Many Americans are getting excess care." According to the center, 20 to 30 percent of health-care spending goes for procedures, office visits, drugs, hospitalization, and treatments that do absolutely nothing to improve the quality or increase the length of our lives. At the same time, the type of treatment that offers clear benefits is not reaching many Americans, even those who are insured.

That's a sobering thought, but it opens the possibility of a new way to look at the conundrum of health-care reform. Lawmakers, insurers, and the health-care industry might be able to save money if they were to concentrate on improving the quality of medicine rather than on controlling costs. Better health care will of course mean more medicine for some Americans, particularly the uninsured; but for many of us it will mean less medicine.

Support for this idea can be found in *The Dartmouth Atlas of Health Care*, a compendium of statistics and patterns of medical spending in 306 regions of the country. The atlas is generated by a group of nearly two dozen doctors, epidemiologists, and health-care economists, using data from Medicare, large private insurers, and a variety of other sources. Wennberg is the group's leader and the patron saint of the idea that more medicine does not necessarily mean better health—a view that has not exactly endeared him to the medical establishment over the years. These days, however, his ideas are bolstered by the Institute of Medicine and other independent researchers, and by new results coming from his Dartmouth research team, which is showing precisely how the nation misspends its health-care dollars.

Take the regions surrounding Miami and Minneapolis, which represent the high and low ends, respectively, of Medicare spending. A sixty-five-year-old in Miami will typically account for $50,000 more in Medicare expenses over the rest of his life than a sixty-five-year-old in Minneapolis. During the last six months of life, a period that usually accounts for more than 20 percent of a patient's total Medicare expenditures, a Miamian spends, on average, twice as many days in the hospital as his counterpart in Minneapolis, and is twice as likely to see the inside of an intensive-care unit.

This type of regional variation would make perfect sense if regions where citizens were sickest were the ones that used the most medical services. After all, it's only fair that we should spend more and do more in places where people need more medical attention. But, as Wennberg and his colleagues Elliott Fisher and Jonathan Skinner point out in a recent paper, "Geography and the Debate Over Medicare Reform," which appeared online in the journal *Health Affairs*, rates of underlying illness do not account for the differences in spending among regions. If they did, the region around Provo, Utah, one of the healthiest in the country, would get 14 percent fewer Medicare dollars than the national average, because its citizens are less likely to smoke, drink, or suffer from strokes, heart attacks, and other ailments. Instead it receives seven percent more than the national average. In contrast, elderly people in the region around Richmond, Virginia, tend to be sicker than the average American, and should be receiving 11 percent more—rather than 21 percent less—than the national average. Nor are regional differences explained by variations in the cost of care. Provo doctors are not, for example, charging significantly more for office visits or lumpectomies than doctors in Richmond, and their patients aren't getting costlier artificial hips.

Rather, much of the variation among regions—about 41 percent of it, by the most recent estimate—is driven by hospital resources and numbers of doctors. In other words, it is the supply of medical services rather than the demand for them that determines the amount of care delivered. Where neonatal intensive-care units are more abundant, more babies spend more days in the NICU. Where there are more MRI machines, people get more diagnostic tests; where there are more specialty practices, people see more specialists. It's probably safe to assume that many people are gravely ill during the last six months of their lives no matter where they live; but Medicare beneficiaries see, on average, twenty-five specialists in a year in Miami versus two in Mason City, Iowa, largely because Miami is home to a lot more specialists.

It would be one thing if all this lavish medical attention were helping people in high-cost regions like Miami to live longer or better. But that doesn't appear to be the case. Recent studies are beginning to show that excess spending in high-cost regions does not buy citizens better health. Medicare patients visit doctors more frequently in high-cost regions, to be sure, but they are no more likely than citizens in low-cost regions to receive preventive care such as flu shots or careful monitoring of their diabetes, and they don't live any longer. In fact, their lives may be slightly shorter. The most likely explanation for the increased mortality seen in high-cost regions is that elderly people who live there spend more time in hospitals than do citizens in low-cost regions, Wennberg says, "and we know that hospitals are risky places." Patients who are hospitalized run the risk of suffering from medical errors or drug interactions, receiving the wrong drug, getting an infection, or being subjected to diagnostic testing that leads to unnecessary treatment.

An obvious way we might cut excess medical care is to change the way we pay hospitals and doctors. "Medicine is the only industry where high quality is reimbursed no better than low quality," says David Cutler, a health economist at Harvard. "The reason we do all the wasteful stuff is that we pay for what's done, not what's accomplished." Although that's clearly the case, figuring out the right incentives for health-care providers is by no means easy. Let's say that Medicare decided to use low-cost regions as a benchmark and told providers in the rest of the country that their compensation would be capped at some level not far above the benchmark. Some doctors in high-cost regions would undoubtedly be encouraged to practice more conservatively, but many others would maintain their incomes by either dropping Medicare patients altogether or giving them even more hysterectomies and CT scans they don't need (thus compensating for lower fees by simply performing a greater number of procedures).

Even if policymakers come up with the right financial incentives, restructuring compensation will constitute only one small component of the reform that's needed to turn medicine into an efficient, effective industry. Think of it this way: at 13 to 14 percent of GDP, health care is the nation's largest single industry, and probably its most complex. Transforming this sprawling behemoth is going to involve a lot more upheaval than, say, the shift that took place in the auto industry when companies adopted the assembly line, or the shake-up that Hollywood and the music industry now face with the advent of Web entertainment.

Step No. 1 toward improving the quality of health care is reducing what the Dartmouth group calls "supply-sensitive" care—the excess procedures, hospital admissions, and doctor visits that are driven by the supply of doctors and hospital resources rather than by need. Organizations such as the American Medical Association and Kaiser Permanente will need to set standards for more-conservative practices, and for measuring patient outcomes. Benchmarks are also needed to ensure that doctors deliver more "evidence-based" medicine: procedures and practices whose benefits are proven. Three recent studies, conducted by the Institute of Medicine, the Rand Corporation, and the President's Advisory Commission on Consumer Protection and Quality in the Health Care Industry, report widespread underuse of evidence-based treatment, such as balloon angioplasty to open blocked arteries in heart-attack victims, even among citizens with gold-plated health insurance.

Probably the hardest part of reforming health care will be persuading policymakers and politicians that improving the quality of care can also save money. The Medical Quality Improvement Act, introduced last July by Vermont Senator James Jeffords, is a step in the right direction. It would call on several medical centers around the country to model high-quality medicine that also reins in costs.

But evidence already exists that improving quality can hold down costs. Franklin Health, a company based in Upper Saddle River, New Jersey, manages so-called "complex cases" for private insurers. Complex cases are the sickest of the sick, patients with multiple or terminal illnesses, who are also the most costly to treat. They typically make up only one or two percent of the average patient population while accounting for 30 percent of costs. Franklin employs a battalion of nurses, who make home visits and spend hours on the phone, sometimes every day, to help patients control pain and other symptoms and stay out of the hospital. For this low-tech but intensive service the company charges insurers an average of $6,000 to $8,000 per patient—but it saves them $14,000 to $18,000 per patient in medical bills.

How much money is at stake? If spending in high-cost regions could somehow be brought in line with spending in low-cost regions, Medicare alone could save on the order of 29 percent, or $59 billion a year—enough to keep the Medicare system afloat for an additional ten years, or to fund a generous prescription-drug benefit for seniors. And there's no reason to believe that doctors and hospitals behave any differently toward their non-Medicare patients. That means the system as a whole is wasting about $400 billion a year—more than enough to cover the needs of the 41 million uninsured citizens.

The last attempt at reforming the U.S. health-care system failed in large measure because of fears of rationing. Reform was viewed as an effort to cut costs, not to improve health, and voters believed, rightly or wrongly, that they would end up being denied the benefits of modern medicine. Future efforts at reform are going to have to persuade Americans and their doctors that sometimes less care is better.

Shannon Brownlee, a senior fellow at the New America Foundation, was formerly a senior writer for Discover *and* U.S. News & World Report. *Her work has appeared frequently in* The New Republic, The Washington Post, *and other publications.*

Stay safe in the hospital

Patients and relatives alike need to take action to get the best care and prevent hospital medical and medication errors.

You may heave a sigh of relief when you or a relative is admitted to a hospital, because you're finally getting help for a difficult medical problem. But it's crucial to remember that what happens in the hospital can sometimes cause additional health problems and that patients and relatives need to exercise caution, ask questions, and be vigilant about the quality of care received.

In the hospital, "You have vulnerable people exposed to powerful medicines and traumatic surgical procedures," says Robert Wachter, M.D., a professor at the University of California, San Francisco, who prepared a major government report on hospital safety. "And that risk is greater when doctors or nurses are rushed or tired, as they often are, or when hospitals haven't instituted comprehensive patient-safety practices, as too few have," Wachter says.

The Institute of Medicine (IOM), which advises the government on health policy, highlighted those dangers in a 1999 study showing that errors made by hospital staff kill up to 100,000 people each year and seriously injure roughly a half-million more. More recent evidence suggests that the problem is either getting worse or is larger than originally thought. A 2004 study of 37 million Medicare patient records suggested that hospital errors killed and hurt roughly twice as many patients as found in the IOM report.

Research has identified four areas of particular concern:

• **Infections,** including those stemming from antibiotic resistant "superbugs"bred often by the improper and excessive prescribing of antibiotics.

• **Drug errors,** caused by staff forgetting to give a needed medication, giving an unauthorized drug, or giving a drug at the wrong time or in the wrong dose.

• **Surgical mistakes,** including operating on the wrong side of the body and forgetting to remove sponges or clamps before sewing up the patient. Also, patients waking up mid-operation because of insufficient anesthesia.

• **Miscommunication,** which not only makes patients feel helpless but also contributes to drug and test errors, lack of a clear recovery plan, and failure to follow people's wishes for end-of-life care.

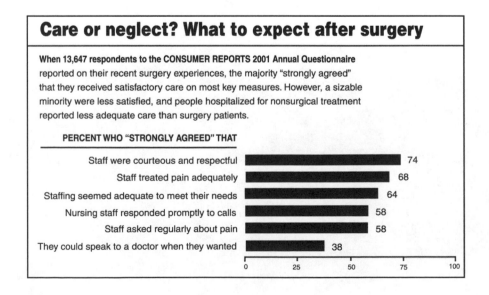

Care or neglect? What to expect after surgery

When 13,647 respondents to the CONSUMER REPORTS 2001 Annual Questionnaire reported on their recent surgery experiences, the majority "strongly agreed" that they received satisfactory care on most key measures. However, a sizable minority were less satisfied, and people hospitalized for nonsurgical treatment reported less adequate care than surgery patients.

PERCENT WHO "STRONGLY AGREED" THAT

Staff were courteous and respectful	74
Staff treated pain adequately	68
Staffing seemed adequate to meet their needs	64
Nursing staff responded promptly to calls	58
Staff asked regularly about pain	58
They could speak to a doctor when they wanted	38

In search of the right surgeon and hospital

Here are some strategies to help you select a qualified surgeon and a hospital with a good safety record.

Seeking a surgeon

Ask your primary-care doctor to recommend a surgeon, if necessary from the list of doctors approved by your insurance company. For complicated or unusual problems, ask for the name of a recognized expert or search the medical literature to find someone who has published major articles about your problem. Then contact that physician and ask him or her to recommend someone in your locale.

If you don't have a solid recommendation, it's wise to learn all you can about the prospective surgeons. Start by contacting the American Board of Medical Specialties (www.certified doctor.org,866-275-2267) to learn whether the surgeon is board certified in a relevant specialty, such as the American Board of Orthopaedic Surgery.

The American Medical Association's "Doctor Finder" Web site (*www.ama-assn.org/aps/amahg.htm*) tells you where the physician underwent residency training. Doctors trained at or working in university medical centers may have more experience with a wider variety of cases than those at smaller hospitals.

Administrators in Medicine (*www.docfinder.org*), an association of state medical-board executive directors, provides state-by-state information about professional misconduct by physicians.

Finally, talk with the prospective surgeon and ask how many operations of the type you need he or she has performed. Studies suggest that experience leads to higher success and lower complication rates. Also ask if the surgeon can provide references from patients willing to speak with you. Find out which hospitals the doctor admits patients to, and check their quality. Better hospitals tend to attract better doctors.

Hospital hunting

For help in finding a hospital in your region that is both high quality and accepted by your insurance, consult one or more of the "hospital report cards" listed below. They provide information on nursing ratios, error-prevention programs, and, perhaps most important, experience with various disorders.

If you need surgery, look for information on volume and outcomes, such as mortality, for the procedure you are going to have. Try to avoid hospitals with volume numbers that seem much lower or death or complication rates much higher than others. Here are some of the places you can find report cards:

- **America's Best Hospitals by U.S.News & World Report** (*www.usnews.com*).
- **Guide to Hospitals by Consumers' Checkbook** (*www.checkbook.org, $19.95 for a two-year subscription*).
- **Health Care Choices** (*www.healthcarechoices.org*).
- **Health Grades Inc.** (*www.healthgrades.com*).
- **The LeapFrog Group** (*www.leapfroggroup.org/ consumer_intro1.htm*).
- **Quality Check by the Joint Commission on Accreditation of Healthcare Organizations** (www.jcaho.org).

In the past five years many hospitals have launched patient-safety initiatives meant to combat those and other problems. Patient and family awareness is another important safety check for heading off problems.

INFECTION PROTECTION

The Centers for Disease Control and Prevention (CDC) estimates that about 2 million people contract hospital acquired infections each year, with nearly 90,000 of those proving fatal. Hospitals are filled with patients who come in with infections and others who are very vulnerable due to weakened immunity. Surgical procedures, needles, and catheters can carry germs into the body. And hospital staff may fail to take the necessary steps needed to stop the spread of infection.

The situation has become more dangerous because of the emergence of bacteria that are resistant to antibiotics. Here are some key steps that can help you reduce your risk.

- **Insist on clean hands.** Some 150 years after scientists demonstrated that hand washing stops the spread of infections, less than half of doctors and nurses adhere to this essential step. Expect anyone who touches you—including your visitors—to first wash his or her hands with soap or an alcohol-based solution. If you don't see them do that, politely ask if they have.

- **Monitor antibiotic use.** The overuse of powerful broad-spectrum antibiotics breeds drug-resistant germs that can infect the blood stream and the gut. Stomach infections are particularly common when antibiotics are paired with potent heartburn drugs, which suppress stomach acid and allow invading organisms to thrive. So if your doctor prescribes antibiotics during your hospital stay, especially along with a heartburn drug, ask if it's really necessary.

Before surgery, on the other hand, antibiotics are sometimes underused or improperly prescribed.While many surgical patients should receive presurgical antibiotics, research suggests that the regimen or the timing of the drug is wrong in up to 50 percent of cases.

Ask your doctor if your operation poses a significant threat of infection; if so, make sure you receive a single dose of an antibiotic in the hour before surgery.

• **Stay warm.** Body temperature drops by several degrees during surgery, a decline that can impair immune function and blood flow and make infections more likely. So ask your doctor if it makes sense in your case to use a special surgical blanket or other techniques to keep you warm.

• **Be aware of the catheter.** About 40 percent of hospital-acquired infections stem from urinary-tract infections. And the risk of those infections increases significantly if the urinary catheter is left in place for more than two or three days. If you're still using a catheter 48 hours after surgery, find out whether removal has been overlooked. If you start feeling urinary discomfort, ask your nurse to check whether the catheter is clogged.

• **Get moving.** That can help prevent bedsores, another cause of hospital-acquired infections, as well as potentially dangerous blood clots in the legs. But since postoperative falls are common, ask your nurse—or a friend or relative —to help you out of bed and, if possible, take a stroll. If you must spend a lot of time in bed, ask for special pads that help prevent bedsores and "pneumatic" stockings that can prevent blood clots.

• **Boost your immunity.** Smokers and people with diabetes are especially prone to infection because of weakened immune function. Smokers should give up cigarettes as long as possible before admission. People with diabetes should make sure their blood sugar levels stay under control before and during their hospital stay.

PREVENTING MEDICATION MIX-UPS

The average hospital patient receives 10 different drugs; some of these may have look-alike labels or sound alike names and may be prescribed by various specialists who leave notes in cryptic handwriting or don't communicate with each other at all. Busy staffers may mistake micrograms for milligrams or mistake one patient for another.

In one study of 36 randomly selected hospitals in Georgia and Colorado, researchers found mistakes in 19 percent of the medication doses given. The following steps can help prevent medication and test errors.

• **Make a drug list.** Make sure your attending doctor knows that you want to be told the name of each new medicine given to you as well as its intended purpose. You can refuse any medication you think is being given to you in error. Be certain that any drugs you've been taking for chronic conditions, such as diabetes or high blood pressure, are continued, because many hospitals routinely stop such medications when patients are admitted. That practice may increase the risk of complications.

• **Check your wristband.** Make sure the information on your wristband—your name plus any drug allergies—is accurate. Hospital staff are supposed to check the band each time they give you a drug, take a blood sample, or perform a test. If they don't, it's wise to mention your name and your allergies.

STOPPING SURGICAL ERRORS

The suggestions listed below may sound like you're asking for special privileges. But surgeons are getting used to such requests and shouldn't mind, provided you ask in a friendly manner.

• **Pay attention to imaging procedures.** It makes no sense for you to have a CT scan of your head if you're in for a hip replacement. Remind your doctor to tell you about X-rays and scans in advance.

Have a friend, relative, or private-duty nurse stay with you if you're too sick to fend for yourself the first night after surgery.

• **If possible, schedule surgery for well staffed times.** Hospital staffing can be skimpy on weekends and at night. Nonemergency procedures slated for Monday sometimes get delayed or bumped because of the spillover of emergency cases from the weekend; when surgery is done on Friday, you may get reduced postoperative care on the weekend. So ask if you can have your surgery on a Tuesday, Wednesday, or Thursday morning. That way the immediate postoperative hours, when you need the most care, will come on the midweek day shift, when staffing is at full capacity.

• **Bank your blood.** Transfusions pose a very slight risk of transmitting an infectious disease. So if your doctor says a transfusion is likely, consider banking your own blood supply ahead of time.

• **Ask the surgeon to autograph your surgery site.** While reports of surgeons operating on the wrong limb or organ are rare, they occur often enough that hospital- safety experts now advise surgeons to initial the surgery site beforehand.

• **Know your heart-attack and blood-clot risk.** Every surgical patient over the age of 50 should be evaluated to see if he or she is at risk of having a heart attack or stroke during the operation. If you are, you should receive a beta-blocker such as metoprolol (*Toprol-XL*) or atenolol (*Tenormin*) before the operation and possibly other medications as well.

And many surgical patients—including nearly all undergoing hip- or kneereplacement procedures—should get blood-thinning drugs, such as warfarin, right after surgery to reduce the chance of getting a blood clot in the leg or lungs.

• **Get enough anesthesia.** Too much anesthesia increases the risk of complications. But up to 40,000 surgical patients a year wake up in the middle of their operation because of too little. That's a particular risk to patients undergoing cardiac, obstetric, and major trauma surgeries. Ask your surgeon or anesthesiologist to make sure you stay under for the entire operation.

CONTROLLING YOUR PAIN

Roughly half of patients say their pain isn't adequately managed during their hospital stay. Patients with uncontrolled pain tend to stay in the hospital longer and suffer more complications. Yet drugs and other techniques can substantially ease most pain.

Some surgeons are reluctant to order morphine or other opiates, the strongest painkillers, even though the chance of addiction is minuscule. Or they fail to consider newer options, such as epidural anesthesia, which controls pain by feeding a nerve-blocking drug into the spine. Nerve blockade may be preferable to opiates after certain operations, such as joint replacement, since it controls pain equally well but doesn't make you groggy. In addition, most hospitals now have patient-controlled intravenous analgesia (PCA), which lets you administer your own medication (while also preventing overdosage) by pushing a button on a computerized pump.

Patients should insist on a pain management plan. That includes asking your admitting doctor to leave standing orders for pain (as well as insomnia and constipation) medication, so if the need arises you won't face a long wait while the nurse puts in a call to your doctor. Also ask if the use of PCA is appropriate and, if so, ask to be trained in its use both before and after surgery.

Certain self-help steps may provide further pain control. Several studies have found that surgery patients who listened to soothing music through headphones while recovering reported less pain than other patients. Other helpful relaxation techniques include deep breathing, muscle relaxation, or listening to guided imagery or self hypnosis tapes.

CLEAR COMMUNICATION

Rushed nurses may barely have enough time to answer your call button, let alone give detailed answers to your questions. Technicians take blood samples or wheel you off for imaging tests but can't always explain what the tests are for. Unfamiliar doctors stop by for brief visits, sometimes with a group of students in tow, and seem to talk about you but not to you. And it's often unclear who, if anyone, is overseeing all your care.

Here are some steps that can help you communicate clearly with hospital staff.

• **Appoint a companion.** Having a friend, relative, or private-duty nurse with you is particularly important the first night after surgery and at other times when you may be too sick to fend for yourself. A companion can help you assert your needs and preferences, articulate your questions, record the answers, retain copies of key medi-

cal documents, including your drug list, and advocate for you if any problems arise.

• **Be polite but assertive when necessary.** Complaining too often or too aggressively about minor inconveniences can alienate the often-overworked staff. But you should expect reasonable and timely responses to reasonable requests and questions. If you're being neglected, ask to speak to the hospital's patient advocate or social-service worker.

• **Find out who is in charge.** To minimize the chance of conflicting orders from specialists, have one doctor coordinate your treatment. Your primary doctor or one of his or her colleagues should visit you daily. Alternatively, your care can be coordinated by a staff hospitalist, a new breed of specialist who focuses on overseeing the care patients receive while in the hospital.

• **Prepare a living will.** Make sure your admitting doctor and the hospital have a copy of your living will and health-care proxy form. This written record of your preferences can help you avoid overaggressive care. Appoint a health-care proxy to make sure doctors follow your wishes and to make decisions not covered in your living will if you're incapacitated. (For details, see the accompanying "For More Information" box.)

• **Plan your discharge.** At discharge time, ask your doctor, surgeon, or discharge planner for a list and instructions for the medications or devices you may need at home. Next, discuss how to prepare your home for your convalescence. For example, you may want to move to a downstairs bedroom, get an elevated toilet seat, move obstructing furniture out of the way, and remove throw rugs.

Finally, find out whether you're likely to need physical therapy, home nursing care, or a stay in a rehabilitation facility. Once you check into the hospital, ask to speak with the hospital's discharge planner (and ask your doctors to do the same), so the hospital can start arranging for the appropriate services.

If the hospital tries to discharge you before you feel ready, insist on talking first with your doctor. You shouldn't go home if you feel disoriented, faint, or unsteady, have pain that's not controlled by oral medication, can't go to the bathroom unassisted, or can't keep food or drink down. If your doctor isn't able to extend your stay, appeal to the discharge planner or the patient advocate. If necessary, contact your insurance carrier and the hospital administration. And ask a companion to take you home and stay there with you for at least a day.

WHAT YOU CAN DO

To optimize a hospital stay:

• Enlist the help of people who can help monitor your care, including a friend or relative, your primary-care doctor, and, if necessary, the hospital's patient advocate or social-service worker.

• Talk with your doctor about the drugs and tests you'll likely need while in the hospital and about your living will.

• Ask your surgeon about the optimal timing for surgery, antibiotics, transfusions, anesthesia, staying warm during the operation, and also pain control.

• Check all medications and ask for an explanation if any are unfamiliar.

• If necessary, remind the nurses and doctors to wash their hands, check your wristband, catheter, and surgical site, assess your risk of complications during surgery, and get you up walking again.

• Object strenuously to attempts at premature discharge and get complete information about convalescing at home.

A HIGH DOSE OF TECH

"Some grocery stores have better technology than our hospitals and clinics."

Tommy Thompson, secretary of health and human services

By Rob Turner

Eyebrows shot up at Thompson's uncharacteristically feisty zinger a couple of years ago. Technologically backward? Hospitals, where multi-million-dollar scanners painted finely detailed images of body parts? Where miniature restorative devices were threaded through tiny tubes into ailing vessels? Surely Thompson was engaging in a bit of hyperbole.

Not so—hospital administrators knew he was right on the money. Humble bar-code scanners, ancient technology at neighborhood supermarkets, had barely dented U.S. hospitals. Most patient records were still kept on paper and stuffed in bulging manila folders. Physicians in different parts of the same healthcare system couldn't send clinical data back and forth. Some doctors were technophobes and proud of it, boasting that real docs don't touch a keyboard.

And change was vital. Hospitals were inefficient—but worse, medical mistakes were killing tens of thousands of hospital patients a year. Available technology could slash the toll. Physicians' scrawled prescriptions could be entered directly into a computer, for example, eliminating errors that were causing complica-

tions and deaths. Thompson's message to hospitals: Make it happen.

And slowly but surely, hospitals are obeying—junking creaky old computer systems, cabling high-speed networks, and pumping up information-technology budgets that had bumped along hand to mouth for years.

But the few Seabiscuits are being trailed by thousands of also-rans, and last week, Thompson unveiled an ambitious 10-year initiative with a blunt bottom line: You're not wiring up fast enough, so we'll light a fire under you. The plan makes Medicare a vehicle for pilot programs ranging from handling prescriptions electronically to moving patient records online so that caregivers—and patients—can refer to them regardless of time or place. New standards, promised Thompson, will mesh the innovations into a seamless nationwide network.

"In most technology, America is the world leader," declared Thompson. "I can use my bank ATM card in Russia. Your pet has records that are likely kept electronically so you get an automatic E-mail reminder to bring in your dog for a checkup. Don't you think we

should do the same in medicine? Isn't it time to bring medicine into the 21st century?"

Percentage of most-wired hospitals that let patients preregister at home:

58.4%

Even minus a federal push, the number of plugged-in medical centers has climbed. Responses to annual "most-wired hospitals" surveys by *Hospitals & Health Networks*, an American Hospital Association trade publication, have risen steadily. The latest survey, released last week, represents nearly 1,300 hospitals, almost 20 percent above 2003.

Already, results are evident. Patients in intensive care, who usually are watched over by nurses during off-times, are being monitored by doctors miles away. Patients are being armed with more of their own medical information as medical records are converted from paper to digital bits. And the boom is spinning off amenities like bedside Web access and E-mail.

Hospital executives talk about saving lives, not saving money, as the reason to wire up. But the corporate community, pounded by rising healthcare costs, has also been pushing higher tech hard. Four years ago, a group of *Fortune* 500 companies and other major employers created the Leapfrog Group to reshape the delivery of hospital healthcare in ways that would save lives and reduce complications—and, not coincidentally, drive down costs. The sheer size of Leapfrog's members has given the group unusual muscle in dictating an agenda that includes a laundry list of 27 safety-related practices, computer entry of prescriptions, and improved ICU staffing.

But while hospitals are starting to embrace technology, many are doing so tentatively, having observed the bruises suffered by early adopters. It's not just high cost, or software that needs further tweaking. Old-fashioned stubbornness has been a source of frequent hiccups and occasional debacles. And notwithstanding Thompson's grand plan, a blueprint remains to be drawn up, so wiring up is being done piecemeal. A healthcare system with a number of small or rural hospitals might opt first to fund remote intensive-care monitoring. California hospitals, on the other hand, must submit detailed plans for reducing medication errors by next January, so they might focus on computerized drug orders.

Three features of wired hospitals are especially meaningful to patients: taking the guesswork out of ordering medications, preventing errors when medications are brought to the bedside, and giving patients access to their medical records through a website. For a closer look, read on.

KILLER PRESCRIPTION PADS

A small piece of paper doesn't look like a deadly weapon, but much of the concern over patient safety and hopes attached to technology have centered on the innocuous prescription pad. No one seriously argues that relying on handwritten drug orders is anything other than antiquated, inefficient, and dangerous. Many of the more than 1 million serious medication errors estimated by Leapfrog to occur in hospitals every year, killing 7,000 patients and driving up healthcare costs by an estimated $2 billion, start with a physician's sloppy scrawl.

The high-tech remedy is computerized physician order entry, or CPOE. Placing orders by computer for medications—and, as a side benefit, for lab tests, special diets, and other procedures—not only eliminates confusion caused by barely legible scrawls but moves medications to patients faster and minimizes the possibility of incorrect dosages and dangerous drug interactions.

In studies, CPOE has cut serious medical errors by 55 percent or more, and Mark Zielazinski, chief information officer for El Camino Hospital in Mountain View, Calif., thinks that may be too conservative. The hospital started using computerized order entry more than 30 years ago—the first in the country to do so, says Zielazinski—working in tandem with Lockheed Martin. Error rates weren't recorded until 1992, but since then, he says, the number of errors per 1,000 patient-days has dropped from approximately 12 to six last year and now stands at four, a decline of 67 percent in a 12-year span.

In a CPOE-equipped hospital, the physician logs in to a computer that might be a terminal in a corridor niche, a laptop on a wheeled cart, or even, as at El Camino, a wireless tablet PC. Depending on the system, the doctor might key in the name of the drug and the dose, or point and click from a list of medications she regularly prescribes. The order is automatically forwarded to the hospital pharmacy and to nurses responsible for administering the medication.

Even a relatively narrow application like CPOE, however, demands a substantial foundation. A database consisting of detailed medical records for each patient in electronic form must be created and scrupulously kept up to the minute. Custom hardware and software packages must be installed. The human beings who will make or break the new system must be trained. Their cooperation is vital, and winning it can be tough.

In 2002, Cedars-Sinai Medical Center in Los Angeles spent millions of dollars on CPOE but quickly scuttled the program because private physicians who sent patients to the hospital rebelled. "It was a noble attempt, but Cedars bit off more than they could chew," says Stephen Uman, an infectious disease specialist who helped organize the movement to dismantle the program, which he believed demanded too much time and attention. Handwritten orders that could be dashed off in a few seconds were taking five to 10 minutes, adding up to hours daily. The system would not allow doctors to prescribe new drugs that hadn't been entered into the computer—and, says Uman, didn't tolerate the smallest misspellings. If a doctor keyed in penicillin with one "l," the computer would respond that no such drug existed. Cedars-Sinai executives did not return repeated requests for details.

"That's the nightmare everybody wants to avoid," says Steve Clark, chief information officer of the University of Colorado Hospital in Denver, which plans to switch to CPOE this fall. "Your success is dependent on the physicians' accepting the technology. It's far easier to just scribble something or tell a nurse what to do." Proper training is a must, says Clark, but it is just as important to demonstrate hospital commitment from the boardroom down.

Clark hopes for a reasonably smooth ride. At a university hospital, the majority of the physicians are on staff, so their choice is to go along or leave. But presumably, as employees they also are more loyal and committed to the hospital than outside physicians typically would be and, Clark agrees, should be easier to persuade. Hospital department

"AMERICA'S BEST" PLUGGED-IN HOSPITALS

Last week Hospitals & Health Networks, *a publication of the American Hospital Association, released its annual list of the "100 most wired hospitals and health systems." Of the 100, the 38 below have additional appeal: They were also ranked in U.S. News's "America's Best Hospitals" this year.*

ADVOCATE LUTHERAN GENERAL HOSPITAL, Park Ridge, Ill*
ARTHUR G. JAMES CANCER HOSPITAL, Columbus, Ohio*
BAYLOR INSTITUTE FOR REHABILITATION, Dallas*
BAYLOR UNIVERSITY MEDICAL CENTER, Dallas*
BETH ISRAEL DEACONESS MEDICAL CENTER, Boston*
BRIGHAM AND WOMEN'S HOSPITAL, Boston*
CHILDREN'S HOSPITAL OF PHILADELPHIA
CHILDREN'S HOSPITAL OF PITTSBURGH*
CLARIAN HEALTH PARTNERS (IU & Meth. Hosps.), Indianapolis
DARTMOUTH-HITCHCOCK MEDICAL CENTER, Lebanon, N.H.
HACKENSACK UNIVERSITY MEDICAL CENTER, Hackensack, N.J.
HAMOT MEDICAL CENTER, Erie, Pa.
HOSPITAL OF THE UNIVERSITY OF PENNSYLVANIA, Philadelphia*
INOVA FAIRFAX HOSPITAL, Falls Church, Va.*
LEHIGH VALLEY HOSPITAL, Allentown, Pa.*
MAGEE-WOMENS HOSPITAL, Pittsburgh*
MASSACHUSETTS GENERAL HOSPITAL, Boston*
MCLEAN HOSPITAL, Belmont, Mass.*
METHODIST HOSPITAL, Houston

NATIONAL REHABILITATION HOSPITAL, Washington, D.C.*
NEW ENGLAND BAPTIST HOSPITAL, Boston*
NORTH CAROLINA BAPTIST HOSPITAL, Winston-Salem*
NORTHWESTERN MEMORIAL HOSPITAL, Chicago
OCHSNER CLINIC FOUNDATION, New Orleans
OHIO STATE UNIVERSITY MEDICAL CENTER, Columbus*
POUDRE VALLEY HOSPITAL, Fort Collins, Colo.
RUSH-PRESBYTERIAN-ST. LUKE'S MEDICAL CENTER, Chicago
SENTARA NORFOLK GENERAL HOSPITAL, Norfolk, Va.*
SPAULDING REHABILITATION HOSPITAL, Boston*
TEXAS HEART INST. AT ST. LUKE'S EPISCOPAL HOSPS., Houston
UNION MEMORIAL HOSPITAL, Baltimore*
UNIVERSITY HOSPITAL OF ARKANSAS, Little Rock
UNIVERSITY OF ALABAMA HOSPITAL AT BIRMINGHAM
UNIVERSITY OF PITTSBURGH MEDICAL CENTER
UNIVERSITY OF UTAH HOSPITALS AND CLINICS, Salt Lake City
UNIVERSITY OF WISCONSIN HOSPITAL AND CLINICS, Madison
WASHINGTON HOSPITAL CENTER, Washington, D.C.*
YALE-NEW HAVEN HOSPITAL, New Haven, Conn.

*In a healthcare system named on the "100 most-wired" list

WHAT TO LIKE ABOUT WIRED HOSPITALS

A big reason hospitals wire up is to reduce prescription mistakes and other medical errors. But patients benefit in other ways, too, according to Hospitals & Health Networks' *yearly surveys.*

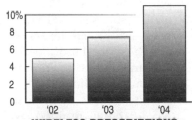

WIRELESS PRESCRIPTIONS
The percentage of hospitals where almost all doctors prescribe using wireless devices is rising, and nearly 22 percent of "most wired" hospitals prescribe that way.

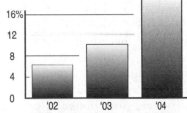

MATCHING DRUG TO PATIENT
Hospitals that use information technology to match most medications and doses with patients are increasing: Almost 35 percent of "most wired" hospitals do so.

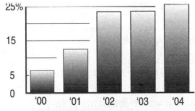

ONLINE SCHEDULING
At a growing number of hospitals, outpatients can book future appointments by logging on to a hospital website. Almost 54 percent of "most wired" hospitals allow it.

heads and other managers also are emphasizing to caregivers the potential for improving patients' safety in ways that will show up in performance numbers.

At Children's Hospital & Regional Medical Center in Seattle, the conversion to CPOE last November was no cakewalk, especially for some older doctors. Tradition was the main obstacle, says Mark Del Beccaro, clinical director of information services—the idea that "I know how to use a pen to write an order— I don't want to spend hours learning a new way and then have to actually get used to doing it." Says Del Beccaro: "I told people,'This [is] going to be one of the hardest things you're ever going to do, because it really, fundamentally, changes the way we practice medicine, and there aren't too many times when you do that in your career.' "

Children's required private doctors to go through training if they wanted to retain their admitting privileges. "There was a little bit of grumbling," says Del Beccaro. "But now we have some people who didn't even open their own E-mail before; now they're doing their own orders. Once they get used to it, they find that it's actually quicker."

At Children's, the system has halved the time for medications to reach inpatients, meaning that critical drugs are reaching sick kids faster. Pharmacy errors due to hard-to-decipher prescriptions have dropped to zero. And orders for lab tests often move more rapidly, sometimes because of innovations made possible by new features that exploit clinical data. "Last night I was admitting a child with a new diagnosis of leukemia, and there's a bunch of labs we always have to get for those," says Del Beccaro. "Well, I can never remember what they are." The new software, however, displays a list of the required lab tests for new leukemia cases. "I pulled it up and bam, I sent it off. I can write those orders now in under two minutes. If I did it the old way, it would take me forever"—about 20 minutes longer, he says, which now seems like forever.

Percentage of most-wired hospitals that let patients query claims online:

30.7%

While adoption of CPOE has been steady, it has a long way to go. Fewer than 5 percent of hospitals in Leapfrog surveys had some form of CPOE in place as of last year. The two biggest barriers are large startup costs—typically from $3 million to $10 million per hospital—and difficulty in showing bottom-line savings, according to an article last month in the journal *Health Affairs*. Fewer errors and higher productivity may more than offset the expense, but the savings are largely pocketed by health insurance carriers, not hospitals, because fewer complications and improved efficiency add up to shorter hospital stays.

Hospitals do benefit from increased patient safety, says internist Eric Poon, a coauthor of the article and a researcher at Brigham and Women's Hospital in Boston, but the high expense of CPOE still has to be justified. "Both the government and the insurance companies need to start thinking about providing financial incentives," he says. Part of the

new federal program, says Mark McClellan, director of the federal Centers for Medicare and Medicaid Services, would do just that. A new Medicare pilot program will test the effect of higher payments to hospitals that meet various technology requirements.

Taking the long view, Leapfrog CEO Suzanne Delbanco is encouraged. About 16 percent of hospitals have told Leapfrog they plan to have some form of the system fully implemented by the end of 2005—which, she observes, "really is a sea change from where it was four years ago."

ONE LAST CHECK

About one third of hospital medication errors happen at the front end, according to studies by Lucian Leape of the Harvard School of Public Health, when a doctor prescribes the wrong drug or the wrong dose. Another one third occur in the middle, because a hospital pharmacist misreads the doctor's handwriting or a transcriptionist writing up the doctor's dictated notes fumbles the name of the drug. That two thirds should shrink as hospitals adopt CPOE.

But then there is the back end: a medication administered to the wrong patient or to a patient who has a reaction because allergies, a health condition, potential drug interactions, or other medical information is missing from the record. To reduce those errors, more hospitals are bar-coding not only drugs but patients and nurses.

Before a medication is administered, the nurse scans in the bar codes on her badge, the patient's identification bracelet, and the medication. The computer alerts her to possible conflicts, such as a potentially dangerous interaction with another drug the patient is taking. It can also alert the nurse if the drug isn't being given at the proper time or at the proper dose.

At Eisenhower Medical Center in Rancho Mirage, Calif., 115 beds are wired for bar coding, and an additional 120 are in the works. "It's pre-

venting medication errors daily," says Mary Ann McLaughlin, administrative director for medical-surgical services. Nurses there have come to rely on the system so much, along with pop-up screen alerts like "check blood pressure," says McLaughlin, that they don't "feel as protected" on floors still lacking the system.

All prescription drugs will have to come bar-coded by 2006 under Food and Drug Administration rules, and most likely before then, McClellan said last week, for Medicare patients. To Susan Bumatay, chief nurse at Sutter Delta Medical Center in Antioch, Calif., that's good news. Sutter currently spends millions of dollars to bar-code uncoded medications because keeping medications straight has become critical, says Bumatay. The number of drugs is burgeoning, and many have names that look or sound similar. More than 17,000 medications are currently marketed in Northern California, and processing 30 million prescriptions a year in Sutter Health's system offers plenty of opportunities for error. "We're human," she says. "That's why we need additional layers of safety." The hospital hasn't used the new system long enough to gauge overall results, says Bumatay, but her staff already can see the near misses that would have resulted without it. "We're dealing with lives here," she says emphatically. "We're not flipping hamburgers."

DIGITAL MEDICAL RECORDS

Bruce Freedman was diagnosed with bladder cancer in 1992. Then, in 2001, he had triple coronary artery bypass surgery. He had a mild heart attack last October. And he has kidney problems on top of it all. As the years passed, Freedman, now 62, acquired new doctors with each new ailment. Each one would give him different drugs, and he couldn't keep track of all the instructions and advice.

Then Danny Sands, an internist at Beth Israel Deaconess Medical Center in Boston, became Freedman's primary-care physician. Sands had spent years developing electronic health records that patients could access at any time from home from a secure website.

It was a radical notion. Thanks to bureaucratic obstacles and physician resistance, patients rarely see their medical records. But Sands believed patients could help manage their own care if they felt more connected to information about their health. Besides, he says, studies show that patients forget 30 percent to 50 percent of what a doctor tells them during an office visit almost as soon as they walk out the door. If patients had their information available at a website, he reasoned, and could E-mail follow-up questions, they would be better informed and ultimately healthier.

So in 2000, Sands launched PatientSite on the Web, intended to contain everything that would go into the usual hospital medical record except for doctors' clinical notes (many doctors weren't comfortable including them and the patients weren't asking for them). Patients now could even see results of lab tests, usually as soon as their physicians got them. And patients could share the information with family members at home. As the site has evolved, Sands has added enhancements—such as the ability to schedule appointments and order refills online for maintenance medications. More than 20,000 patients at Beth Israel currently have access to their health records online, he says.

Freedman, a commercial real-estate broker, especially likes the E-mail feature. Before, he had trouble

reaching Sands by phone, or they would play phone tag for days. Now he can fire off a message with a question and usually get an answer within a few hours to a day. "It saves me a lot of aggravation and time and effort," he says.

Not all doctors are as enthusiastic. About two thirds of doctors in national surveys would want to participate only if they were compensated, says Sands. The Beth Israel site doesn't charge for messaging capabilities, but that could change. (The Palo Alto Medical Foundation in California charges patients $60 a year for unlimited E-mailing.)

"Consumers have a right to know about their health," says Leapfrog's Delbanco. "That's why we are working so hard to promote a more transparent healthcare system, where we have as much information about our healthcare choices as we do about choosing a car or a dishwasher."

That's a theme heard repeatedly at hospitals that switch to electronic records and open them up to patients. At Palo Alto Medical, more than 25,000 patients now have 24-hour access. "In my mind, it levels the playing field," says Paul Tang, chief medical information officer, "so patients, not just their providers, are armed with information." He plans to launch a disease-management component on his site this fall to give diabetics specialized tools to help them monitor their own progress interactively—by, say, entering their cholesterol and glucose results. "It's one thing to be told your LDL cholesterol is 120," says Tang. "It's another to look at a graph and know what your target is."

Besides involving patients more directly, putting health records in electronic form makes patients safer. At Brigham and Women's Hospital in Boston and its many clinics scattered throughout the area, all patient records are electronic. A patient who comes to one hospital has her record available online at all of them. Perhaps an elderly woman from the suburbs breaks her hip and is taken to Brigham and Women's. The emergency physician calls up her records, says Robert Goldszer, vice chair of medicine, "and sees right away not to give her certain medications because she has a heart condition."

The University of Colorado Hospital in Denver experimented with the ultimate step in 2002, giving 54 regular outpatients at the hospital's heart center full access to their medical records, including clinical notes. Their behavior over the next year was compared with that of 53 other patients matched by age, sex, medical condition, and other qualities. Several physicians resisted, fearing they would have to censor themselves to keep from being E-mailed to death.

"Some of my colleagues may have felt a little threatened," says clinic cardiologist Gene Wolfel. "My philosophy is that these people should know what's going on. ... If they don't understand something, that's an opportunity for dialogue." Moreover, the feared hounding didn't happen. The 54 patients sent their seven doctors a total of 60 E-mails over the next year, barely more than one per patient. At the end of the study, the 53 other patients got total access, too.

Putting a Value on Health

The way to arrest spiraling costs is to admit that we already do what we say we never will—ration health care—and then figure out how to do that better

By Don Peck

For all its flaws, medical care in the United States has improved enormously over the past several decades. Deaths from heart disease have fallen by 40 percent since 1970. In the mid-1980s HIV was an automatic death sentence; it's not anymore. Since 1990, thanks to better detection and treatment, cancer mortality rates have been falling. (Breast-cancer mortality is down by 20 percent since 1990.) Altogether, medical advances have helped to raise U.S. life expectancy from an average of sixty-eight years in 1950 to seventy-seven years today.

Not only have American lives grown longer, but their quality has improved. The proportion of people over sixty-five with one or more chronic disabilities—such as the inability to walk, or to get dressed, without aid—declined from greater than 25 percent in 1982 to less than 20 percent in 1999. And the development of Viagra and vision-correction surgery, among many other drugs and procedures, has allowed many Americans to prolong pleasures historically associated with youth.

Of course, not all the recent improvements in American health and longevity can be directly attributed to our health-care system; some are as much the result of adopting healthier habits (exercise, better diet) or of dropping unhealthy ones (smoking, excessive alcohol consumption). And even though life expectancy has been rising in America, it remains lower than in many other advanced nations—probably because those nations have lower rates of obesity, broader access to health care, and lesser degrees of wealth inequality. Still, better medical care is the principal cause of improvements in American health and life-span over the past fifty years.

The problem, of course, is that since 1960 health-care spending has grown significantly faster than the economy, meaning that we're spending an ever larger portion of our incomes on medical care. In 1960 health care constituted 5.1 percent of the U.S. economy; in 1980 it constituted 8.8 percent; today it constitutes 13.3 percent. The Centers for Medicare and Medicaid Services (CMMS) projects that healthcare spending will grow by an average of more than seven percent a year until 2012, even after adjusting for in-

flation. Meanwhile, private health-insurance premiums—which rose by 14 percent last year alone—are becoming unaffordable for ever more Americans.

It seems that cutting costs should be relatively easy. After all, health-care delivery in the United States is notoriously inefficient. Consumers lack sufficient information or expertise to make informed choices of physicians, hospitals, and treatments. Also, because most of their health care is paid for by insurance, they tend to overuse the system. Physicians, for their part, usually profit from the tests and procedures they order and perform—whether or not those tests and procedures are truly necessary. Shouldn't it be a simple matter to reduce waste and abuse?

Up to a point, yes. The frequency of a major surgical procedure such as coronary bypass surgery varies widely from physician to physician and region to region, with no discernible difference in health outcomes, on average, between patients who receive such treatments and those who don't. According to one study, 20 to 30 percent of health-care spending goes for tests, treatments, and visits that have no positive effect on either the quality or the length of our lives. If we could identify and prevent even half this spending, we would save some $25 billion to $35 billion each year on Medicare alone.

But this would do little to address the fundamental problem. That's because the largest driver of growth in health-care spending is not waste or price gouging or the slow aging of the population but, rather, the cost of technological innovation. Even when technological improvements make some treatments less expensive and more effective, overall spending often rises. Cataract surgery, for example, used to require up to a week in the hospital and offer only uncertain results. Now it's a quick, highly effective outpatient surgery. Per-procedure costs of this surgery have fallen, on average, by about one percent a year over the long term, alter controlling for inflation. But because so many more people opt for cataract surgery today, real total spending on the procedure has risen by four percent a year over the same period. Given the over-

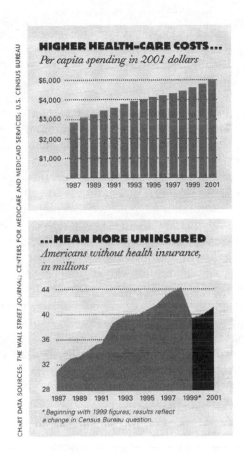

HIGHER HEALTH-CARE COSTS...
Per capita spending in 2001 dollars

[Bar chart showing values from $5,000 down to $1,000, years 1987, 1989, 1991, 1993, 1995, 1997, 1999, 2001]

...MEAN MORE UNINSURED
Americans without health insurance, in millions

[Line/area chart with values 44, 40, 36, 32, 28, years 1987, 1989, 1991, 1993, 1995, 1997, 1999*, 2001]

* Beginning with 1999 figures, results reflect a change in Census Bureau question.

CHART DATA SOURCES: THE WALL STREET JOURNAL; CENTERS FOR MEDICARE AND MEDICAID SERVICES; U.S. CENSUS BUREAU

not every health plan covers every test or treatment, but most health-insurance plans have been rapidly expanding what they cover. The result is a system in which patients with insurance can order up an expensive test that is one percent more effective than a test costing one third as much—indirectly pushing health-care premiums beyond the reach of many others.

- **THE NUMBER OF THINGS WE CAN DO TO PRESERVE HEALTH IS EXPANDING FASTER THAN THE ABILITY OF AMERICANS TO PAY FOR THEM.**

- **KEY FACTOR MISSING FROM REFORM EFFORTS IS RELIABLE INFORMATION ABOUT WHAT MEDICAL TREATMENTS WORK.**

- **THE SIMPLEST WAY TO ACHIEVE UNIVERSAL HEALTH INSURANCE IS TO REQUIRE AMERICANS TO BUY IT.**

Is there anything we can do about this? Unfortunately, the most obvious way to significantly reduce health-care costs without substantially decreasing the quality of care is rationing—that is, limiting the range of treatments and tests that insurance will cover in certain circumstances, a practice that runs counter to the prevailing any-care-at-any-cost ethos. Hardly a politician dares even to mouth the word "rationing," save as an expression of opprobrium.

Yet the fact is that the system already rations; we just don't acknowledge it openly. Every day on the front lines and in the back offices of the health-care profession ICU nurses, hospital executives, and Medicare and insurance-company administrators make difficult cost-versus-value decisions. How long should a man in a coma be allowed to linger in an expensive ICU bed while others who could benefit from the specialized care wait? Is it worth $7,000 to give Xigris—a drug to treat virulent infections that can develop in hospital settings—to an uninsured patient with less than three months to live? In a recent survey of 620 critical-care physicians, 68 percent said they had rationed medications or procedures in the preceding year. Such decisions are often morally complex, even agonizing—and often benefit patients with money: overall, people who have health insurance receive about twice as much medical care as those who lack it.

Without intervention this gap will most likely widen: a majority of Americans will continue to receive state-of-the-art care, whereas a growing minority will be shut out of the insurance system, finding themselves without access either to the cutting-edge treatments of 2004 or to proven forms of medical care that have been available for decades.

So the key question is not *whether* health care should be rationed in the United States; it already is. Rather, the question is *how* health care should be rationed. How

all growth in health-care spending currently projected by the CMMS, even an immediate drop, through waste reduction, of 20 percent in nationwide spending—which would be highly difficult to achieve—would be undone by new technology-fueled spending in just four years.

Most of the growth in health-care spending has produced real improvements in the scope of medical services and the quality of care. But the number of things we can do to cure disease, eliminate discomfort and stave off aging is expanding faster than the ability of many Americans to pay for them. Indeed, it appears very likely that growth in medical spending will continue to outpace growth in personal income or GDP over the next few decades—even if we introduce temporary cost-saving measures.

That we spend enormous sums of money for even tiny improvements in health-care quality reflects a social ethos to which most Americans implicitly subscribe: anything that might improve health or extend life, however marginally, should be made available to everyone, at whatever cost. That may seem morally proper. But because of the way that health care is bought and financed in this country, we tend to be blind to the costs, both economic and moral, of taking this ethos too far. Because neither patients nor physicians pay for them directly, expensive tests, treatments, and procedures of only marginal value are routinely ordered, and expensive new technologies that barely improve the ability to detect or treat a disease are widely and rapidly adopted. Of course,

Insurance Required

If mandatory insurance is good enough for your car ...

Believe it or not, there is a politically appealing way to achieve universal health-care coverage: simply require all U.S. residents to buy insurance, with government help if necessary.

To understand why and how this might work, consider that the majority of those who lack health insurance are not unemployed. Nearly 60 percent of uninsured Americans work full time; another 16 percent work part time. These tend to be workers whose employers don't offer them health insurance (because they are low-wage or newly hired), or who cant afford to pay a share of the premiums.

In addition, about a third of the uninsured live in families with household incomes greater than $50,000 a year; many of these people could afford the costs of health insurance if they chose. Moreover, many of the uninsured are relatively young and healthy; about 40 percent are aged eighteen to thirty-four, and another 20 percent are under eighteen. This provides an opportunity. Requiring all these young, healthy Americans—who are currently gambling that they'll stay healthy—to enter the risk pool would drive down premiums for those Americans who currently have health insurance while lowering the cost of entry for those who don't.

Here's how it might work. States would establish insurance polls that would offer every American a choice among competing private insurance plans. Insurers offering coverage through these polls would be required to offer a core benefits package and could not discriminate on the basis of pre-existing conditions. Individuals could purchase more-comprehensive coverage if they wished.

Each year, according to a recent study published in the *Annals of Family Medicine*, 20 percent of people with insurance are forced to change health plans, resulting in higher costs and lower-quality care. A citizen-based (as opposed to employer-based) universal insurance program would eliminate this problem by enabling workers to keep their doctors and health plans when they changed jobs. And rather than being limited to the health plans chosen by their employers, workers could choose plans and levels of coverage from among competing private providers.

Under a universal citizen-based plan those employers who wished to continue administering health-care benefits could do so; but those who wanted to shed the administrative burden could choose instead to contribute a fixed amount (currently employers contribute more then $300 billion to employee health coverage each hear) to an insurance pool or to the plans of their employees' choosing.

This proposal would cost the federal government somewhere on the order of $80 billion a year, with most of that money going to provide subsidies to those who couldn't afford the minimum cost of coverage themselves. But the plan would also save the nation the cost of uncompensated care (currently some $35 billion, which is passed on to employers and insured employees in the form of rising premiums), and it would recoup some of the $65 billion to $130 billion of labor productivity that is lost to untreated health problems each year.

Won't Americans balk at a radical proposal that forces even those who don't want health insurance to buy it? Actually, it's hardly radical: Americans are already well accustomed to the idea of mandatory insurance. After all, almost anyone who wants to drive a car is required to buy car insurance, and anyone who wants to carry a mortgage must buy homeowner's insurance. The details are different, but the idea is the same. Applying this principle—universal coverage in exchange for universal responsibility—makes economic, moral, and practical sense.

—LAURIE RUBINER

Laurie Rubiner is the director of the Universal Health Insurance Program at the New America Foundation.

should the potential benefits of reduced pain, improved quality of life, or extended life be weighed against the high costs of the medications or procedures involved? And who should weigh them? These are hard questions with high moral stakes. We do ourselves a disservice by dismissing them with a platitude like "You can't put a value on health." That may be true in the abstract, but one *can* put a value on different treatments and practices. When we decline to do so, we are automatically putting a lower value on other areas, such as education and security, in which increased spending might in fact add more to life expectancy and quality of life. By refusing even to countenance sensible limits on the health care citizens have a right to demand, we make universal health-care coverage—a worthy goal that we are long overdue in attaining—nearly impossible. It would be un-American to suggest that those who can afford truly comprehensive insurance—call it "Cadillac insurance"—should be prevented from buying it. And no one is suggesting that. But if we will not consider that perhaps not everyone who pays premiums should be *guaranteed* Cadillac insurance, more Americans each year will be left unable to afford any coverage at all. At the very least we need to begin a national conversation about the meaning of "medical necessity"—for instance, does it include knee surgery for someone who is not in acute pain but wants to continue playing recreational tennis or touch football? what about bariatric surgery (stomach stapling) for those who are not morbidly obese?—and to launch an honest discussion about what kind of rationing would be fairest and most efficient.

To start the conversation, here's one scenario: Imagine a system in which everyone has insurance (including prescription-drug coverage) offering a basic standard of care almost equal to what the insured enjoy today, but people who want the very latest and most expensive treatments must eidier buy supplemental insurance or pay out of pocket. (For one vision of how coverage might be extended with little disruption, see Insurance Required.) As innovations prove to offer dramatically better care, or somewhat better care at roughly equal cost, basic coverage would be extended to include them; but the standard for what could be included would be set high (perhaps with the help of an institute like the one proposed by Shannon Brownlee on the facing page). With fewer patients opting for expensive new treatments that are only marginally more effective than older ones, research doctors, drug companies, and medical-hardware makers could devote more of their R&D resources to making existing treatments cheaper and more effective. Though health-care spending will never stop growing completely, it would grow more slowly under this scenario. Similarly, although the rate of improvement in health-care quality might slow marginally, improvement would continue. America would still have care equal to the best in the world—and the system would cover more people. Would that sort of rationing really be so bad?

Don Peck is the director of The Atlantic's *editorial-research staff.*

UNIT 9

Consumer Health

Unit Selections

Key Points to Consider

- What are the risks associated with tanning parlors?

- What are some concrete examples of actions you can take to ensure that you get what you want from your doctor's visit?

- What should women know before they consider breast implants?

Student Website

www.mhcls.com/online

Internet References

Further information regarding these websites may be found in this book's preface or online.

FDA Consumer Magazine
   http://www.fda.gov/fdac/796?toc.html
Global Vaccine Awareness League
   http://www.gval.com

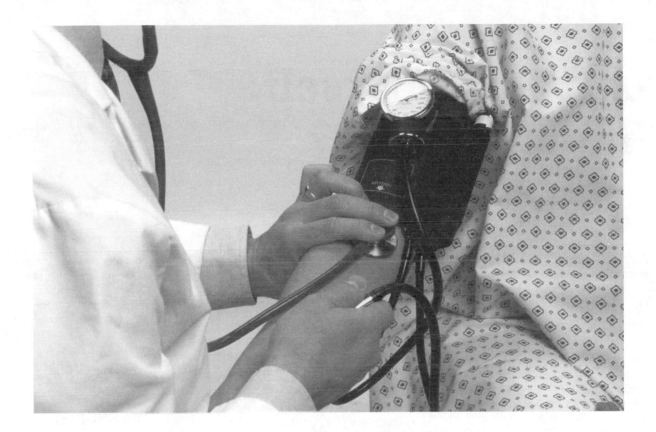

For many people the term "consumer health" conjures up images of selecting health care services and paying medical bills. While these two aspects of health care are indeed consumer health issues, the term consumer health encompasses all consumer products and services that influence the health and welfare of people. A definition this broad suggests that almost everything we see or do may be construed to be a consumer health issue. In many ways, consumer health is an outward expression of our health behavior and decision-making processes and as such is based on both our desire to make healthy choices, be assertive, and to be in possession of accurate information on which to base our decisions. "Doctoring Yourself: When is it Wise?" provides consumers with several useful tips that will help ensure that they seek medical help when needed and avoid it when unnecessary. Fortunately many people have turned to their doctors following the withdrawal of the pain medication Vioxx from the market. This, and other pain treatments, were found to increase the risk of cardiovascular disease. In "How to Ease Your Pain," consumers are offered advice on managing acute and chronic pain.

Breast implants are another known health risk that consumers demand. Many women want to increase their breast size via implants, while mastectomy patients seek implants to restore their breasts. For whatever reason, choosing implants is a decision that should be made only after a woman fully understands and acknowledges the potential harm and the importance of follow up medical care. While researchers have found that implants do not contribute to life-threatening systemic illnesses, there are many other concerns. Some of the risks of implants include pain, hardening of the scar tissue that forms around the implant, rupture of the saline-filled breast, nerve damage, and the potential inability to breast feed children. Most women with implants will also need at least one additional surgery over the course of their life for a variety of complications such as rupture or asymmetry.

The health-conscious consumer seeks to be as informed as possible when making dietary and medical decisions—but the best intentions come to no avail when consumers base their decisions on inaccurate information, old beliefs, or media hype that lacks a scientific basis. Knowledge (based on accurate information) and critical thinking skills are the key elements required to become proactive in managing your daily health concerns.

Doctoring yourself: When is it wise?

The promise and pitfalls of self-care.

Today's consumers are taking on many tasks that previous generations were content to leave to their doctors. It's now increasingly easy and common for people to:

- Do their own medical research by reading medical literature over the Internet.
- Self-diagnose by buying tests for various disorders. Or they can get the same blood and urine tests as their doctors would request by referring themselves to the many labs that accept patients without a doctor's order. They can even walk into certain radiology clinics and choose imaging scans of their organs.
- Self-medicate with an ever-expanding array of over-the-counter drugs. When nonprescription medications don't suffice, patients are increasingly telling their doctors which prescription drugs they need, often in response to ads pitching pills directly to consumers. If their doctor balks—or if they don't want to bother with an office visit—they can buy some of those drugs online without ever communicating with a doctor.

Surveys show that consumers appreciate the convenience and sense of control that self-care brings. Some research suggests that involved, self-directed patients get sick less often and recover faster than others. And bypassing the doctor can save you money. For example, you can buy the new over-the-counter (OTC) version of the allergy drug loratadine (*Claritin*) without paying for an office visit—and for less than one-fourth the cost of the older brand-name prescription version.

"But along with those benefits come new opportunities for improper and dangerous care," says Gene Herbek, M.D., a

Safe self-treatment with OTC drugs

Just because you can buy over-the-counter drugs without a prescription doesn't mean they're safe (see main report). To protect yourself:

- **Check the directions and heed warnings.** Ask your pharmacist or doctor about anything you don't understand.
- **Avoid "shotgun" remedies,** which contain multiple ingredients. You may not need those ingredients, and they raise the risk of side effects and of overdoses if you're using more than one remedy.
- **Choose by active ingredient,** not brand name, to avoid getting either the wrong ingredient or unnecessary ones.
- **If symptoms persist,** stop the drug and call your doctor. You could be masking or mistreating a serious underlying problem or becoming dependent on the drug.
- **Ask you doctor about precautions** if you're pregnant or have a chronic disease.
- **Start at the lower end** of the recommended dosage if you're over 65 or so, to reduce the risk of side effects.

pathologist and researcher who has followed the self-care movement.

Several recent studies have found that much of the health information online is plain wrong—and what's right is often hard to decipher, even for trained professionals. Similarly, many home and self-referred tests have little if any medical value; those that do work need to be interpreted and put in context. Even diagnosing prob-

lems with seemingly straightforward symptoms, such as headaches or back pain, can be surprisingly difficult. And self-medicating sometimes poses serious risks, especially since people can often overlook or disregard directions and warnings.

This report will help you determine when you need a doctor's help and when you can handle problems yourself.

SELF-DIAGNOSIS: RECOGNIZING DANGER

Most people feel comfortable identifying familiar and relatively harmless problems that have obvious symptoms, such as a runny nose and cough from a cold. But those and other common symptoms can sometimes signal more serious problems. For example, coldlike symptoms can stem from flu or pneumonia, and back pain can indicate kidney infection or even spinal-cord cancer. Such misdiagnoses are especially worrisome when they lead to treatment that masks a more serious problem. Someone who successfully controls headaches with painkillers, for example, may not realize the attacks stem from uncontrolled hypertension.

Potentially dangerous mix-ups occur more often when the symptoms are less common or clear-cut. For example, a recent study in the journal Obstetrics and Gynecology found that most women who've diagnosed themselves with a presumed yeast infection actually have other problems, most often a bacterial infection that can lead to obstetric complications and possibly cervical cancer. Other research found that women need a doctor to diagnose a yeast infection twice before they can accurately diagnose it themselves. Similarly, people who self-diagnose presumed jock itch—a rash caused by a fungus in warm, dark regions of the groin—may actually have a sexually transmitted disease.

Recommendation: To safely diagnose even common symptoms, you need to know when they may require professional attention (see When common symptoms signal serious problems). Don't try to self-diagnose less common conditions unless your doctor has previously made the same diagnosis.

SELF-TESTS: HIDDEN RISKS

Today's confident consumers are using various home and direct-access lab tests as well as self-referred X-rays and CT scans to screen themselves for unseen problems, such as elevated blood-pressure or cholesterol levels as well as cancer and clogged arteries. "Consumers can now glimpse the hidden workings of their body, something that used to be the sole and mysterious ability of doctors," says Herbek. Such tests can also be more convenient, more private, and less expensive than the same tests done in the doctor's office. "But it pays to choose carefully," Herbek cautions, "since some don't work and many require a doctor's experienced eye."

Here's what to look for:

- **Home tests.** Tests for detecting pregnancy, evaluating fertility, and monitoring blood-pressure and blood-sugar levels are clearly useful. Recent analyses by CONSUMER REPORTS identified several products in each of those categories that are accurate and easy to use.

However, many other home tests are of dubious value. For example, a scratch-and-sniff home test for Alzheimer's disease works on the premise that an impaired sense of smell precedes onset of the disease. But a recent study found no solid evidence to support that notion. Moreover, home versions of even scientifically validated tests may not work well; a recent CONSUMER REPORTS analysis of five home-cholesterol tests found that all were inaccurate, incomplete, or inconvenient. Similarly, the maker of an "instant" home-HIV test—available only online and not approved by the Food and Drug Administration (FDA)—couldn't provide us with any proof of the test's accuracy or reliability.

Still other valid home tests may be accurate but hard to interpret. For example,

home fecal-occult blood tests can detect traces of blood, a possible sign of colon cancer, in a small sample of stool smeared onto a special testing card. "But untrained individuals often have difficulty distinguishing the subtle color changes on the card that can indicate a possible problem," says John Bond, M.D., an expert on the test at the University of Minnesota.

Recommendation: The worthwhile home tests listed above should be used in tandem with a doctor, who can determine if you need to make any changes to control your blood pressure or blood sugar, confirm a pregnancy, or possibly recommend simpler ways of tracking your fertility. If you want to try other home tests, make sure they're approved by the FDA by checking the label or asking the store's pharmacist; approval suggests it's at least plausible, fairly accurate, and easy to use.

- **Self-referred lab tests.** You can get these by walking into one of the many labs that now offer them or by ordering a kit online that lets you gather your own sample and ship it to a lab for analysis. Such tests can avoid some problems of home tests, since they're identical or very similar to doctors' versions and are generally analyzed by qualified professionals.

Even moderate overdoses of presumably safe drugs can cause harm.

But there are serious limitations. Some tests require you to decipher the results largely on your own, either with basic information from the lab or with resources you track down. Others will forward the results to your doctor. But doctors often can't determine their significance without examining you or gathering other medical information. And getting a test on your own may mean skipping the step of first discussing it with your doctor. That's essential, since many tests offer unproven benefits and can lead to unnecessary and harmful treatment.

Recommendation: Consider direct access lab testing only if convenience is paramount or it will save you money because you lack insurance. Even then, limit the tests to those recommended by your physician and insist that the lab forward the results to your doctor.

- **Walk-in radiology clinics.** Random CT scans performed on the heart, lungs, or other organs of apparently healthy people—who can now order these powerful tests on their own—occasionally uncover potentially serious problems, such as an early-stage cancer. But a recent analysis of that growing trend, published in the journal Radiology, warned that random CT scans pose considerable risks that probably far outweigh the benefits: They often reveal minor abnormalities that have no clear significance but that prompt follow-up tests and treatments, some of which are potentially dangerous; and they can expose you to high doses of radiation that theoretically increase cancer risk.

Recommendation: CT scans should be done only when you and your doctor conclude that your symptoms, signs, or medical history make it likely that the test will yield useful information.

OTC DRUGS: KNOW THE LIMITS

Self-treatment usually involves over-the-counter drugs. The recent prescription-to-OTC switches of two top-selling medications, loratadine (*Claritin*) and omeprazole (*Prilosec OTC*), are part of the FDA's effort to increase the number of drugs patients can use on their own. Such switches can indeed benefit consumers; OTC loratadine, for example, is safer and more effective than other nonprescription allergy drugs. But all OTC drugs can pose risks, particularly if they're used improperly. Here are the common problems that OTC drugs can pose.

- **Overuse.** Most OTC labels warn patients to discontinue the drug after two weeks at most and to see a doctor if symptoms don't improve, because that may signal a more serious problem. In addition, frequent, repeated use of certain OTC drugs—including drugs for headache, insomnia, nasal congestion, or eye inflammation—can cause dependency: After the drug wears off, you can develop "rebound" symptoms worse than the original ones.

- **Inadequate treatment.** The ability to buy a drug over the counter sometimes persuades patients to treat themselves when they need prescription drugs. People may try to control asthma symptoms by taking the OTC bronchodilator epinephrine (*Bronkaid Mist, Primatene Mist*), for example. But prescription

When common symptoms signal serious problems

Common symptoms usually indicate common problems that can be safely and effectively self-treated with non-prescription drugs or common sense self-help measures. But sometimes they stem from serious causes that require a trip to the doctor—or the emergency room. Note that some of the indicators in the first column below become increasingly important starting at age 50 or so, when the chance of serious problems starts to rise.

SEE A DOCTOR WHEN ...	POSSIBLE CAUSE
Headache	
Is much more painful than any you've had before, or is sudden and severe.	Hemorrhagic stroke, cerebral aneurysm, or severely inflamed artery
Follows an accident.	Head injury or other trauma
Lasts longer than 24 hours.	Severely inflamed artery
Is provoked by exertion.	Hyertension
Occurs most mornings.	Sleep apnea or hypertension
Often impairs daily function, usually affects one side of the head, or is accompanied by nausea or other symptoms.	Migraine
Is accompanied by fever, stiff neck, vomiting, confusion, loss of consciousness, loss of balance, convulsions, changes in vision or speech, or numbness and weakness in a limb or on one side of the body.	Hemorrhagic stroke or, possibly, infection such as menigitis or encephalitis
Back pain	
Includes severe or progressive leg weakness, or pain radiating down from the buttock to below the knee, usually with numbness or tingling.	Herniated or fragmented disk, or spinal tumor
Follows a recent accident or is accompanied by history or high risk of osteoporosis.	Spinal fracture
Is accompanied by fever, night sweats, or a recent bacterial infection, particularly if the immune system has been weakened.	Spinal infection
Is accompanied by unexplained weight loss, history of cancer, or incontinence.	Spinal-cord cancer
Hearburn	
Is accompanied by painful or difficult swallowing.	Schatzki's ring, a benign growth in the esophagus; esophageal or stomach cancer
Doesn't improve with OTC drug use, occurs more than once a week, or requires chronic drug use.	Diabetes, stomach ulcers (Chronic heartburn can lead to asthma, bronchitis, pneumonia, precancerous growths, or esophageal cancer.)
Rash	
Spreads rapidly.	Unclear, but likely severe
Appears as red streaks on a leg or an arm.	Infection of lymph vessels
Accompanies fever, chills, sweats, or other symptoms.	Rocky Mountain spotted fever, Lyme disease, measles, meningitis, or other infection
Is painful and limited to one side of the body.	Shingles
Is on or around the eye.	Unclear, but may injure or scar the cornea
Is on or near the genitals.	Sexually transmitted disease or drug reaction
Cough, runny nose, or congestion	
Accompanies fever over 100 degrees plus one or more of these groups: muscle aches, chills, or fatigue; very sore throat or swollen glands; wheezing or cough with grayish or rust-colored phlegm.	Flu; strep throat or tonsillitis; bronchitis or pneumonia
Accompanies pain above or below the eyes or thick, yellow nasal discharge.	Sinusitis

bronchodilators such as albuterol (*Proventil, Ventolin*) are safer and more effective. And most asthma sufferers also need prescription inhaled steroids such as becomethasone (*Beclovent, Vanceril*) to prevent attacks.

- **Overdoses.** Some people treat themselves with more than the recommended dosage because they want the potency of a prescription dose. But that raises the risk of adverse effects, too, including the rarer, more worrisome ones. Self-medicating with multiple drugs makes overdoses particularly likely, since many products with different brand names contain the same active ingredient. And even moderate overdoses of single, presumably safe drugs can cause harm. For example, consuming more than three times the maximum recommended dose of acetaminophen (*Panadol, Tylenol*) can produce early signs of liver toxicity.

- **Side effects.** Even recommended doses pose risks. For example, all OTC pain killers except acetaminophen can upset the stomach and, less often, cause stomach bleeding. Side effects are especially common in people with certain chronic diseases, notably of the kidney or liver, as well as in people over 65 or so.

- **Drug interactions.** Without professional supervision, you're more likely to take drugs that can interact adversely with other medications. Even food, drink, or dietary supplements can complicate drug use. For example, repeatedly trying to calm your stomach by drinking lots of milk and taking calcium antacids can eventually cause kidney failure.

RX DRUGS: WATCH WHAT YOU ASK FOR

Direct-to-consumer ads for prescription drugs can provide potentially useful information about drugs and diseases. But such ads are obviously designed mainly to sell drugs, not to educate patients. So do some investigating before you ask your doctor for a specific drug:

- **Seek unbiased information.** Check the caveats and dosage information in Consumer Reports' Consumer Drug Reference or in an online drug reference such as that available through the National Library of Medicine (www.medline-plus.gov).

- **Be especially wary of new drugs,** which have the shortest safety record. For the latest updates, visit the FDA's Web site (www.fda.gov/med-watch/safety.htm).

- **Ask your doctor the key questions.** Do I have the condition this drug treats? What are its benefits and risks compared with other treatments? If it's a newer drug, do its benefits justify the possible risks and the often greater cost?

- **Don't pressure your doctor into prescribing a drug unless you have strong evidence that you truly need it,** such as a clear-cut recommendation from a leading medical journal or other reputable source. Even then, keep an open mind; your doctor may have good reasons for avoiding it. Your health plan may also encourage your doctor to first consider medications listed on a formulary of drugs shown to be cost-effective.

- **Resist the temptation to order online any drug that your doctor hasn't approved.** Some Web sites will sell consumers prescription drugs after conducting an online "consultation" that usually involves filling in a basic questionnaire. That cursory check can't replace a face-to-face visit with your doctor, who can confirm that you need the drug and that it won't interact with your other medications or worsen any other problems. Some sites, generally based overseas, are even more lax, requiring only your credit-card number.

But it's generally safe—and sometimes cheaper—to fill legitimate prescriptions through reputable online drugstores. Seek sites that participate in the Verified Internet Pharmacy Practice Site (VIPPS) program; they're licensed by the appropriate regulatory agencies, have no current trouble with those agencies, and are approved by the National Association of Boards of Pharmacy.

Summing up

It's possible to safely diagnose and treat many of your own health problems, provided you take certain precautions:

- **Self-diagnosis.** Be alert to the warning signs that indicate when common symptoms may stem from serious problems, and don't try to diagnose uncommon symptoms unless your doctor has previously identified them at least once. In general, use only those home diagnostic tests that clearly offer health advantages and work reliably, notably those for high blood-pressure or blood-sugar levels, pregnancy, and fertility. Use labs or radiology clinics where you order your own tests only if your doctor approves.

- **Self-treatment.** Recognize that over-the-counter medications pose risks, especially when taken longer or in higher doses than recommended, and by older people or those with certain chronic conditions. While it's fine to ask your doctor about prescription drugs, don't insist on getting them without solid support from a reputable source and only buy drugs online that your doctor has prescribed.

Making an
INFORMED DECISION
About Breast Implants

Carol Rados

Despite more than a decade of controversy over their safety, breast implants are more popular than ever among women who want to build upon what nature gave them or who want to restore what disease has taken away. Whatever the reason, opting for breast implants is a personal decision that should be made only after a woman fully understands and accepts the potential risks of the devices and the importance of follow-up evaluations with her physician.

Some people see an enormous benefit to getting implants and are willing to accept associated risks. They say that using breast implants to rebuild the breast (reconstruction), or change its size and shape (augmentation), significantly improves the quality of life for many women. Advocates of breast implants also say that a woman's consent to the surgery should be considered valid as long as she weighs the risks and benefits of the procedure.

While every surgical procedure has potential risks, such as infection, bleeding, and scarring, there are risks that are specific to breast implants. Learning about them is key to being properly informed about the procedure.

A Primer on Breast Implants

According to the American Society of Plastic Surgeons (ASPS), there were nearly 255,000 breast enhancement implant surgeries in 2003, nearly twice the number done in 1998. Another 68,000 women received breast implants for reconstruction following mastectomy due to cancer or other disease.

But also in 2003, 45,000 augmentation patients and 17,000 reconstruction patients had their breast implants removed. The medical community and others, including the Food and Drug Administration, would like to better understand why.

Breast implants are designed for augmentation, a cosmetic procedure; reconstruction; and replacement of existing implants, called revision. There are two primary types: saline filled and silicone gel-filled. Depending on the type of implant, the shell is either pre-filled with a fixed volume of solution or filled through a valve during the surgery to the desired size. Some allow for adjustments of the filler volume after surgery. Breast implants vary in shape, size, and shell texture.

While every surgical procedure has potential risks, such as infection, bleeding, and scarring, there are risks that are specific to breast implants.

At this time, there are two manufacturers with approved saline-filled breast implants. No manufacturer has yet received FDA approval to market a silicone gel-filled breast implant.

Questions to Ask a Surgeon About Breast Augmentation

- What are the risks and complications associated with having breast implants?
- How many additional implant-related operations can I expect over my lifetime?
- How will my breasts look if I choose to have the implants removed without replacement?
- What shape, size, surface texturing, incision site, and placement site is recommended for me?
- How will my ability to breast-feed be affected?
- How can I expect my implanted breasts to look over time?
- How can I expect my implanted breasts to look after pregnancy? After breast-feeding?
- What are my options if I am dissatisfied with the cosmetic outcome of my implanted breasts?
- What alternate procedures or products are available if I choose not to have breast implants?
- Do you have before-and-after photos I can look at for each procedure and what results are reasonable for me?

Source: FDA

The Silicone Controversy

Breast implants were first marketed in the early 1960s, before the 1976 Medical Device Amendments to the Federal Food, Drug, and Cosmetic Act required a reasonable assurance of safety and effectiveness to be shown for certain medical devices. The 1976 law gave the FDA authority over such devices, but breast implants were "grandfathered" into the regulatory scheme, meaning that manufacturers were not required to provide the agency with scientific evidence of product safety unless questions arose about the safety and effectiveness of these already-marketed devices. Silicone was initially assumed by manufacturers to be biologically inactive and, therefore, to have no harmful effects.

But over the years, questions did arise about the effects of silicone on the body. In 1991, the FDA published a regulation that required manufacturers of silicone gel-filled breast implants to submit premarket approval applications (PMAs). This requirement meant that the FDA needed to agree that the manufacturer has presented data showing a reasonable assurance of safety and effectiveness in order for the devices to remain on the market.

In January 1992, the FDA called for a voluntary moratorium—a delay on the use of these implants—until new safety information could be thoroughly reviewed. The moratorium was not intended to "ban" the implants, but instead to allow time to review the new safety information.

In April 1992, the agency decided that no PMA yet submitted contained sufficient safety and effectiveness data to support approval. However, access to these silicone gel-filled breast implants would continue for women enrolled in certain clinical studies.

In the years that followed that decision, thousands of women filed lawsuits against the manufacturers of silicone gel-filled implants, claiming the devices had caused serious ailments, such as connective tissue diseases, neurological diseases, and cancer. Consumer groups repeatedly filed petitions urging more studies on the implants. But many women said they were pleased with their implants, including cancer patients who had pleaded for the opportunity to choose silicone gel-filled implants for reconstruction.

A Turn of Events

In October 2003, the FDA held a two-day advisory panel meeting to discuss a manufacturer's PMA for a silicone gel-filled breast implant. Some people complained that the meeting was premature in light of the fact that long-term studies had not been completed, but the FDA proceeded because the agency was required by law to consider the pending PMA within a specified time frame. The meeting also provided patients and others with timely access to information and expert analyses on the issue. The issues before the panel reflected much of the decades-long debate over the implants. Moreover, the meeting provided a valuable public forum for discussing the issue from many diverse perspectives and for raising important additional questions.

As a panel member, Benjamin O. Anderson, M.D., voted with the majority to recommend that the FDA approve the new PMA, but only with specific conditions. Anderson says he wants to avoid getting into the business of determining how a woman defines the value of breast reconstruction or augmentation.

"The use of implants and augmentation conjures up some social judgments that may well be unfair," says Anderson, a professor of surgery and director of the University of Washington's Breast Health Center. Rather than deciding that no woman can have access to silicone gel-filled implants because a small number may be at risk for certain illnesses, he says, "I believe the better approach is to make the devices available and inform all women of the degree of risk involved."

That, according to Anderson, "is reasonable informed consent."

In January 2004—contrary to the recommendation of the agency's advisory panel—the FDA determined that the new silicone gel-filled breast implant PMA was "not approvable" at that time. This meant that the implants were not approved for marketing pending additional information, but that women would continue to have limited access to them by enrolling in clinical studies.

"The public scientific process that has been used to consider these devices is fully consistent with the FDA's mission —to use the best available science to protect and promote the public health interests of the American people," says Linda Kahan, deputy director of the FDA's Center for Devices and Radiological Health (CDRH).

Also in January 2004, the agency released a draft of its new guidelines for companies submitting breast implant PMAs, explaining the scientific issues that the FDA recommends be addressed as part of their applications. The guidance document reflects the FDA's current thinking about new scientific information that the agency, manufacturers, and the clinical community have gained over the last 10 years, including information learned at the October 2003 advisory panel meeting. Consistent with the FDA's good guidance practices, the agency has asked for public comments on the breast implant guidance. The guidance is not intended for implementation until it is finalized.

"Current testing doesn't reflect reality," says Michael A. Choti, M.D., an associate professor of surgery and oncology at the Johns Hopkins University School of Medicine in Baltimore, and also an FDA advisory panel member. The implants, he says, are extremely durable when tested outside the body. "You can virtually run a truck over them and they'll hold up. But the question is, what happens when implanted long-term in a woman's body?"

The FDA's draft guidance document says that two to three years of follow-up data may not be enough to allow the agency to evaluate the safety and effectiveness of breast implants. The agency recommends the use of tests that can predict clinical outcomes, such as how long breast implants will last before rupturing in the body, as well as tests that explain how and why the breast implants rupture. In addition, the agency recommends that more data be gathered regarding the rate of rupture over time, as well as the health consequences of rupture.

Breast Implant Risks

In 1999, the Institute of Medicine (IOM) issued a report on a review of information related to health effects associated with silicone breast implants, both gel-filled and saline-filled, in humans. An important goal of the IOM was to provide women with detailed information about the potential risks of silicone breast implants.

One risk is capsular contracture, which is a tightening and squeezing of the scar tissue that naturally forms around the implant. This contracture may result in hardening of the breast tissue, rippling of the skin, and changes in breast shape. It also may cause pain, which, if severe, can require surgery to remove the scar tissue or replace the implant.

In addition, a rupture can occur at any time. While saline-filled breast implants leak only salt water when they rupture, the health effects of leaking silicone gel-filled implants remain controversial. Women sense a change more easily when saline-filled breast implants rupture. But the silicone gel-filled implants are more likely to maintain their shape after they rupture, which can make it more difficult to detect a break.

Questions to Ask a Surgeon About Breast Reconstruction

- What are all my options for breast reconstruction?
- What are the risks and complications of each type of breast reconstruction surgery and how common are they?
- What if my cancer recurs or occurs in the other breast?
- Will reconstruction interfere with my cancer treatment?
- How many steps are there in each procedure? What are they?
- How much experience do you have with each procedure?
- What is the estimated total cost of each procedure?
- How long will it take to complete my reconstruction?
- Do you have before-and-after photos I can look at for each procedure and what results are reasonable for me?
- What will my scars look like?
- What kind of changes in my reconstructed breast can I expect over time?
- What kind of changes in my implanted breast can I expect with pregnancy?
- What are my options if I am dissatisfied with the cosmetic outcome of my implanted breast?
- How much pain or discomfort will I feel and for how long?
- How long will I be in the hospital? Will I need blood transfusions, and can I donate my own blood?
- When will I be able to resume my normal activities?

Source: FDA

Called "silent ruptures," these breaks involving silicone gel implants may occur without a visible change. And a woman may not feel any sensation, says Sahar M. Dawisha, M.D., a medical officer in CDRH who has reviewed data submitted by implant manufacturers. Magnetic resonance imaging (MRI) with equipment specifically designed for imaging the breast may be used for evaluating women with suspected rupture of their silicone gel-filled implant. The FDA considers MRI to be the best method at this time. There are no standards on how often to screen for silent rupture with MRI, and the costs of this procedure must be considered when choosing a silicone gel-filled breast implant. Physicians usually recommend removal of the implant if it has ruptured, regardless of whether it is saline-filled or silicone gel-filled.

Another potential complication of implant surgery is nerve damage, which can cause some women to experience a loss or increase in sensation in their nipples and breast tissue. These symptoms may disappear eventually, but can be permanent in some cases. It is unclear at this time whether insufficient milk production to breast-feed—another reported problem—is due to damaged nerves or to other reasons.

Women should know that, regardless of the type of implant, it is likely they will need to have one or more additional surgeries (reoperations) over the course of their lives, because of complications from breast implants. Reasons for reoperations include any of the potential complications, such as capsular contracture, wrinkling, asymmetry, rupture, or implant malposition.

The IOM committee also found that women with silicone breast implants are no more likely than women without implants to develop the life-threatening systemic illnesses that some people have claimed might be related to the implants.

But many women disagree. They have reported health problems related to their immune systems or neurological symptoms that they believe are caused by ruptured or intact breast implants. And some women who have received breast implants claim they weren't fully informed of the risks.

Lynda Roth, who was diagnosed with breast cancer in 1990, says she was forced to make a quick decision, based on very little information, about getting breast implants following a mastectomy.

"I trusted what my highly respected doctors were telling me was true," says the 63-year-old social worker in central Colorado. "You're in shock, you think you're going to die, so what kind of informed decision can you possibly make about what you want your breasts to look like if you're lucky enough to survive?"

Roth did survive—both breast cancer and two silicone breast implants gone bad. But the ruptured devices, she believes, caused her to lose her good health, her job, and eventually her health insurance over the next 11 years. "I found out the hard way," she says. "There were many risks with the implants that I didn't know about.

Other women are pleased with their implants. Clara Filion underwent reconstruction in 1993 after having a breast removal that included the lymph nodes under the arm (modified radical mastectomy) due to cancer. The 67 year old Bedias, Texas, resident says she's thrilled with the outcome of her saline filled implant, as well as with her surgeon, even though her original implant will need replacing soon due to scar tissue—a local complication that Filion says she always knew could occur, Filion has experienced no other complications related to the implant in 11 years.

Other Considerations

"My doctor told me that these implants would go with me to my grave," says 44-year-old Patty Faussett of Henderson, Nev., who chose to augment her breasts with saline breast implants in 1997, after years of breastfeeding distorted their shape.

Faussett had her implants removed a year after implantation because she believes they caused a mixed bag of health problems, including disturbed vision, heart palpitations, muscle twitching, and an autoimmune thyroid disease. She says, "The risks were much greater than my surgeon led me to believe."

Experts caution that breast implants do not last a lifetime. Women should be prepared for long term follow up and additional surgeries to treat complications. They also should be prepared for the accompanying additional costs. One of the biggest problems Faussett says she hears from women in her breast implant support group is that "most don't plan for the money it takes to fix what goes wrong."

In addition, women should be aware that hard pressure on the breast (compression) during mammography may cause implant rupture. Breast implants also can interfere with finding breast cancer during mammography. Doctors say the implant can hide breast tissue and, as a result, hide lesions as well. Extensive scarring and calcium deposits in tissue surrounding an implant can mimic the appearance of cancer, making the deposits difficult to distinguish from tumors on a mammogram.

Another consideration is the choice of a surgeon. Patient advocates, professional groups, and others agree that it's important to choose a plastic surgeon who has been trained in breast implant surgery and who has performed it successfully on many women.

After switching to a new, firmer silicone gel-filled implant through a clinical study only a year after experiencing rippling with her saline implants, Kathy Bracy says it's important that women who are considering breast implants do their homework.

"I love my breast implants, but I also spent six months researching the devices, which included picking the best doctor for me," says Bracy, a 38- year-old self-employed bookkeeper from Tampa, Fla. "It's not necessarily the product, but who is doing the surgery." The key to breast implant satisfaction, she says, is to "find a doctor who is willing to answer all your questions and take all your concerns seriously. And the relationship with your doctor doesn't end after the surgery."

Experts also advise women to have realistic expectations about breast implants. There is no guarantee that the results will match those of other women. Overall health, age, chest structure, the shape and position of the breast and nipple, skin texture, the tendency to bleed, prior breast surgeries, and the surgical team's skill and experience all figure into the outcome of breast implant surgeries.

The Teen Scene

In addition to safety issues, there is concern about the growing use of breast implants among teen-agers. Health officials worry that teen-agers and their parents may not realize the relative permanence of the changes caused by the devices. They also want to be sure that teens are physically ready—that is, they're finished developing —and that they are psychologically mature enough to handle the outcome of surgery.

"I didn't know my breasts were still growing when I signed up for the surgery," admits Kacey Long, who got saline-filled breast implants in July 2001, when she was 19. Prior to her surgery, the college student from Ennis, Texas, was a 34B—a breast size she thought would be with her for life.

Teen-agers who are dissatisfied with their bodies see breast implants as a harmless—and, according to Long, "fun"—thing to do to improve their self-image. Long says she felt that her body was too "bottom heavy" for her breasts and wanted to "even out" her figure. "But I never thought about my implants being dangerous," she says. A friend's mother worked for a plastic surgeon for 12 years and told Long she knew of no problems with patients who had gotten the implants. "I really thought that I had inside information, and that these devices were completely safe and maintenance-free."

Following implantation, Long went to a 34D. But complications convinced her to have the implants removed a short time later. "I had shooting pains in my arms, excruciating pain in every joint, bone, and muscle of my body, I was exhausted all the time, had no energy, lost my hair, and had pains in my chest, heart, and ribs. I had trouble remembering things and thinking clearly,

and the list goes on," she says. "Before the implants, all I had was allergies."

Many of the changes to the breast that occur with an implant cannot be undone. If a teen chooses to have her implants removed, she may experience dimpling, puckering, wrinkling, or other cosmetic changes.

Three years later, Long's breasts measure 36C—one size larger than before she was implanted—suggesting that her own breasts continued to develop even after the implants were removed. "When you're making a decision that can impact your life at 19," Long advises other young women, "you need to research the subject like you're 50 years old."

Ongoing clinical studies for unapproved saline-filled and silicone gel-filled breast implants do not allow for those younger than 18 to receive the implants for augmentation purposes. Some of these clinical studies even limit reconstruction and revision uses to women 18 and over.

Consumers can get a copy of the "FDA Breast Implant Consumer Handbook 2004," which provides in-depth information on both saline and silicone breast implants, by visiting www.fda.gov/cdrh/breastimplants/, or by writing to: FDA, Office of Device Evaluation, Division of General, Restorative, and Neurological Devices, 9200 Corporate Blvd., HEZ-410, Rockville, MD 20850.

From *FDA Consumer,* September/October 2004, pp. 33-37. Published 2004 by the U.S. Food and Drug Administration. www.fda.gov/cdrh/breastimplants/

How to ease your pain

Here's what you need to know to get safe relief.

The withdrawal in late September 2004 of the painkilling drug rofecoxib (*Vioxx*) because of increased heart-attack risk—plus subsequent concerns raised about celecoxib (*Celebrex*), naproxen (*Aleve, Naprosyn*), and valdecoxib (*Bextra*)—left millions of Americans scrambling for a safe and effective way to control their pain. But it's not just users of those drugs who face that predicament.

Virtually all prescription and nonprescription pain relievers pose some risks, even when used properly. Many people multiply the risks by overusing such drugs. And even high doses may not quell the pain if the doctor or patient chooses the wrong drug. Indeed, studies suggest that roughly half of people with chronic or recurrent pain fail to get adequate relief despite drug therapy.

> "Over-the-counter **acetaminophen** is often a good first choice for relieving chronic pain."

That's a huge amount of needless suffering. "Even when pain can't be completely eliminated, we now have numerous ways to rein it in so it doesn't interfere with your daily life," says Morris Levin, M.D., a pain-control expert at the Dartmouth-Hitchcock Medical Center in Hanover, N.H.

The key is knowing when and how to use nonprescription drugs, such as acetaminophen (*Tylenol*) or ibuprofen (*Advil, Motrin IB*), and, when prescription drugs are needed, being aware of the choices your doctor should consider. While the withdrawal of rofecoxib and concerns about its cousins celecoxib (*Celebrex*) and valdecoxib (*Bextra*) have made picking prescription drugs more difficult, there are several other good options, provided you and your doctor can overcome certain misconceptions.

For example, too many people refuse to consider opioids, such as codeine, because of excessive concerns about addiction. Others fail to consider drugs not normally considered painkillers, such as certain antidepressants and anticonvulsants, despite growing evidence that they're effective against some types of pain. Equally important, proper pain management means knowing which nondrug measures can sometimes relieve pain and even treat the underlying cause.

The accompanying table, "Targeted Pain Relief," describes proven or possible treatments for several common kinds of pain. Below we describe the proper use of over-the-counter (OTC) pain relievers and advise when to see a doctor for prescription drugs or other options.

ACUTE PAIN: RATE IT AND TREAT IT

For occasional or sudden pain (from common headaches, menstrual cramps, or injuries, for example), appropriate treatment starts with assessing the pain's severity. The best way is to grade your pain along a scale from 0 (no pain) to 10 (the worst pain you've ever had).

For mild-to-moderate pain, rated 5 or less, nonprescription drugs usually suffice. Though some evidence suggests that nonsteroidal anti-inflammatory drugs (NSAIDs), such as ibuprofen and, to a lesser extent, ketoprofen (*Orudis KT*) and naproxen (*Aleve*), may provide slightly faster and greater relief than aspirin or acetaminophen, all are often adequate. But certain individuals may want to choose or avoid specific pain relievers:

- Avoid aspirin if you're breast-feeding, since aspirin might cause bleeding or other problems in the baby.
- Avoid acetaminophen if you're a heavy drinker or have liver disease; even modest doses can harm the liver in such cases.
- Choose acetaminophen if you have hypertension, heart failure, ulcers, or kidney disease, which may be worsened by the other drugs. Also stick with acetaminophen if you take a daily aspirin to protect your heart. Additional aspirin might cause bleeding, while ibuprofen and possibly other NSAIDs have been shown to undermine aspirin's coronary benefits. And pick acetaminophen if you're pregnant, since the other drugs may harm the fetus and prolong labor.

If your pain is relatively severe (rated 6 or more) or persists despite the recommended doses of nonprescription medication, it's important to see your doctor for several reasons.

Targeted pain relief

Most people should treat each kind of pain listed below by trying lifestyle changes and the first treatment option. If those don't help, talk with your doctor about other options. You could also consider alternative therapies, though the evidence is usually weaker and the possible benefits smaller.

Condition	Lifestyle measures	First choice	Second choice	Alternative therapies	Cautions
Osteo-arthritis	• Lose excess weight and do low-impact exercise.	• Acetaminophen (*Tylenol*). • Capsaicin cream (*Capsin, Zostrix*).	• Ibuprofen (*Advil*). Combine with stomach-protecting drugs such as misoprostol (*Cytotec*) or omeprazole (*Prilosec, Prilosec OTC*) if you've had ulcers or gastrointestinal bleeding or have signs of GI reactions to ibuprofen.	• Glucosamine and chondroitin supplements. • Relaxation techniques, such as biofeedback, guided imagery, progressive muscle relaxation, or massage.	• Acetaminophen can harm liver when used in high doses or by heavy drinkers or liver patients. • Ibuprofen and related drugs in high doses or with extended use can cause ulcers and stomach bleeding, increase blood pressure, trigger asthma attacks, and worsen kidney problems and heart failure.
Rheumatoid arthritis	• Low-impact exercise. • Avoid triggers, such as stress, infection, and insufficient sleep.	• Ibuprofen. Combine with stomach-protecting drug such as misoprostol or omeprazole if you've had ulcers or gastrointestinal bleeding. • Capsaicin cream.	• Corticosteroids, such as prednisone (*Deltasone*), for short-term relief of acute pain. • New immunosuppressants, such as adalimumab (*Humira*), etanercept (*Enbrel*), or infliximab (*Remicade*). • Older drugs, such as gold (*Solganal*) or methotrexate (*Rheumatrex*).	• Fish oil or gamma-linolenic acid, though risks (including upset stomach, diarrhea, and increased risk of bleeding) may outweigh slight benefit.	• Steroids can cause weight gain, bruising, thin bones, cataracts, and diabetes. • Immunosuppressants can increase chance of infection. • Older drugs cost less but are riskier and less effective.
Headache	• Identify possible triggers (such as red wine, chocolate, or stress) or underlying causes (such as sleep apnea, sinus infection, or caffeine withdrawal) and try to avoid or control them.	• Acetaminophen, aspirin, or ibuprofen.	• One or more first-choice drugs combined with caffeine (*Anacin, Excedrin Migraine*). • Triptans, such as sumatriptan (*Imitrex*) or zolmitriptan (*Zomig*), for migraines. Nasal sumatriptan works fastest but is more expensive. • Ergot alkaloids, such as dihydroergotamine (*Migranal Nasal Spray*) or ergotamine (*Ergomar*).	• Relaxation techniques. • The herb feverfew (products contain variable amounts of possible active ingredient). • Botulinum toxin (*Botox*) (requires up to 30 injections, must be repeated every few months, and isn't reimbursible).	• Triptans and caffeine drugs more likely to cause "rebound" headaches as drug wears off. •Triptans can cause flushing, dizziness, tightness in chest; can't be used if you have heart disease. • Ergot alkaloids cost less but are less effective. Can cause nausea, vomiting, diarrhea, and muscle cramps.
Back pain	• Apply cold pack for first day or two, then heating pad; resume gentle exercise as soon as possible. • Strengthen muscles in the abdomen and back to prevent pain.	• Aspirin. • Ibuprofen. Combine with stomach-protecting drugs such as misoprostol or omeprazole, or take acetaminophen, if you've had ulcers or gastrointestinal bleeding. • Capsaicin cream.	• For acute, severe pain, possibly opioids, such as oxycodone (*Oxycontin*) or fentanyl (*Duragesic*); muscle relaxants, such as cyclobenzaprine (*Flexeril*) or methocarbamol (*Carbacot, Robaxin*); or, for pinched nerve, steroid injections. • For chronic pain, tricyclic antidepressants, such as amitriptyline, or possibly surgery.	• Hands-on care, including chiropracty, massage, or physical therapy. • Botulinum (*Botox*) injections.	• Opioids, muscle relaxants, and tricyclic antidepressants can cause sedation, dizziness, confusion, urinary retention, and other problems, especially in older people.
Muscle or joint injury	• Rest, ice, compression, and elevation for first 24-48 hours or until inflammation subsides, then heat. • Resume gentle activity as soon as possible.	• Acetaminophen, aspirin, or ibuprofen.	• Physical therapy for chronic muscle pain and possibly surgery.	• Massage • Acupuncture.	• Acetaminophen can harm liver when used in high doses or by heavy drinkers or liver patients. • Ibuprofen and related drugs in high doses or with extended use can cause ulcers and stomach bleeding, increase blood pressure, trigger asthma attacks, and worsen kidney problems and heart failure.
Irritable bowel syndrome (IBS)	• Drink more fluids, limit triggering foods, and eat more high-fiber foods (except beans and cabbage, which can cause gas). • Regular physical activity.	• For IBS with constipation, high-fiber supplements or, for short-term use, nonprescription laxatives such as docusate (*Colace, Sof-lax*). • For IBS with diarrhea, OTC loperamide (*Imodium A-D*).	• For IBS with constipation, tegaserod (*Zelnorm*). • For IBS with diarrhea, diphenoxylate (*Lomotil*); cholestyramine (*Questran*); antispasmodics, such as hyoscyamine (*Levsin*); combination products, such as *Donnatal*; or tricyclic antidepressants.	• Relaxation techniques, especially stress management.	• Tegaserod for short-term use only; can cause severe diarrhea and intestinal problems. See doctor immediately if rectal bleeding, bloody diarrhea, or new or worse abdominal pain develops. • Frequent laxative use can worsen constipation.
Neuropathy (from diabetes, shingles, fibromyalgia, other causes)	• Treat underlying condition, such as diabetes.	• Tricyclic antidepressants; anticonvulsants, such as gabapentin (*Neurontin*); lidocaine patch (*Lidoderm*); or capsaicin cream.	• Nerve-block injections or surgery, especially for face and head pain caused by nerve damage. • Psychotherapy to develop pain-management strategies.	• Relaxation techniques. • Acupuncture.	• Consider seeking referral to pain clinic if pain persists.

Treating yourself by boosting the doses increases the risks, particularly with acetaminophen, since more than 4 grams a day—the daily maximum for adults—can damage the liver. And the drug you've chosen may not work against your type of pain, regardless of the dosage. Moreover, it's essential to stop acute, severe pain early because it becomes harder to control as it worsens.

Prescription NSAIDs, some of them stronger versions of the corresponding OTC drug, may yield additional relief. However, the risks generally increase along with the benefits as the dosage rises. A better approach to severe, acute pain is often a prescription opioid, such as codeine or hydrocodone. With proper dosing, you can remain reasonably alert, and short-term treatment carries little risk of addiction.

Drugs that pair an opioid with acetaminophen, aspirin, or ibuprofen may be an even better choice: They provide greater relief, since the two ingredients work in different ways, and they reduce the risk of side effects because the combination permits smaller doses of each one.

CHRONIC PAIN: LIMIT THE RISKS

You should also see your physician if you've taken a nonprescription analgesic regularly for more than about 10 days, regardless of the pain's severity. Drug risks rise with prolonged use, and your doctor may be able to recommend a better treatment. Tell him or her how severe the pain is and what it feels like—a steady ache, a sharp pain, or a burning or shooting sensation, for example—because different types respond to different drugs.

People with osteoarthritis or other chronic pain should first try the nondrug measures described in the accompanying table that may reduce or even eliminate the need for medication. If those steps don't help, their physician may first recommend a nonprescription drug. Acetaminophen is a good initial choice because even frequent, prolonged use is reasonably safe if you stick with the recommended doses and have no increased risk of liver damage.

However, many people with arthritis or other chronic pain need greater relief, which NSAIDs may provide. In theory, celecoxib (*Celebrex*) and valdecoxib (*Bextra*), like their banished cousin rofecoxib (*Vioxx*), may be less likely to cause gastrointestinal bleeding than the other, older NSAIDs. But some research has raised concerns about celecoxib and valdecoxib, too. For now, at least, our medical consultants advise people with elevated cardiovascular risk to avoid those drugs; other people should take them with considerable caution and only after careful consultation with their physician.

One alternative is ibuprofen, since some research suggests it may be gentler on the stomach than most of the NSAIDs unrelated to *Vioxx*. Those who've had ulcers or bleeding or who have any gastrointestinal reactions to ibuprofen should consider taking it with a stomach protecting drug, such as misoprostol (*Cytotec*) or omeprazole (*Prilosec*, *Prilosec OTC*). And try to use the pills just to treat flare-ups, not continually to prevent them.

If NSAIDs don't control chronic pain, opioids may, though the risk of addiction with frequent use generally makes them a last resort. A better choice is often an antidepressant such as amitriptyline or an anticonvulsant such as gabapentin (*Neurontin*). They can substantially relieve the burning or shooting pain from certain common neurologic disorders, such as diabetic nerve damage, apparently by interfering with certain brain chemicals.

People with unresolved chronic pain despite treatment should ask for a referral to a pain clinic. Such facilities take a multidisciplinary approach, with neurologists, anesthesiologists, psychiatrists, and other specialists collaborating on a treatment plan that eases pain, avoids drug dependency, and helps people resume a normal life.

WHAT YOU CAN DO

- For our latest recommendations on pain-relieving drugs, go to our new health-letter Web site

- For short-term relief of mild to moderate pain, use nonprescription drugs, such as acetaminophen or ibuprofen; for severe pain, see your doctor, who may prescribe an opioid.

- For chronic pain, try nondrug steps when possible and see your doctor, who may prescribe a treatment described in the accompanying table.

- Avoid celecoxib and valdecoxib if you have increased cardiovascular risk; if you don't, use those drugs with considerable caution. Consider taking ibuprofen plus a stomach-protecting medication if you need an NSAID but have elevated gastrointestinal risk.

UNIT 10

Contemporary Health Hazards

Unit Selections

Key Points to Consider

- What connection, if any, exists between bacterial and viral infections and the development of chronic illness such as cancer, cardiovascular disease, asthma, and multiple sclerosis?

- Why was there a shortage of flu vaccine in the 2004-2005 season?

- Why do you think many Americans avoid getting a flu shot?

- What can you do to protect yourself from mad cow disease?

- How does exposure to loud noise affect your health?

- What diseases are most likely to have an environmental link?

- What is autism?

- Why do you think autism has increased so dramatically in the past 20 years?

Student Website
www.mhcls.com/online

Internet References
Further information regarding these websites may be found in this book's preface or online.

Centers for Disease Control: Flu
http://www.cdc.gov/flu

Center for the Study of Autism
http://www.autism.org

Noise Pollution Clearinghouse
http://www.nonoise.org

Food and Drug Administration Mad Cow Disease Page
http://www.fda.gov/oc/opacom/hottopics/bse.html

Environmental Protection Agency
http://www.epa.gov

This unit examines a variety of health hazards that Americans must face on a daily basis and includes topics ranging from environmental health issues to newly emerging infectious illness. During the 1970s and 1980s Americans became deeply concerned about toxic substances in our air, water, and food. While some improvements have been observed in these areas, much remains to be done as new areas of concern continue to emerge. In "What's at Risk?" John Eyles and Nicole Consitt address issues related to health and the environment. Newly recognized diseases such as Severe Acute Respiratory Syndrome (SARS), AIDS, West Nile Virus, and Mad Cow Disease may have environmental relationships. Another disease that may have environmental relationships is autism though doctors truly don't know the exact cause. They do know, however, that autism cases continue to rise which may be due to better diagnoses or to an increase in whatever it is that is causing this vexing brain disorder that now affects one in 166 children in the United States.

One other environmental issue that can affect our health is noise pollution. While many people consider it to be merely an annoyance, author Jeffrey Kluger identifies several health risks related to loud noise exposure. These include hearing loss, sleep disturbances, and high blood pressure.

Mad cow disease has been present in the British beef supply since the early 1980s. Recently, the organism responsible for the disease was discovered in Washington State causing a ban on U.S. beef exports. Prions, the agent at the root of the condition, cannot be killed off by cooking or other conventional means. The organism is transmitted to cattle via feed mixed with tissue from sheep and other animals. Humans who eat contaminated beef may develop the fatal neurological disease known as Creutzfeldt-Jakob. In "Agencies Work to Corral Mad Cow Disease," Linda Bren discusses ways to avoid eating contaminated beef.

While emerging diseases such as Mad Cow Disease make headlines, the latest strain of influenza virus hits the country with the vengeance. Between October 2003 and January 2004, 93 children under 18 died from the flu. Most were not vaccinated. When consumers flocked to doctors and clinics demanding flu shots, they were told that supplies were not adequate. During the 2004-2005 season, consumers again tried to get flu shots only to again be turned away. One of the two suppliers of influenza vaccine was forced to discard the serum due to contamination. This led to calls for reform of the development and distribution system of influenza vaccination.

While this unit focuses on exogenous factors that influence our state of health, it is important to remember that health is a dynamic state representing the degree of harmony or balance that exists between endogenous and exogenous factors. This concept of balance applies to the environment as well. Due to the intimate relationship that exists between people, animals, and their environment, it is impossible to promote the concept of wellness without also safeguarding the quality of our environment, both physical and social.

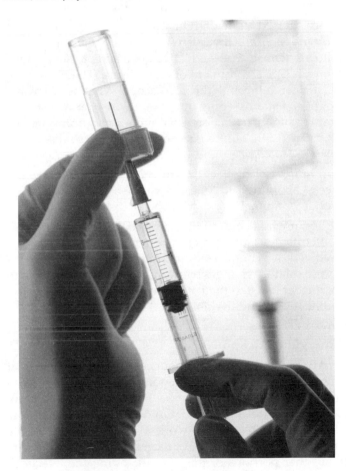

Agencies Work to Corral Mad Cow Disease

Linda Bren

When he entered his lab on Dec. 23, 2003, Allen Jenny, D.V.M., knew right away that something was wrong. He recalls the solemn expression on the face of a fellow scientist, who said, "I've got a slide to show you." Jenny, a U.S. Department of Agriculture (USDA) pathologist, peered through the microscope. What he saw was a bright red stain seeping into the gray matter of a slice of brain tissue—a telltale sign of bovine spongiform encephalopathy (BSE), otherwise known as mad cow disease.

"Are you sure it's a cow?" Jenny asked, a logical question in light of the fact that the National Veterinary Services Laboratory in Ames, Iowa, also tests sheep, deer, and other animals for mad cow-like diseases.

Yes, it was a cow, and this first diagnosis of BSE in the United States launched an emergency investigation that involved two countries—the United States and Canada—and regulatory changes by two U.S. government agencies to further bolster their effective safeguards to protect public health and livestock.

Emergency Response

After U.S. authorities announced on the same day that a single dairy cow in Washington state was infected with the fatal brain-wasting disease, BSE, the Food and Drug Administration and the USDA took immediate action. While the USDA went to work to trace the origin of the cow and to initiate a recall of its meat, the FDA made sure that other portions of the cow, including the infectious brain and spinal cord, didn't get into animal feed or other FDA-regulated products. It is believed that BSE spreads when cows eat feed containing remnants of infected cattle. The FDA, which regulates animal feed, has banned the use of these remnants in feed for cattle and other ruminants, such as sheep and goats, since 1997. Canada implemented a similar ban at the same time.

USDA investigators and Canadian health officials found the herd the infected cow originally came from, identified her former herd mates, and then traced many of them to the herds they were later sent to.

"BSE does not spread from cow-to-cow contact," says Stephen F. Sundlof, D.V.M., Ph.D., director of the FDA's Center for Veterinary Medicine. "But we wanted to find these cows because they may have shared a common feed source when they were young," he says, and might also be infected.

An exhaustive search uncovered no other infected cows.

By the time the BSE investigation was completed in February 2004, the USDA had examined the identification tags and other devices on 75,000 cattle in three states—Washington, Oregon, and Idaho—and had humanely slaughtered 255 adult cattle and tested them for BSE.

Previously, in May 2003, Canadian authorities had reported finding the first native BSE cow in North America. Records indicated that this cow and the one found in Washington were more than six years old. "We now have very good evidence that both of these animals were born prior to the feed ban" in the United States and Canada, says Ron DeHaven, chief veterinarian at the USDA.

New Safeguards

Beginning as far back as 1989, the FDA and the USDA had set up a series of safeguards to protect against the spread of BSE. The two agencies have continually evaluated these safeguards and other possible measures to protect public health. After finding the BSE-infected cow in Washington, the agencies introduced some additional measures to further safeguard human and animal health. [Photos Omitted]

The FDA and the USDA work in complementary roles to protect the food supply, and both have regulatory responsibilities. The FDA's responsibility in the human food area generally covers all domestic and imported food except meat, poultry, and frozen, dried, and liquid eggs, which are under the authority of the USDA. But the FDA does regulate certain foods that contain a small amount of meat, such as soups, gravies, and pizza with meat topping. In addition, the FDA regulates animal feed. The USDA also protects and improves the health of the

Cow Parts Banned From the Human Food Chain

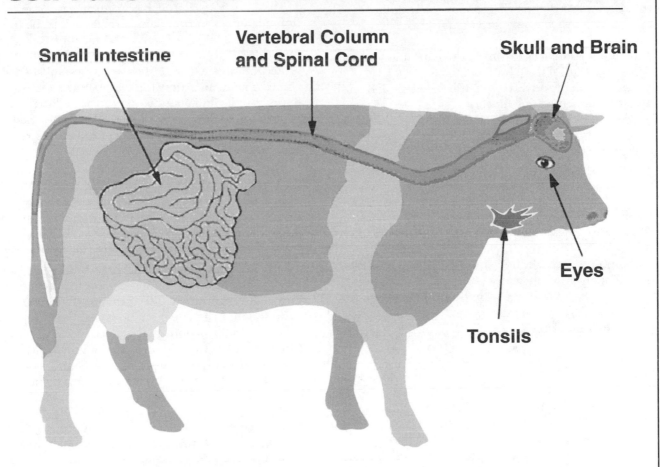

Parts of cattle at high risk for harboring the infectious agent for bovine spongiform encephalopathy (BSE), or mad cow disease, include the skull, brain, eyes, vertebral column, and spinal cord of cows at least 30 months of age. The tonsils and a portion of the small intestine of all cattle also may contain the agent. Federal agencies protect public health by prohibiting these cow parts in the human food supply.

Infographic: FDA/Michael Ermarth

nation's animals by preventing, controlling, and eliminating animal diseases.

Agriculture Secretary Ann M. Veneman announced the USDA's additional measures to protect against BSE on Dec. 30, 2003. These measures include prohibiting all material from non-ambulatory cattle in human food, removing certain cattle tissues from the human food chain, and banning certain nervous system tissues in meat products obtained by an industrial technology to cut meat from bones called advanced meat recovery.

On Jan. 26, 2004, Health and Human Services Secretary Tommy G. Thompson announced the FDA's new measures, including banning certain additional materials from animal feed. "These actions will make strong public health protections against BSE even stronger," said Thompson.

Previous Safeguards

The recent measures to protect against BSE add strength to the federal government's already effective series of safeguards, or "firewalls." If one firewall fails, multiple backup safeguards are in place to continue protecting the public.

The first firewall is the USDA's 1989 ban on importing live ruminants and subsequent USDA and FDA import controls over most ruminant products from countries with BSE or considered to be at risk for BSE.

USDA's Additional Safeguards

On Dec. 30, 2003, the USDA announced additional measures to bolster safeguards against mad cow disease:

• Banning all material from cattle that cannot walk ("downer" cattle) from human food.

• Holding all products from cattle tested for BSE until tests are confirmed negative.

• Prohibiting from human food certain "high-risk" organs and tissues from cattle older than 30 months, and the small intestine from cattle of all ages.

• Prohibiting the use of certain materials in advanced meat recovery, an industrial technology that scrapes muscle tissue away from the bone of beef carcasses. This ban will ensure that spinal cord and other high-risk tissues are not included in products for human use.

• Prohibiting air-injection stunning. This is a method of humanely stunning cattle during slaughter, but it poses the possibility that brain tissue, at high risk for BSE, could contaminate cow parts that become food or people or animals.

The second firewall, the USDA's surveillance program to look for BSE in cows, began in 1990. It was through this program that the BSE-infected cow in Washington was found. The USDA has tested more than 20,000 cows for BSE in each of the last two years, and plans on significantly increasing its testing to test every animal in the high-risk cattle population in 2004 and 2005.

Despite this rigorous surveillance program, some people have called for testing all slaughtered cows. But many of these cows are young and the BSE agent doesn't usually show up in animals until after 30 months of age, says DeHaven. "This is a disease with a very long incubation period—typically three to eight years," he says. "To suggest that we would test all animals regardless of age at slaughter is not consistent with the science and what we know about the disease."

"Animals may get exposed at a very young age," says Linda Detwiler, D.V.M., adjunct professor at the University of Maryland. "During the incubation period, the BSE agent replicates in certain tissues of the body and usually after three years makes its way to the brain." The tests used today can detect the infection only in the brain—not in other tissues or blood, so BSE cannot be diagnosed in very young animals, says Detwiler. "The animal may be infected, but it just can't be detected."

Detwiler uses the analogy of looking for a human disease, such as Alzheimer's, to explain the rationale for the current BSE surveillance system. "If you didn't know that Alzheimer's was in the United States, what population would you concentrate on to be able to find it?" asks Detwiler. "Would

you start taking brain biopsies from teen-agers, middle-aged, or older people? Testing older folks with dementias increases your chance of finding the disease."

The FDA's 1997 feed rule, which bans most protein from mammals in ruminant animal feed, is the third BSE firewall. In 2001, the Harvard Center for Risk Analysis concluded that the feed rule provided the nation's major protection against BSE becoming established in the United States. In August 2003, Harvard reaffirmed the findings of its initial study and concluded that if infected animals or feed material entered the United States from Canada, the risk of spreading extensively within U.S. herds was extremely low.

The fourth firewall is the additional protective measures recently taken by the FDA and the USDA, and the fifth firewall is the emergency response plan that the agencies initiated immediately after finding the BSE-positive cow in Washington state.

Some critics have suggested that the federal government take further actions, such as tightening slaughter controls and feed regulations, similar to practices used by European governments in their efforts to combat BSE. "You shouldn't equate the actions that the Europeans had to take with the actions that we need to take because the situation in the two continents was very different when BSE was discovered in each continent," says Murray Lumpkin, M.D., the FDA's deputy commissioner for special programs. "In Europe, BSE was at an epidemic stage in their cattle population with ultimately thousands of cases identified. So they had to put in place measures not only to keep BSE from spreading but to contain an epidemic. Based on their experience, we put many BSE firewalls in place before we had any evidence of disease in this country."

Feed Ban Enforcement

Since the feed rule went into effect in 1997, FDA and state inspectors have conducted more than 26,000 inspections involving more than 13,000 firms that handle animal feed.

'Regulations are only as good as your enforcement activities.'

"Regulations are only as good as your enforcement activities," says Sundlof. When violations are found, the firm must quickly address them and undergo a prompt follow-up inspection. Depending on the nature of the violation, a firm's products could be recalled, it could receive an FDA warning letter that demands a response from the firm about how it will correct the violations, or it could find itself in court. Renderers, feed mills, and protein blenders that process materials prohibited for ruminants are inspected at least annually, and more frequently if they are not in compliance with the rule, says Sundlof.

From 1997 to the end of 2003, 47 feed firms had recalled a total of 280 feed products, the FDA had issued 63 warning letters, and the court had ordered one permanent injunction against a feed company. The recall track record is improving: Only 12 of the 280 recalls occurred during 2003.

Sundlof says a strong education program on the feed rule for industry and inspectors has contributed to the high rate of compliance, which has climbed from 75 percent when inspections first began in 1997 to more than 99 percent today.

"The compliance rate is the highest of any FDA compliance program in all of the categories of products that we regulate," says Acting Commissioner of Food and Drugs Dr. Lester M. Crawford. "It is probably the most effective regulatory program that FDA has had in its 100-year history."

All of the firms involved in the investigation of the BSE-infected cow in Washington were in compliance with the FDA's feed rule.

The agency is stepping up its inspections of feed facilities to further ensure compliance. The FDA, along with state agencies, plans to conduct 6,600 inspections in 2004, several hundred more than the previous year.

Protecting Foods and Cosmetics

Protecting the food supply from BSE includes ensuring not only the safety of meat, but also of milk and other foods, including dietary supplements, which may contain ingredients from cows.

There is no scientific evidence that milk and dairy products pose any risk for transmitting BSE to humans, and people should not be concerned about consuming milk and milk products, says the FDA's Center for Food Safety and Applied Nutrition.

Other cow-derived foods, such as gelatin, are also protected from BSE through FDA regulations and guidance to manufacturers. And since 1992, the FDA has advised dietary supplement manufacturers and distributors to take steps to ensure that supplement ingredients come from BSE-free herds. The agency also has directed manufacturers of soaps, lipsticks, and other cosmetics that may contain fat or other ingredients from cows to use only ingredients from BSE-free cattle.

Protecting the Blood Supply

Until recently, the possibility of getting the human form of mad cow disease, called variant Creutzfeldt-Jakob disease (vCJD), through tainted blood was only a theory. But in December 2003, authorities in the United Kingdom announced the death of an adult from vCID whom they believe was infected by a blood transfusion during surgery seven and a half years earlier. The blood had been donated by a young, apparently healthy person in 1996, who died three years later from vCJD.

"We've taken the theoretical risk of blood-borne infection seriously for years, even before the U.K. transfusion case appeared," says David Asher, M.D., head of an FDA laboratory that studies contaminants in blood and tissues. Although there are no rapid, reliable tests to screen the blood supply for vCJD, the FDA has worked with blood centers since 1999 to exclude blood donations by people who lived in the U.K. during a high-risk period for BSE. In 2002, the agency added exclusions of people who might have been exposed to BSE while living elsewhere in Europe.

Protecting Medical Products

Certain cattle parts are used to produce a variety of medical products regulated by the FDA, including some blood products, drugs, devices, vaccines, and human cell- and tissue-based products. For example, some oral medications contain amino acids from cow tissues. Vaccines may be made by growing viruses in cell cultures using a highly diluted cow blood product called fetal bovine serum. And diseased heart valves in people may be replaced with medical devices made from tissues surrounding the heart of a cow.

In regulating these and other medical products, the FDA has advised manufacturers to use cow materials only from BSE free herds and has recommended that non-animal materials be used in their products whenever possible. Human medical products—whether they're devices or biologics or drugs—have preapproval requirements, says Lumpkin. When companies come to the FDA for approval, "we work with them on their manufacturing processes, what materials go into the products, and where those materials come from," he says.

The FDA continues to evaluate its regulations and guidances and seeks advice from experts outside the agency to help keep pace with the evolving science relating to transmissible spongiform encephalopathies (TSEs), the family of degenerative diseases of the nervous system that includes BSE and vCJD.

One forum for soliciting independent opinions is the TSE Advisory Committee, a group of scientists and medical experts who met most recently in Silver Spring, Md., in February 2004. In this two-day public meeting, the committee discussed additional measures that the agency might take to further minimize the risk of getting a TSE disease from FDA-regulated medical products. The agency will consider the recommendations of this committee in its regulatory decision-making to keep medical products safe.

Better BSE Science

No one knows for certain what causes BSE, but the leading scientific theory is that an abnormal form of a protein called a prion is responsible. All humans and other mammals have prion proteins in their cells that are harmless in their normal form, but become potentially

CJD and vCJD: Two Different Diseases

As of February 2004, 156 cases of the human form of mad cow disease, known as variant Creutzfeldt-Jakob disease (vCJD), have been reported worldwide, according to the Centers for Disease Control and Prevention (CDC). But there has never been a case of vCJD contracted in the United States. One resident of Florida was diagnosed in 2002 with a probable case of vCJD, but it is believed she acquired it in the United Kingdom, where she lived for more than 12 years during an epidemic of bovine spongiform encephalopathy (BSE), or mad cow disease. It is believed that the vCJD victims got the human variant by eating beef products that came from BSE-infected cattle.

The classic form of CJD has been found in the United States. Unlike the variant, the classic form is not known to be food-related. "CJD and vCJD are best thought of as two different diseases," says Lawrence Schonberger, M.D., M.P.H., epidemiologist and assistant director of

the CDC's National Center for Infectious Diseases. "CJD was around long before the emergence of BSE in cattle." Both diseases are brain disorders, but the patterns of the brain lesions they leave are distinct.

Variant CJD is found in younger patients and the length of illness is longer. There is no treatment for either disease, and they always result in death. The average age for death of vCJD is under 30 years versus the mid- to late 60s for classic CJD.

Neither vCJD nor CJD is spread through direct contact with others with the infection. The classic form of CJD may be inherited (familial), transmitted by infectious surgical instruments or tissues (iatrogenic), or occur among people with no known environmental risk factors (sporadic). The sporadic form generally occurs at a rate of about 1 case per million people per year, and familial and iatrogenic cases are even rarer, according to the CDC.

damaging when they fold into a different shape, clump together, and accumulate in brain tissue. In BSE, abnormal prions are believed to enter the bodies of mammals when they eat tissues contaminated with these prions.

Researchers worldwide are studying how prions cause BSE and other TSEs and how to block the conversion of normal prion protein to the abnormal form, which may lead to methods to prevent or treat these deadly diseases.

Other areas of research focus on developing tests to diagnose TSEs in humans and animals and developing methods to detect the abnormal prions in animal feed and human food. Scientists are trying to find ways to detect BSE in live cattle, since current tests can detect it only by examining brain tissue after death.

Diagnosis of the human form of BSE, vCJD, is also confirmed by looking at brain tissue. In humans, this tissue may be collected through a biopsy while the person is ill or collected after the person has died.

Probable cases can be diagnosed in living people based on their symptoms and the results of either a tonsil biopsy or two non-invasive tests of the brain, electroencephalogram and magnetic resonance imaging. The tonsil biopsy is invasive and requires anesthetizing the patient, says Lawrence Schonberger, M.D., M.P.H., epidemiologist and assistant director of the Centers for Disease Control

and Prevention's National Center for Infectious Diseases. "What we're really looking for is a urine or blood test," he says, and research continues to identify less invasive tests.

FDA researchers are developing tests to detect the prohibited proteins in animal feed for cows. These tests will help the agency enforce the feed ban, allowing samples of feed from processing facilities to be checked to ensure that they do not contain the protein that may carry the BSE agent.

FDA scientists are also evaluating decontamination techniques to try to rid TSE agents from surgical instruments, hospital rooms, and other areas where patients and health care workers may be accidentally exposed. Using an evaluation method they developed, FDA scientists have found that conventional decontamination procedures, such as heating with steam augmented by soaking in solutions of lye or using chlorine bleach, "are extremely effective in removing most of the infectivity," says Asher. "This is contrary to the mythology that boiling, heating, or other sterilization doesn't kill the agent," he says. "They don't remove 100 percent of infectivity under worst-case circumstances, but they are successful in removing huge amounts of infective material."

From *FDA Consumer*, May/June 2004, pp. 29-35. Published 2004 by the U.S. Food and Drug Administration. www.fda.gov/oc/opacom/hottopics/bse.html

Just Too LOUD

Car alarms! Boom boxes! Leaf blowers! If the noise isn't making you crazy, it may be making you sick

By JEFFREY KLUGER

TED RUETER ISN'T JOKING ABOUT possibly moving to New Zealand. And if he does go, it won't be the frenzy or the expense of living in the U.S. that drives him away. It will be the leaf blowers. Americans now own more than 90 million of the infernal things, he says, each of them making the job of lawn clearing much easier—and much, much louder. Rueter, a onetime political-science professor at UCLA who is head of the advocacy group Noise Free America, already fled Los Angeles to get away from the leaf-blower blight, only to move to New Orleans and find the problem just as bad there. "Everywhere has turned into leaf-blower hell," he says.

It's not just the blowers that are driving Rueter daft. It's the boom cars—those high-decibel, low-frequency speakers on wheels that cause your windshield to buzz and your eardrums to pulse when they pull up next to you at a stoplight. It's the car alarms too, as well as the barking dogs and the banging garbage trucks and the screaming airplanes and the roaring highways and the plaster-cracking sound tracks in action movies that shake the seats not only in the theater where an action movie is being shown but in the one on the other side of the multiplex wall where *some* people are trying to watch a Merchant-Ivory film, if you don't mind. It's the explosion of ambient noise that seems to be everywhere, costing more and more people not only their sleep and their sanity but increasingly their hearing and health as well.

According to the National Institutes of Health, more than 10 million Americans already suffer some permanent noise-induced hearing loss. The National Institute of Occupational Safety and Health (NIOSH) reports that some 30 million are exposed to daily noise levels that will eventually reduce their ability to hear. One in eight children between the ages of 6 and 19 already have some degree of hearing loss, and adults who are going deaf are doing so earlier and earlier. "The greatest increase [in noise-related hearing loss] occurs for people 45 to 64 years old," says Dr. James Battey, director of the National Institute on Deafness and Other Communication Disorders. "This is almost 20 years younger than we would expect."

And it's not just our ears the noise is hurting. It takes sounds in excess of 85 decibels (db) to damage hearing, but noise at less than 75 db may be linked to hypertension, and that at just 65 db leads to stress, heart damage and depression. Think the noise in your environment doesn't rise to that level? Think again. A ringing telephone can reach 80 db; a hair dryer hits 90 db; an ambulance siren can top out at an excruciating 120 db. "Noise pollution is truly a public health threat," says Representative Nita Lowey of New York, who has reintroduced a bill in Congress to turn down the volume. "It's critical," she says, "that we work to diminish the impact [noise] has on our communities."

The booming of America has many causes. Population growth in city centers, loss of rural land to suburban sprawl, and the soaring number and size of cars on the highways all play a role. So too does the entertainment industry, with Walkmans, iPods and surround-sound theaters pouring noise into consumers' ears. Even sports stadiums, always noisy places, have got louder as earsplitting commercials fill the comparatively quiet interludes that used to prevail during pauses in the action. Also to blame are moves made in Washington more than a generation ago. In 1972, the Office of Noise Abatement and Control (ONAC) was created to identify sources of noise and combat them. But in 1981, Congress and the Reagan Administration eliminated ONAC funding, removing one federal blanket that had been thrown over the din.

Whatever the roots of the problem, the clamor is now everywhere—and the workplace may be the worst place of all. At least 20% of U.S. workers do their jobs in environments that could endanger their hearing, according to NIOSH. The U.S. government estimates that more than 90% of coal miners suffer hearing impairment by age 50. Even farms are not exempt: according to the New York Center for Agricultural Medicine and Health, a staggering 75% of farmers now exhibit some hearing impairment, mostly as a result of noisy equipment. "Hearing loss is one of the most common workplace conditions," says audiologist Ted

Madison, president of the National Hearing Conservation Association.

For kids, the racket starts in the cradle. A squeaky toy held close to the ear—which is precisely where babies may put them—can reach 94 db. A toy xylophone can ring in at 92 db. And since babies' ear canals are so small, a sound that gets in them may knock around harder than it does in an adult's ears and do commensurately more damage. When these battered baby ears make it to high school they only suffer more abuse as kids start listening to music at full volume and going to dance clubs where wall-to-wall reverberation is the point.

A single noisy motor scooter **driving through Paris in the middle of the night can wake up** as many as 200,000 people

Noise can be controlled to an extent, depending on the source. Some of the biggest sources of ambient noise are highways and roads, but the cause is less honking horns or gunning engines—though those play a role—than tires hitting pavement. Pliable rubber making contact with asphalt doesn't seem as if it would produce a lot of noise but in fact it does, and in a lot of ways. As any spot on the tire strikes the highway, it hits with the thunk of a little rubber hammer. Also, the patch of tire that's in contact with the ground at any instant—the so-called tread block—can squeak like a sneaker on a gym floor and pop like a suction cup when it pulls back off the surface. Air pumping through tire grooves makes noise of its own.

The solution, says engineer Bob Bernhard, co-director of Purdue University's Institute for Safe, Quiet and Durable Highways, is to change not the tires but the road surface. "You can make the pavement porous," he says, "which affects the air-pumping

mechanism. You can also mix a little rubber in with the asphalt, which changes the road's stiffness." Porous surfaces are already being rolled out in parts of Georgia, Florida and Arizona, as well as in Europe.

Road noise that cannot be eliminated can be muffled. More and more highways are being framed by high walls, additions that do little for the view but an awful lot for the peace and quiet of the people living nearby. The walls reduce noise by either reflecting or absorbing it. This low-tech though pricey fix—about $1 million a mile—reduces sound levels only as much as 7 db, but given the exponential way noise propagates, that's a lot. "A 10-db reduction may work out to a halving of loudness," says Nicholas Miller, head of Harris Miller Miller & Hanson, a noise-consulting firm in Burlington, Mass.

Airport noise is harder to stifle but not impossible. An airport can determine which of its runways require a plane to fly over the least populated area and use those as its default approaches. Miller's firm recommends that noisy banking on takeoffs and landings occur over water where possible. Other studies suggest that pilots eliminate the stair-step method of descending from flight and instead ease down at a smooth angle to eliminate a lot of noisy throttling.

Local governments have also started to step in. In 2002, New York City launched what it calls Operation Silent Night, a campaign to crack down on noise in 24 high-volume neighborhoods. Police officers with noise meters impose fines from $45 to $25,000—the highest ones going to scofflaw businesses like nightclubs. Noise summonses jumped 20% in the first year, making the city not only quieter but safer too, since some of the noisiest offenders turned out to have outstanding warrants for more serious offenses.

The European Union has been somewhat more aggressive in com-

batting noise. Calls for explicit limits on noise were rejected by the European Parliament, but compromise legislation does require all member countries to produce color-coded, 3-D noise maps of all major cities, enabling planners to spot the biggest problems at a glance. The maps, which must be completed by 2007, can then be used for computer models to test the noise impact of a new building or street design before construction begins. In a city like Paris, where a single noisy motor scooter in the middle of the night can wake up more than 200,000 people, a little planning can go a long way.

In the U.S., there is still no comparable program. Representative Lowey's bill, now pending in Congress, would provide $20 million a year for noise reduction and reopen the shuttered noise-abatement office. Some appliances are now designed for reduced noise, and a uniform-labeling program could enable consumers to compare decibel levels the same way they compare energy efficiency in a toaster or dishwasher.

Ted Rueter's Noise Free America is pushing a more aggressive approach, filing class actions against makers of boom-car equipment, for example. "The ads that companies run to encourage kids to invest in these things are despicable," he gripes. He hopes that restaurants and other establishments will be required to post noise levels at the door alongside no-smoking, occupancy-limit and alcohol-warning signs.

Such micromanagement of noise may never be entirely possible, but it may be the best of an imperfect array of options. The alternative—walling ourselves off behind a thickening barricade of earplugs, triple-glazed windows and white-noise machines—may keep down the noise, but it will also deafen us to much of the world, not just the parts we don't want to hear.

What's at Risk?

Environmental Influences on Human Health

JOHN EYLES AND NICOLE COSITT

How important is the environment when it comes to human health? The 1962 publication *Silent Spring* not only rippled throughout the scientific community and public conscience but initiated a growing wave of research into the linkages between environment and human health.[1] Yet there is limited hard scientific proof that adverse health outcomes are caused by the contaminant load that human activities add to the environment. Most scientists remain concerned about the emerging epidemic of lifestyle diseases and are committed to genetic research as the next magic bullet, while the relations between human health and environmental exposures remain highly contentious.

For example, dichlorodiphenyltrichloroethane (DDT) was indicted as an extreme risk to human health in spite of a significant lack of human toxicological or epidemiological evidence.[2] Despite the chemical's proven ability to control, if not eradicate, the spread of mosquito borne malaria in human populations, animal studies were deemed sufficient to warrant the ban on the use of DDT-containing agents. But recent research does not support any association between DDE (p,p'-dichlorodiphenyldichloroethylene, the predominant DDT metabolite) and, for example, breast cancer.[3] Whether or not the ban on DDT was premature or in fact beneficial to human health is still debatable. DDT remains a significant part of mosquito-control programs in malaria-endemic countries and undoubtedly saves thousands of lives.

In fact, there is much scientific debate about the causes of all cancer. Lifestyle and behavioral factors such as tobacco use and unhealthy diets are the main drivers of the cancer burden, with the World Health Organization (WHO) estimating that just 2 percent of all cancers are attributable to air pollution and only 5 percent due to occupational exposures.[4] Diseases and conditions such as diabetes, cardiovascular disease, and certain cancers have emerged as what has been coined "the epidemic of lifestyle disease."

So why worry about the environment? Environmental exposure is difficult to delineate. Scientific evidence to support associations between environmental contaminants and human disease is often limited to very high exposures resulting from occupational or accidental exposures. For the general public, evidence remains circumstantial that what we eat, drink, and breathe are major risk factors for disease. Yet there are significant fears that these factors outside our control adversely affect us, making the environment-health linkage intensely political.

The Skeptical Environmentalist, the recent antithesis to *Silent Spring*, asserts that the state of the global environment and pollution is improving and refutes much of the research that implies any connection between our environment and human disease.[5] In addition, the physical environment was notably absent as an important factor in WHO's 2003 report, *Social Determinants of Health*.[6] Trying to quantify the disease burden borne by environmental factors is complicated not only by changing definitions and parameters but also by the unknown impacts of emerging risks. One recent study evaluating the role of environmental pollutants on human health stated that only 8-9 percent of the total disease burden is attributable to environmental pollutants, with unsafe water, poor sanitation, and hygiene occupying the most significant sources of exposure along with indoor air pollution (see Table 1).[7] A study that followed looked specifically at the effects of water, sanitation, and hygiene and concluded that these environmental factors accounted for 4 percent of global mortality and 5.7 percent of total disability adjusted life years.[8]

But despite these statistics, there is still considerable concern regarding environmental influences on human health—not only because these factors are outside the control of individuals, but because there is still so much that science does not know. Significant unexplained connections remain between death and disability for many diseases—cancer, heart disease, diabetes, neurological conditions—that may be filled by "environment."

Table 1. Global burden of disease attributable to selected sources of environmental and occupational pollution

Risk factor	Deaths		Disability-adjusted life years	
	Thousands	Percent	Thousands	Percent
Total (all risk factors)	55,861		1,455,473	
Water, sanitation, and hygiene	1,730	3.1	54,158	3.7
Urban outdoor air pollution	799	1.4	6,404	0.4
Indoor smoke from solid fuels	1,619	2.9	38,539	2.6
Lead	234	0.4	12,926	0.9
Occupational carcinogens	118	0.2	1,183	0.1
Occupational airborne particulates	356	0.6	5,354	0.4
Occupational noise	0	0.0	4,151	0.3
Total (pollution-related)	4,856	8.7	122,715	8.4

SOURCE: M. Ezzati, A. D. Lopez, A. Rodgers, S. Vander Hoorn, and C. J. L. Murray, "Selected Major Risk Factors and Global and Regional Burden of Disease," *The Lancet*, 30 October 2002, http://image.thelancet.com/extras/02art9066web.pdf (accessed 18 June 2004).

This is particularly worrying, as startling body burden evidence reveals that our bodies are harboring pesticides, flame retardants, nicotine-metabolites, lead, and other toxic human-made chemicals. A particularly illuminating product of this research already has shown that women in San Francisco have 3-10 times the levels of flame retardant in their breast tissue than European or Japanese women.[9] Similar research reported that women and infants in Indiana and California had 20 times the levels of flame retardant present in women of Sweden or Norway.[10] (It is useful to note that Sweden and Norway have both recently banned flame retardants.) Researchers link flame retardants with accumulating "e-waste" of old technology products—something present in large quantities in parts of California, specifically Silicon Valley. Coincidence? Not likely. Debatable and unproven? Unfortunately, yes. Because females on average carry 10 percent more body fat than their male counterparts and are able to absorb and carry more fat soluble toxic material, women are particularly at risk for this toxic loading. This new research is yet another piece in the evolving, complex story of how the environment is related to human health. Indeed, its salience is that the environment now appeal's to be inside our bodies.

Such "invasions" add to our worries. Furthermore, the interconnectedness of the world through trade, travel, and migration means that risk appears to be democratized, with all the world apparently at risk and little protection from such environmental exposures.[11] The most common public health risks are indeed mundane and thus not newsworthy. High profile outbreaks of infectious disease grab the public's attention and often fuel our risk perceptions. In a recent poll of U.S. voters, 78 percent agreed or strongly agreed that no amount of environmental pollution was tolerable if it adversely affected human health.[12] Our most common exposures to risk come from areas over which we seem to have little control: the quality of water, food, and air. Such a perceived glut of risks makes their understanding particularly challenging for the public. What should we worry about?

As Severe Acute Respiratory Syndrome (SARS) has illustrated, the danger of new diseases is merely a plane ride away. Also, localized public health triumphs, such as the North American control of tuberculosis, can collapse with the return of such diseases as global population movements make health problems borderless. Taken together, these forces may amplify a "culture of fear," fueled by media attention and scientific uncertainty.[13] This can be exemplified by Bovine Spongiform Encephalopathy (BSE, also known as "mad cow disease"), wherein discordance still exists as to whether BSE is the causal link to cases of new variant Creutzfeldt-Jakob Disease (nvCJD)—a fatal neurological disorder—in humans. Human health risks, specifically those related to environmental exposures, are often biopolitical in nature in that political reasoning underlies which health issues are addressed and which ones are not. Even without strong scientific evidence, political and public concerns can put environmental health linkages in the spotlight.

Environmental Links and Health

So how exactly is environment related to health? What is meant by the term "environment"? What is meant by "health"? It is useful here to limit the definition of environment to the biophysical and chemical surroundings that affect individuals or populations. Mostly they are human influenced or produced and have despoiled the natural environment for decades. But while most concern has been expressed about synthetic chemicals, naturally occurring factors, such as ultraviolet (UV) radiation and radon, may adversely affect humans. As for health, this may be broadly defined too in terms of physical, mental, and spiritual well-being but is limited here to physical health outcomes such as respiratory and gastrointestinal illnesses and cancer. To bring order to this vast, complex picture, it is helpful to emphasize those exposures emanating from the environment that are hazardous to human health. For the hazard to become real, it must travel to humans along or through a medium or pathway—most commonly air, water, or food—or it must be helped along its way by human movement or by animal or insect vectors.

WHO identifies two sets of hazards that lead to human vulnerability.[14] Traditional hazards are associated with a lack of development: They are related to poverty, lack of access to safe drinking water, inadequate basic sanitation in the household and community, indoor air pollution from cooking and using biomass fuel, and inadequate solid waste disposal. Modern hazards are associated with unsustainable development practices and include water pollution from populated areas, industry, and intensive agriculture; urban air pollution from vehicular traffic, coal power stations, and industry; climate change; stratospheric ozone depletion; and transboundary pollution. In a follow-up to its burden of disease report, WHO refines these hazards into risk factors.[15] Of the 26 identified, 6 are environmental: ambient air; indoor air; lead; water, sanitation, and hygiene; climate change; and selected occupational risks (see Figure 1).

Many of these hazards, or risk factors, involve several exposure pathways. For example, changes associated with climate and weather and affecting air, water, and animal populations have direct impacts on human health and disease burdens. The World Bank suggests that such change is occurring at unprecedented rates as large quantities of carbon dioxide, methane, and other greenhouse gases continue to be released into the atmosphere, a suggestion confirmed by Intergovernmental Panel on Climate Change summaries of the scientific evidence.[16] Direct effects are primarily altered rates of heat- and cold-related events. For example, the death tolls attributed to heat stress can be surprisingly high. In Chicago in July 1995, heat stress was implicated in the deaths of 726 people during a 4-day heat wave.[17] Some 15,000 are estimated to have died during August's blistering heat in France in 2003.[18] For industrialized countries such as the United States and Canada, the greatest direct impacts lie in the contribution of greenhouse gases to smog and air pollution and hence respiratory diseases. The indirect effects of climate change stem from climate's association with other driving forces of environmental change, including population dynamics, urbanization, and production and consumption patterns (see Figure 2). For

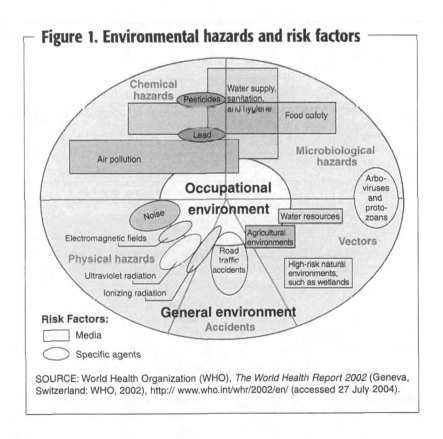

Figure 1. Environmental hazards and risk factors

SOURCE: World Health Organization (WHO), *The World Health Report 2002* (Geneva, Switzerland: WHO, 2002), http:// www.who.int/whr/2002/en/ (accessed 27 July 2004).

Figure 2. Climate change and health pathways

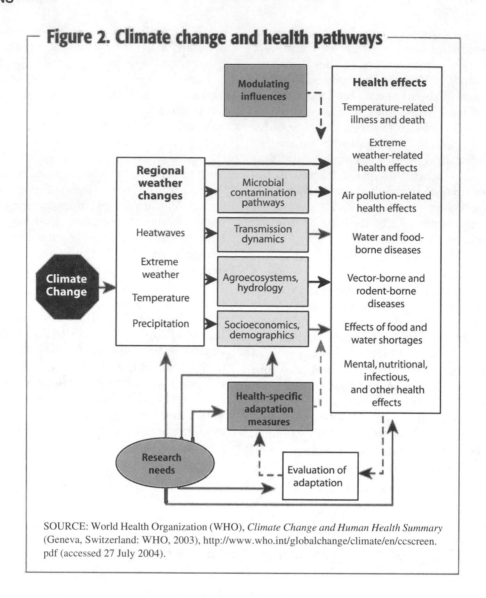

SOURCE: World Health Organization (WHO), *Climate Change and Human Health Summary* (Geneva, Switzerland: WHO, 2003), http://www.who.int/globalchange/climate/en/ccscreen.pdf (accessed 27 July 2004).

example, one study, published in 1994, shows how climate variability led to the appearance in humans of hantavirus pulmonary syndrome (a rodent borne disease) when long-lasting drought was punctuated by heavy rains in the U.S. Southwest.[19] An explosion of rodent numbers enabled the virus to take hold, and when drought returned, rodents sought food in human dwellings, bringing the disease with them. Earlier episodes in China have been associated with increased urbanization and inadequate waste treatment or removal, allowing garbage to proliferate. Urban services and pest control were inadequate, leading to more than 100,000 reported cases in China in the early 1990s.[20]

The spread of West Nile (WN) virus—which can result in a type of Japanese encephalitis—across North America also illustrates several pathways. WN virus may have reached America through an individual returning from an endemic country, the importation of an infected bird, or the accidental importation of an infected mosquito.[21] WN encephalitis was unknown in Europe until 1996,

when more than 500 cases were observed in the Bucharest region of Romania with high rates of neurological disorder and death (up to 10 percent of those affected). It was not detected in the Western Hemisphere until 1999, when 56 cases of WN encephalitis were confirmed in New York City. Of these, 7 died. Russian scientists report a particularly virulent outbreak in Volgograd City in Russia, where about 480 suspected overt WN virus cases were found. There were 84 cases of acute aseptic meningoencephalitis, 40 of which were fatal.[22] Most of the cases in Romania, Russia, and the United States were among the elderly. Another commonality is that these three affected areas are located near large bodies of water and are on bird migration routes. All had unusually dry summers in the year of the outbreak. Similar characteristics may yet be implicated in the 2002 North American episodes that saw Louisiana and Georgia particularly affected. Since then, WN virus has established itself as a persistent public health concern, spreading throughout most of North America. In 2003, there were nearly 10,000 cases of WN

Figure 3. 2003 West Nile virus activity in the United States

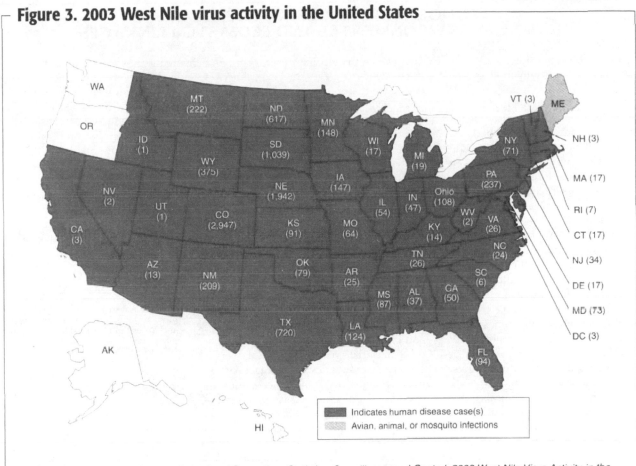

Indicates human disease case(s)
Avian, animal, or mosquito infections

SOURCE: U.S. Centers for Disease Control and Prevention, *Statistics, Surveillance, and Control: 2003 West Nile Virus Activity in the United States (reported as of May 21, 2003)*, http://www.cdc.gov/ncidod/dvbid/westnile/surv&controlcasecount03_detailed.htm (accessed 17 August 2004).

virus infection in the United States with 262 consequent deaths.[23] In Canada, there were 1,388 clinical cases, which resulted in 14 deaths.[24] The rapid expansion of this vector-borne disease from the Queens borough of New York City in 1999 and the eventual spread across virtually the entire North American continent by 2003 exemplifies the speed with which our environmental and social systems can disperse disease (see Figure 3).[25] Although WN encephalitis is apparently a tropical disease, a complex relationship—through trade and travel—between mosquitoes, birds, and human activities may have been what led industrialized and newly industrialized countries to be affected by it.

To better understand the environment human health link, however, it is useful to examine exposure pathways and media: water, air, and food.

Water, Sanitation, and Infectious Diseases

For many years, water quality has been regarded as a prime indicator of health and well-being, as it plays a crucial role in determining the cause and transmission of disease. While access to water is vital to human life, it also serves as a ubiquitous pathway for illness and disease. Approximately 10 million people die each year from water-related diseases or inadequate sanitation. Put another way, 4 percent of deaths worldwide are due to poor water systems and inadequate sanitation.[26] However, a WHO *Burden of Disease* study came to a more conservative estimate, attributing 1.7 million deaths worldwide to unsafe water, sanitation, and hygiene.[27] Global environmental change affects pathogens (such as viruses, bacteria, protozoa, and fungi), vectors, and hosts by influencing their survival, abundance, and dispersal. Waterborne disease outbreaks can be local (in a particular city or village), national, or international in shape. Increased temperatures, flooding, and runoff are some examples that enhance the transmission route of microorganisms to humans.

Water is a significant route for disease transmission, especially in the tropical world: Typhoid fever, cholera, dysentery, enteritis (bacteria), infectious hepatitis (viruses), amoebic dysentery, giardiasis (protozoa), and schistosomiasis (worms) are all transmitted via water. Disease outbreaks and their associated transmission routes that are linked to water can be categorized in the

ENDOCRINE-DISRUPTING CHEMICALS:
COMPLEX ENVIRONMENTAL AND ECOSYSTEM LINKAGES

Brought to public attention by wildlife toxicologist Theo Colbum and her colleagues, endocrine-disrupting chemicals point to complex relationships between industrial processes, the environment, and human health. A growing body of scientific evidence indicates that a number of chemicals with which humans are in contact may interfere with the endocrine system. This interference, attributed to such chemicals as natural and synthetic hormones, organometals, pesticides, persistent environmental pollutants, monomers, and additives used in the plastic industry, has the potential to cause adverse effects to wildlife and humans. There are indications for an increase in the incidence of some hormonally sensitive carcinomas, decrease in sperm count and quality, and increased obesity and earlier puberty occurring in girls, as well as altered physical and mental development in children.[1] The levels of chemicals in the environment and the consequent burden of exposures appear to coincide with the incidence and trends of many of these adverse health outcomes. There is growing evidence to suggest that exposure to endocrine-disrupting chemicals may be associated with a predisposition to obesity later in life.[2] Although endocrine disruption in humans by pollutant chemicals remains largely undemonstrated—due in large part to the surreptitious nature of endocrine disruption—the underlying science is solid and the potential for such effects is real. Endocrine-disrupting chemicals are diverse and cut across chemical classes, and they include persistent organic pollutants (for example, dichlorodiphenyl-trichloroethane (DDT), polychlorinated biphenyls (PCBs), and bisphenol A), methoxychlor, alkyiphenols, and phthalates. A survey by the U.S. Centers for Disease Control and Prevention revealed that toxicological characteristics of these chemicals were shown to produce developmental toxicity, carcinogenicity, mutagenicity, immunotoxicity, and neurotoxicity. Regarding the hormone-disrupting effects of the 48 endocrine-disrupting chemicals, estrogenic effects were the most predominant in pesticides, while effects on thyroid hormone were found for heavy metals. Endocrine-disrupting chemicals showing estrogen-modulating effects were closely related to carcinogenicity or mutagenicity with a high degree of sensitivity.[3]

Reproductive effects have also been noted. In men, hypospadias, cryptorchidism, cancer of the prostate, testicular cancer, and semen quality; and in women, breast cancer, cystic ovaries, and endometriosis have all been suggested as indicators of adverse trends in reproductive health.

1. G. M. Solomon and T. Schettler, "Environment and Health: 6. Endocrine Disruption and Potential Human Health Implications," *Canadian Medical Association Journal* 163, no. 11 (2000): 1471-76.
2. J. J. Heindel, "Endocrine Disruptors, and the Obesity Epidemic." *Toxicological Science* 76, no. 2 (2003): 247-49.
3. K. C. Choi and E. B. Jeung, "The Biomarker and Endocrine Disruptors in Mammals," *Journal of Reproduction and Development* 49, no, 5 (2003): 337-45.

following manner: waterborne (infections spread through water supplies); water-washed (infections spread through lack of water for personal hygiene); water-vectored (infections spread by insects that depend on water); and water-based (infections spread though an aquatic invertebrate host). Most of these are exacerbated by human activities that pollute the water.

Waterborne Diseases

Cryptosporidiosis is prevalent both in the temperate and tropical world, where it can be found in untreated surface waters, as well as swimming and wading pools. It is a zoonosis—a disease transmitted from animals to humans—in that infection is associated with fecal-oral contamination through exposure to farm or wild animals, such as beavers. With increased precipitation and higher temperatures, as seen in patterns in North America, oocysts from these organisms found in fecal matter may be washed into drinking-water supplies, thus exposing the populations to risk through ingestion of contaminated water. These oocysts are of particular concern as they are resistant to chlorine treatment in regular municipal water treatment facilities and are small and difficult to filter. The largest known recorded waterborne outbreak of cryptosporidiosis in U.S. history occurred in 1993 in Milwaukee, Wisconsin, where approximately 400,000 individuals were infected.[28]

Another large outbreak occurred in Saskatchewan, Canada, in 2002 and affected 7,000 people.[29]

Transmission of the microorganism *Vibrio cholerae*, which causes cholera, occurs by bathing in or drinking contaminated water or by ingesting contaminated food. Movements of tidal waters toward land as well as river flows bring cholera bacteria in contact with humans. Cholera outbreaks occur seasonally and are associated with monsoon seasons, warm temperatures, heavy rainfall, and increased plankton populations. New major outbreaks of cholera are continuing to occur, especially in the wake of climate changes. Depending on environmental conditions, however, numbers do vary from year to year: For example, in 1998 there were 293,121 cases and in 2002 there were 123,986.[30]

Water-Washed Diseases

Water-washed diseases, such as shigella, salmonella, *E. coli*, and pseudomonas, are transmitted primarily through inadequate supplies of water for basic hygiene practices, thus exposing individuals to risk through the fecal-oral route. Most often in developing countries, the only source of water available to populations for drinking, bathing, washing clothes, and for animal care is contaminated with pathogens from raw sewage, industrial activities, and human and animal feces. The survival rates of the pathogenic organisms that cause water-washed diseases are enhanced in warm, moist environments and in situations such as increased flooding that facilitate the transportation of the organism. However, lack of water through environmental change also plays an important role in the transmission of pathogenic microorganisms to individuals. In the developed world, inadequate treatment of drinking water has led to an *E. coli* outbreak in Walkerton, Ontario, affecting 2,000 people (7 deaths) in 2000.[31]

Water-Vectored Diseases

Malaria is the world's most important tropical parasitic disease, killing more than one million people each year and causing more cases of morbidity and mortality than any other tropical infectious disease. Malaria's death toll far exceeds the mortality rate from AIDS: It kills a child every 30 seconds and is a public health problem in more than 90 countries with 40 percent of the world's population. Yet more than 90 percent of all malaria cases are in sub-Saharan Africa, where it particularly affects poor people in rural areas. The total economic cost in this region has been calculated at $2 billion (a 1997 estimate).[32]

Its reach, however, is spreading. Malaria is specific to the ecosystem that breeds it. Human infection is caused by protozoans *Plasmodium falciparum* (the most common and virulent strain), *P. malariae, P. vivax,* or *P. ovale*. It is a vector-borne disease, in which an intermediate vector organism is needed to pass the infectious parasite to and between humans. Water plays a crucial role in the transmission of malaria: The infected female *Anopheles* mosquito that carries the disease requires high humidity and standing water in which to breed. Thus, flooding or heavy rainfalls largely determine disease rates. However, global environmental change is affecting the virulence of the parasite and the life cycle of the intermediate host. Thus, as the production of greenhouse gases and global temperatures rise, malaria may spread into new regions of the globe—for example, North America or Europe. In addition, as climate and weather change, as new dams, canals, and irrigation channels are dug, and as people travel and migrate, different reservoirs for mosquitoes to breed are created in airports, industrial sites, agricultural projects, and city waste dumps. These varieties of reservoirs make control difficult and costly.

Water-Based Diseases

One of the most commonly known water-based diseases is dracunculiasis, or guinea worm disease, caused by the parasite *Dracuricuhis medinensis*. This disease is contracted by drinking water contaminated with the infected intermediate hosts of the parasite, called cyclops. Due to significant multilateral aid and research efforts, it is close to being eradicated but remains a significant threat in sub-Saharan Africa. Ensuring safe water supplies is key to controlling dracunculiasis. Also of signifi-

cance is schistosomiasis, a debilitating disease spread by water snails (as intermediate hosts) in stagnant water. It affects a total of 200 million people, causing chronic urinary tract disease; it can be spread to new areas through dam and irrigation projects. River blindness—a parasitic disease transmitted by blackfly—currently affects more than 85 million people in Africa, Latin America, and the Middle East.[33]

It's in the Air: Air Quality and Respiratory Health

Environmental exposures often have the most dramatic impacts on our respiratory systems: Although there has been obvious progress made in air quality in developed countries, WHO reports that outdoor air pollution accounts for more than 800,000 deaths a year worldwide.[34] Air pollution affects people outdoors and indoors, at workplaces and in homes. The environmental consequences of air pollution tend to be noticed in haze and reduced visibility. For example, average visibility in Mexico City has been reduced from 11 kilometers to 1.6 kilometers since the late 1940s. Environmental monitoring shows where the worst air quality is found, but much depends on the pollutants that are measured. The U.S. Environmental Protection Agency (EPA) notes that the worst urban areas for ozone nonattainment targets within the United States are the Los Angeles basin; Chicago-Gary, Houston-Galveston, and New York-New Jersey metro areas; and the southeast desert in California.

Because different pollutants have different health effects, what is measured and controlled is important.[35] In general, exposure to low levels of such pollutants as ozone, sulfur oxides, nitrogen oxides, and particulate matter can irritate the eyes and cause inflammation of the respiratory tract. Many air pollutants may also suppress the immune system, increasing susceptibility to infections. Following the nearly 2,500 deaths that occurred in London in December 1952, attention has been focused on particulate matter (PM).[36] In the last 30 years, consistent association has been found between PM and increases in mortality, hospital admissions, and morbidity. Most recently, in a study of 20 U.S. cities, increases in the relative rate of death from all causes and respiratory and cardiovascular causes were found with each increase in PM level.[37] A detailed study of Montreal found increases in daily mortality and most measures of particulate air pollution of the order of 1-2 percent.[38] While this seems small, it is a serious public health issue on a population level: For example, in cities of more than one million people, 1-2 percent equates to 10,000-20,000 people.

Recent studies are revealing relationships between air quality and many adverse health outcomes, including asthma, lung cancer, cardiovascular disease, diabetes, stroke, and chronic obstructive pulmonary disease.[39] WHO officials stated in a 2000 Air Quality and Health meeting in Geneva that overall, air pollution from various sources contributes to 3 million deaths worldwide.[40] Because of the complexities of causation, this is merely an estimate; the actual death toll may be anywhere from 1.4 million to 6 million. Air pollution's influence on chronic morbidity is much more dramatic. One study concluded that there is an association between fine particulate matter, common in the air of most metropolitan areas, and increased risk of death due to lung cancer and cardiopulmonary disease.[41] A 2002 Dutch study found that people living near a main road were twice as likely to die of heart or lung disease more than those who did not.[42] Increases in and exposure to particulate air pollution have been shown to exacerbate asthma sufferers, symptoms, increasing rates of asthma attacks 3-5 days after coincident increased pollution levels.[43] Although most studies of the relationship between poor air quality and human health have been carried out in developed countries, it is a worldwide problem. For example, studies in São Paulo, Brazil, have shown that an increase of 75 micrograms per cubic meter in concentrations of nitrogen dioxide was related to a 30 percent increase in deaths from respiratory illness in children under 5 years of age.[44]

Is ambient air quality getting worse? In many instances, yes. Despite overall trends of decreasing emissions for the major pollutants in North America, regional disparities still exist that are often obscured by national averages. Fine particulate matter and ground-level ozone levels have shown no appreciable decrease, with many counties along the northeastern seaboard and in California having levels of these pollutants consistently exceeding EPA standards. European health officials state that a large proportion of the morbidity and mortality experienced in last summer's heat wave was attributable to poor air quality, specifically record levels of ground-level ozone during much of August 2003.[45] On a local level, mobile emissions are considered to be the most important contributor to urban air pollution. Although recent regulations and clean air initiatives have greatly reduced emissions in North America and continue to head off projected increases of sulfur dioxide levels in industrializing countries like China and South Korea, rapid urbanization coupled with increasing vehicle populations will continue to have adverse effects on urban air quality.[46] Much of the vehicle fuel efficiency obtained and technology used in industrializing nations such as China are similar to North American vehicles of the late 1960s. In addition, EPA recently announced that in 2002, the volume of toxic pollutants emitted into the atmosphere increased by 5 percent, doubling the last increase in 1997.[47]

Emissions from fossil fuel combustion continue to influence the trend of increasing annual average smog levels in Ontario and the rest of Canada. In 2003, Ontario recorded 34 smog alert days—a record high. Smog is created primarily when sunlight interacts with pollutants released by fossil fuel combustion and industrial processes and products: namely, nitrogen oxides, sulfur dioxide, volatile organic chemicals, and carbon dioxide. Ground-level ozone, which can irreparably harm lung function, is a result of these photochemical reactions and thus a major component of smog. These concentrations are increasing not only in the summer but also in the winter and in rural and urban areas. Overall increasing temperatures—which have been attributed to some of the same smog-producing pollutants (as well as others) acting as greenhouse gases—have also influenced smog levels. Warmer temperatures put increased demands on electrical sources, primarily from the use of air conditioners. Thus, coal-fired power plants, significant greenhouse gas contributors, will be required to produce more and more electricity.[48] Another contributor to the air pollution equation is diesel exhaust. Diesel-powered engines account for 26 percent of the total hazardous particulate pollution emitted into the atmosphere; 90 percent when further broken down for on-road contributors. Diesel exhaust contains 40 toxic chemical pollutants, 26 of which are known carcinogens or reproductive toxicants.[49]

Poor indoor air quality is as significant as outdoor or ambient air pollution: Soot from burning wood, dung, crop residues, and coal for cooking and heating affects about 22 million people worldwide, mostly women and girls. Poor indoor air quality is estimated to kill more than 2.2 million people each year, nearly all in developing countries.[50] In countries such as the United States and Canada, indoor air quality is also a growing concern.

The indoors—homes, shopping malls, offices, and factories—is an important environment in which we spend between 50 and 90 percent of our time, depending on age and occupation.[51] Colds, influenza, headaches, and stomach upsets are common illnesses, often associated with common indoor pollutants, including radon, cigarette smoke, carbon monoxide, nitrogen dioxide, formaldehyde, solvents, pesticides, and ozone. Also found indoors are fungi, bacteria, viruses, mites, pollens, and animal dander, all of which can exacerbate ailments, especially in closed, often air-tight buildings. In fact, the epidemic of childhood asthmas is frequently associated with these indoor contaminants. Asthma is the leading chronic illness of children in the United States, responsible for many school absences, hospitalizations, and visits to the emergency room. EPA estimates that 17 million Americans (children and adults) suffer from asthma, costing $7 billion-$9 billion annually in direct and indirect costs.[52] Furthermore, some of the pollutants in indoor air lead to nonrespiratory problems—such as cancer (caused by radon and tobacco smoke) and reproductive and developmental effects (from lead) and may act as an amplifier of other conditions, particularly heart disease.[53] (As the box on the next page shows, despite regulatory measures, lead remains a concern.)

LEAD AND HUMAN HEALTH

Lead is the most abundant heavy metal in the Earth's crust. It is common in industrial and commercial usage, specifically printing, painting, smelting, and plumbing activities, lending to high levels of occupational and environmental exposure.[1] Lead in petrol fuel and the processing of lead ores are considered the largest exposure sources. Lead is the most common form of pediatric heavy-metal poisoning. Childhood exposure is common through contaminated soil and dust. Environmental exposure to lead is expected to decline due to the phasing out of its usage in many industries, including gasoline, automobiles, and paint. However, recent soil surveys reveal that many regions, specifically downtown cores of older North American cities with histories of leaded gasoline and coal combustion and lead-based paint use have lead concentrations 10-100 times greater than similar neighborhoods in smaller cities.[2] In addition, a 1996 U.S. Environmental Protection Agency study of privately owned housing built prior to 1980 found that 23 percent of homes (18 million) had elevated soil-lead levels. Much of this lead load can be attributed to past car exhaust emissions.

Thus, lead toxicity remains a significant health threat. It is primarily associated with adverse neurodevelopment in those exposed in early life stages. Too much lead in the body can cause serious damage to the brain, kidneys, nervous system, and red blood cells. Those at greatest risk, even with short-term exposure, are young children and pregnant women. A child's mental and physical development can be irreversibly stunted by overexposure to lead. More recent research links lead exposures during infancy and childhood to attention deficits, hyperactivity, impulsive behavior, IQ deficits, reduced school performance, aggression, and delinquent behavior.[3]

1. S. Tong, Y. E. von Schirnding, and T. Prapamontol, "Environmental Lead Exposure: A Public Health Problem of Global Dimensions," *Bulletin of the World Health Organization* 78, no. 9 (2000): 1068-77.
2. H. W. Mielke, C. R. Gonzales, M. K. Smith, and P. W. Mielke, "The Urban Environment and Children's Health: Soils as an Integrator of Lead, Zinc, and Cadmium in New Orleans, Louisiana, U.S.A.," *Environmental Research* 81, no. 2 (1999): 117-29.
3. H. L. Needleman, J. A. Reiss. M. J. Tobin. G. E. Biesecker, and J. B. Greenhouse, "Bone Lead Levels and Delinquent Behaviour," *Journal of the American Medical Association* 275, no. 5 (1996): 363-69.

Health effects from ingesting and breathing lead

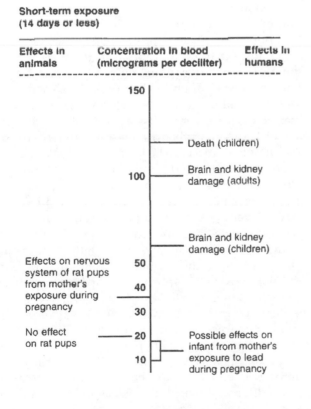
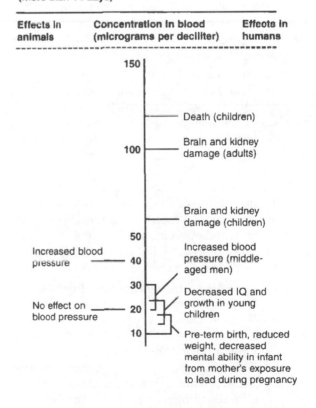

A Murky Environmental Link? Food and Poor Health

The linkage between food consumption, environment, and health is a complex and important one. For example. WHO'S 2004 *Inheriting the World: The Atlas of Children's Health and the Environment* gives credence to the importance of safe food as one of the most important preventive measures to protecting children's health.[54] In the developing world, food security is seriously affected by environmental practices, farming styles, water availability, land ownership patterns, and the tensions between subsistence and export-based agriculture. Food insecurity can result in malnutrition and illness. A massive study of the global burden of disease released in 1996 calculated that malnutrition is responsible for 11.7 percent of all deaths worldwide and 15.9 percent of disability-adjusted life years. For malnutrition, the contribution rises to 31.9 percent of total deaths for sub-Saharan Africa (32.7 percent of disability-adjusted life years).[55] As the United Nations Food and Agriculture Organization (FAO) points out, malnutrition remains significant in many countries of Southeast Asia and Africa: In Mali, nearly half the population was malnourished in 1996-1998, a 30 percent increase in the proportion from 1979-1981. It has become a significant fact of life (and disease) in the republics of the former Soviet Union, with almost a third of the populations of Azerbaijan and Tajikistan undernourished in 1996-1998. In a previous report, FAO notes the devastating impact that poor nutritional status can have on the health status of children. In much of West Africa, for example, one-fifth of all children die before the age of five; in Nigeria this increases to almost one-third. Malnutrition makes people, especially children, susceptible to illnesses such as pneumonia and diarrheal sicknesses.[56]

Globally, changes occurring in the environment (pesticides, antibiotics, and the changing balance of animal and insect populations) are translated into the food we eat. A few examples of the increasing links between imported raw fruits and vegetables that weigh heavily in the minds of consumers include a hepatitis A outbreak linked to Mexican green onions, the *E. coli* and salmonella outbreaks associated with alfalfa sprouts, and the high profile cyclosporiasis outbreak of the late 1990s caused by Guatemalan raspberries. According to the U.S. Centers for Disease Control and Prevention, since 1995 there have been 13 food-borne outbreaks linked to alfalfa sprouts, with 10 of those occurring in the United States.[57]

There are also possible linkages between humans, animals, and disease. Crowding—the result of urbanization and dense population clusters enable favorable conditions of disease transference and proliferation. In China, Guangdong's population of 80 million people live in close contact with the animals, poultry, and fish they consume. Cross pollution between animals and the close proximity of humans with these animals increases the ability of viruses to jump species and infect humans. Zoonotic diseases are known to proliferate in overcrowded populations wrought with pollution and unhygienic conditions. Research is revealing that all mammalian influenza strains originate in aquatic birds, specifically ducks—a staple of Asian diets.[58] Transmission between birds, as well as across species to mammalian populations, occurs through fecal contamination of water—a hallmark of urban slums and wet markets (live-animal markets). The avian flu reported in human populations in China this year is one recent example. Another important mode of transference is the practice of feeding pigs scraps of garbage and dead birds.[59]

Modern factory farming practices have helped the emergence of antibiotic resistance; outbreaks of food-borne illness and disease; and the contamination of water supplies, degradation of land, and loss of biodiversity. Foods expose us to pesticide residues directly and indirectly though air and water. (Pesticides can be carried through air currents during their application to vegetable and fruit crops, and they can pass into drinking water supplies through farm runoff.)

The bioaccumulation of toxins in the food chain has been known in the scientific community for years. Recently, the news media has drawn the public's attention to this increasing threat to human health. Research sampling tissues in Arctic animals first revealed the bioaccumulation of chemical pollutants in the local food chains of relatively nonindustrial regions.[60] Now, however, research is revealing high levels of toxins in food animals farmed in controlled settings, removed from the wild environment. One study, published in 2003, raised alarm in the public when it reported that farmed salmon were more toxic than salmon found in the wild.[61] The study points to the bioaccumulation of toxins as a factor in the increased levels found in farm-raised salmon, which are fed chopped-up fish and oil. Previous research has revealed that carnivorous fish accumulate much higher levels of toxins than their herbivore counterparts, a direct result of their place in the food chain.[62] The salmon, sampled from North and South America and Europe, were analyzed for 14 specific organochlorine toxins. Measurements revealed a prevailing overall trend of elevated toxin levels. Specifically, North American farm-raised salmon showed increased levels of all 14 measured toxins compared to wild Pacific salmon. Of the 14 measured toxins, the study highlights polychlorinated biphenyls (PCBs), dioxins, toxaphene (anticipated human carcinogens), and dieldrin as the most dangerous related to their potential impact on human health. However, the authors of the study also point to the proven health benefits of eating salmon, which is high in omega-3 fatty acids, known to protect against heart disease. Without further human impact assessments, the benefits of salmon related to heart disease outweigh the risk associated with potential cancer-causing toxicants.

There also remains concern over the use of malachite green in trout and salmon farms in the United Kingdom.

Despite being banned two years ago, surveillance shows that the chemical, used in fish farms to disinfect eggs, continues to contaminate farmed fish. Government toxicological officials are expected to announce malachite green as a proven human carcinogen.

Conclusion: Global Linkages and Health

As examples of the human health risks posed by contaminated water, air, and food suggest, it is not just the complex interactions among environmental factors that are responsible for a particular pattern of death and disease. Economic, political, and cultural systems play a large role as well. Another recent case—of the relationship between pollution, famine, malnutrition, and ill health in parts of the tropical world—is illustrative. Large areas of industrial haze have been found over the northern Indian Ocean and western Africa. In the former case, air quality degradation covers, during the winter monsoon, an area in excess of 10 million km^2, largely produced by biofuel use and agricultural burning.[63] This problem is likely to worsen as more fossil fuels are used, leading to photochemical reactions. The impacts of this global plume await study, but some clues can be taken from the African experience. According to Australian researchers, air pollution is likely to have contributed to the catastrophic Sahel drought as sulfate aerosol makes cloud droplets smaller.[64] Smaller droplets in turn make the clouds bigger and longer lasting, reflecting more sunlight into space, cooling the surface below. As a result, the tropical rain belt is weakened in the Northern Hemisphere. Since the 1960s, the Sahel has experienced devastating drought, leading to widespread famine and death.[65] Such complex natural reactions to human activity lead to a double jeopardy for citizens of the developing world: Activities to assist economic development lead to problems, compounding those from the routine hazards of living in such places.

In some ways, as all these examples attest, dealing with potential environmental insults on health seems even more intractable. Environment impacts human health and well-being at many different scales—from the global, with climate change and trade relations—to the local and personal, with the existence of contaminated communities and the personal impacts of the environment through UV-radiation and food and water consumption. But the apparent pervasiveness of environmental effects suggests we cannot stand still as our own health and that of our children and grandchildren is affected. And in our interconnected world our prosperity and security may also be threatened.[66] The intractability of action and intervention does not imply or mean impossibility. At a macroscale, there is a need for international actions, agreements, and cooperation. The fact that the environment is on the agenda of many wealthy nations means that it will be addressed before long at G8 and G20 summits (most likely through its impacts on health). Only then will environmental concerns be given teeth.

Multinational agreements are hard to engineer, as the Kyoto Protocol demonstrates. Yet there are good bilateral collaborations to point to, especially the Great Lakes agreements between the United States and Canada, which have resulted, until recent alarming news about Lake Erie, in cleaner, safer, and healthier lakes, catchments, and drinking water systems. (In 2001, a significant dead zone, resulting from severe oxygen depletion was discovered, extending from Sandusky, Ohio, to Erie, Pennsylvania.[67]) At the local level, there is need for local cleanups and changes in personal behavior to make our cities and industrial places cleaner and healthier. In all, there is a continued need for monitoring, surveillance, research, and education—the bulwarks of a public health system that protects our health. All these actions, it is hoped, will lead to greater respect for the global commons.

It is now almost trite to say we have one Earth, which we despoil at our peril. But now we recognize the Earth or nature, through our activities, adversely affects humans, redistributing disease and death across space. German astronaut Ulf Merbold said, "For the first time in my life, I saw the horizon as a curved line. It was accentuated by the thin seam of dark blue light—our atmosphere. Obviously, this was not the 'ocean' of air I had been told it was so many times in my life. I was terrified by its fragile appearance."[68] The stakes are therefore high for the planet with respect to human activities. Despite the scientific uncertainties in the linkages between environmental exposures and health outcomes, there are serious grounds for concern for human health. In fact, some authorities suggest that such exposures are important mediating factors explaining the relationship between low socioeconomic status and ill-health and premature mortality.[69] Furthermore, agencies such as U.S. Centers for Disease Control and Prevention continue to enhance their monitoring of environmental influences on health.[70] Genetics, lifestyle, and sociodemographics matter and shape health. So, too, does environment directly, indirectly, and in combination with other factors. And it threatens our most precious resource—our children: More than five million die each year from environment related conditions. The biggest threats lurk in the places that should be safe—home, school, and community.[71] Thus, striving for a healthy environment matters for our own health and future.

John Eyles, formerly director of the Institute of Environment and Health at McMaster University in Ontario, Canada, is University Distinguished Professor at McMaster. He is also a professor of geography with cross-appointments in clinical epidemiology and biostatistics and sociology. His main research interests include environmental quality and human health, global health, and the role of science in the policy process. He is author or coauthor of more than 200 publications. He may be reached at eyles@mcmaster.ca. Nicole Consitt is a research assistant at the McMaster Institute of Environment and Health. Her research interests focus on globalizing forces and their role in environmental change and the impacts on global health risks and security. She may be reached at consittn@mcmaster.ca.

NOTES

1. R. Carson, *Silent Spring* (Boston: Houghton Mifflin Co., 1962).

2. A. Attaran and R. Maharaj, "Ethical Debate: Doctoring Malaria, Badly: The Global Campaign to Ban DDT," *British Medical Journal* 322, no. 7287 (2000): 676-77.

3. M. Lopez-Cervantes, L. Torres-Sanchez, A. Tobias, and L. Lopez-Carrillo, "Dichlorodiphenyldichloroethane Burden and Breast Cancer Risk: A Meta-Analysis of the Epidemiologic Evidence," *Environmental Health Perspectives* 112, no. 2 (2004): 207-14.

4. World Health Organization (WHO), *Health and Environment in Sustainable Development,* WHO (Geneva, Switzerland: WHO, 1997). http://www.who.int/docstore/peh/archives/execsume.pdf (accessed 17 April 2004).

5. B. Lomborg, *The Skeptical Environmentalist: Measuring the Real State of the World* (Cambridge, U.K.: Cambridge University Press, 2001). For a review of this controversial book, see P. H. Gleick, "Is the Skeptic All Wet? *The Skeptical Environmentalist* by Bjørn Lomborg," *Environment,* July/August 2002, 36-40.

6. WHO, *Social Determinants of Health: The Solid Facts,* WHO (Geneva, Switzerland: WHO, 2003), http://www.who.dk/document/e81384.pdf (accessed 26 June 2004).

7. M. Ezzati, A. D. Lopez, A. Rodgers, S. Vander Hoorn, and C. J. L. Murray, "Selected Major Risk Factors and Global and Regional Burden of Disease," *The Lancet,* 30 October 2002, http://image.thelancet.com/extras/02art9066web.pdf (accessed 18 June 2004).

8. A. Prüss, D. Kay, L. Fetrell, and J. Bartram, "Estimating the Burden of Disease from Water, Sanitation and Hygiene at a Global Level," *Environmental Health Perspectives* 110 (2002): 537–42. The disability-adjusted life year (DALY) is the only quantitative indicator of burden of disease that reflects the total amount of healthy life lost, to all causes, whether from premature mortality or from some degree of disability during a period of time. One DALY can be thought of as one lost year of "healthy" life. Using DALYs as a measure of disease burden allows major causes of disability such as mental health conditions, hearing loss, and osteoarthritis to be recognized as major causes of disease burden, despite the fact that mortality from these conditions is generally low. See C. J. L. Murray and A. D. Lopez, *The Global Burden of Disease* (Cambridge, MA: Harvard School of Public Health, 1996).

9. M. Petreas et al., "High Body Burdens of 2,2'– 4,4' –Tetrabromodiphenyl Ether (BDE-47) in California Women," *Environmental Health Perspectives* 111, no. 9 (2003): 1175-79.

10. A. Schecter et al., "Polybrominated Dipehnyl Ethers (PBDEs) in U.S. Mothers' Milk." *Environmental Health Perspectives* 111, no. 14 (2003): 1723-29.

11. U. Beck, *Risk Society: Towards a New Modernity* (London: Sage, 1992).

12. Public Agenda, *The Environment: People's Chief Concerns* (Reston, VA: Wirthlin Worldwide, 1999), http://www.public agenda.org/issues/pcc_detail.cfm ?issue_type=environment&list=8 (accessed 13 May 2004).

13. B. Glassner, *The Culture of Fear: Why Americans Are Afraid of the Wrong Things* (New York, NY: Basic Books, 1999) and F. Furedi, *The Culture of Fear: Risk Taking and the Morality of Low Expectation* (London: Continuum, 2002).

14. WHO, *Protection of the Human Environment* (Geneva, Switzerland: WHO, 1999). http://www.who.int/peh/index2.htm (accessed 17 April 2004).

15. WHO, *Global Estimates of Burden of Disease Caused by the Environment and Occupational Risks* (Geneva, Switzerland: WHO, 2002), http://www.who.int/peh/burden/globalestim.htm (accessed 17 April 2004).

16. World Bank, *World Development Report 1999-2000,* World Bank (Washington, DC, 2000); and Intergovernmental Panel on Climate Change, *Climate Change 2001: The Scientific Basis,* http://www.meto.gov.uk/sec5/cr_div/ipcc/wgl/WG1-SPM.pdf (accessed 17 April 2004).

17. "Heat-Related Mortality Chicago July 1995," *MMWR* 44 no. 31 (1995): 57-59; and World Resources Institute, *World Resources 1998-9: Environmental Change and Human Health* (New York: Oxford University Press, 1998).

18. "France Ups Heat Tolls." *CBSNEWS.com,* 25 September 2003, http://www.cbsnews.com/stories/2003/O8/29/world/main570810.shtml (accessed 26 July 2004).

19. P. R. Epstein, "Is Global Warming Harmful to Health?" *Scientific American.Com,* 20 August 2000, http://www.sciam.com/print_version.cfm?articleID =0008C7B2-E060-1C73-9B81809EC588EF21 (accessed 17 April 2004).

20. J. W, LeDuc, J. E. Childs, G. E. Glass, and A. J. Watson, "Hantaan (Korean Hemorrhagic Fever) and Related Rodent Zoonoses," in S. S. Morse, ed., *Emerging Viruses* (New York, NY: Oxford University Press, 1993), 149-58.

21. Health Canada, *West Nile Virus: History,* http:// www.hc-sc.gc.ca/english/westnile/history.html (accessed 17 April 2004).

22. A. E. Platonov et al., "Outbreak of West Nile Virus Infection, Volgograd Region, Russia, 1999,"' *Emerging Infectious Diseases* 7 (2001): 128-32.

23. Center for Disease Control and Prevention, *Statistics, Surveillance, and Control: 2003 West Nile Virus Activity in the United States (reported as of May, 21, 2004),* http://www.cdc.gov/ncidod/dvbid/westnile/surv&controlCase Count03_detailed.htm (accessed 17 August 2004).

24. Health Canada, *West Nile Virus: Human Surveillance: Results of 2003 Program,* http://www.hc-sc.gc.ca/pphb-dgspsp/wnv/pdf_sr-rs/2004/surveillance_table_042904_htm.pdf (accessed 17 April 2004).

25. B. Nosal and R. Pellizzari, "West Nile Virus," *Canadian Medical Association Journal* 168, no. 11 (2003): 1443-44.

26. Prüss, Kay, Fetrell, and Bartram, note 8 above.

27. Ezzati, Lopez, Rodgers, Vander Hoorn, and Murray, note 7 above.

28. P. S. Corso et al., "Cost of Illness in the 1993 Waterborne Cryptosporidium Outbreak, Milwaukee, Wisconsin," *Emerging Infectious Diseases* 9, no. 4 (2003), http://www.cdc.gov/ncidod/EID/vol9n04/02-417.htm (accessed 26 July 2004).

29. S. E. Hrudey and E. J. Hrudey, "Walkerton and North Battleford—Key Lessons for Public Health Professionals," *Canadian Medical Association Journal* 93, no. 5 (2002): 332-33.

30. WHO, *Cholera Cases Officially Reported to WHO: 1 January 2002 to 31 December 2002,* http://www.who.int/emc/diseases/cholera/choltbld2002.html (accessed 26 June 2004); and WHO, "Cholera, 1998," *Weekly Epidemiological Record,* 74 (1999): 257-64.

31. C. N. Perkel, *Well Of Lies: The Walkerton Water Tragedy* (Toronto: McLelland & Stewart Limited, 2002).

32. WHO, *Malaria* (Geneva, Switzerland: WHO, 1998), http://www.who.int/inf-fs/en/fact094.html (accessed 26 July 2004).

33. WHO, *Report on Infectious Diseases* (Geneva, Switzerland: WHO, 1999), http://www.who.int/infectious-disease-report/pages/textonly.html (accessed 26 July 2004).

34. Ezzati, Lopez, Rodgers, Vander Hoorn, and Murray, note 7 above.

35. A. J. McMichael, *Human Frontiers, Environment and Disease* (Cambridge, UK: Cambridge University Press, 2001).

36. J. Schwarz, "What Are People Dying Of on High Air Pollution Days?" *Environmental Research,* 64 (1994): 26-39.

37. J. M. Samet, F. Dominici, F. C. Curriero, I. Coursoc, and S. L. Zeger, "Fine Particulate Air Pollution and Mortality in 20 US Cities: 1987-94," *New England Journal of Medicine* 343, no. 24 (2001): 1742-49.

38. M. S. Goldberg et al., "The Association between Daily Mortality and Ambient Air Particle Pollution in Montreal, Quebec 1. Nonaccidental Mortality," *Environmental Research* 86, no. 1 (2001): 12-25.

39. K. Katsouyanni, "Ambient Air Pollution and Health," *British Medical Bulletin* 68 (2003): 143-56.

40. "Air Pollution Kills, but Deaths Can Be Prevented," *CNN.com,* 30 August 1999, http://www.cnn.com/NATURE/9908/30/air.pollution.enn (accessed 26 July 2004).

41. C. A. Pope III et al., "Lung Cancer, Cardiopulmonary Mortality, and Long-Term Exposure to Fine Particulate Air Pollution," *Journal of the American Medical* 287, no. 9 (2002): 1132-41.

42. G. Hoek, B. Brunekreef, S. Goldbohm, P. Fischer, and P. A. van den Brandt, "Association between Mortality and Indica-

tors of Traffic-Related Air Pollution in the Netherlands: A Cohort Study," *The Lancet* 360, no. 9341 (2002): 1203-9.

43. H. Desqueroux, J.-C. Pujet, M. Prosper, F. Squinazi, and I. Momas, "Short-Term Effects of Low-Level Air Pollution on Respiratory Health of Adults Suffering from Moderate to Severe Asthma," *Environmental Research Section A* 89 (2002): 29-37.

44. WHO, "Air Pollution: Fact Sheet No. 187" (Geneva, Switzerland: WHO), http://www.who.int/mediacentre/factsheets/fs187/en/ (accessed 17 April 2004).

45. P. H. Fischer, B. Brunekreef, and E. Lebret, "Air Pollution Related Deaths during the 2003 Heat Wave in the Netherlands," *Atmospheric Environment* 38 (2004): 1083-85.

46. G. R. Carmichael et al., "Changing Trends in Sulfur Emissions in Asia: Implications for Acid Deposition, Air Pollution, and Climate," *Environmental Science & Technology* 36, no. 22 (2002): 4707-13; and Z. Klimont et al., "Anthropogenic Emissions of Non-Methane Volatile Organic Compounds in China," *Atmospheric Environment* 36, no. 8 (2002): 1309-22.

47. "Toxic Pollution Rose 5 Percent in 2002," *ABCNEWS.com*, 22 June 2004, http://www.wjla.com/news/stories/0604/154758.html (accessed 27 July 2004).

48. Environment Canada, *Clean Air: What is Smog?* (Gatineau, Quebec: Environment Canada, 2002), http://www.ec.gc.ca/air/smog_e.shtml (accessed 27 March 2004).

49. H. Decker, V. Patton, J. Scott, and N. Spencer, *Closing the Diesel Divide: Protecting Public Health from Diesel Air Pollution* (New York: Environmental Defense, 2003), http://www.edf.org/documents/2748_DieselDivide ExecSumm.pdf (accessed 17 April 2004).

50. United Nations Population Fund (UNFPA), *The State of World Population 2001: Footprints and Milestones: Population and Environmental Change* (New York: UNFPA, 2001), http://www.unfpa.org/swp/2001/english/index.html (accessed 17 April 2004). See also K. R. Smith, "Air Pollution: Assessing Total Exposure in the United States," *Environment*, October 1988, 10-15, 33-38; and K. R. Smith, "Air Pollution: Assessing Total Exposure in Developing Countries," *Environment*, December 1988, 16-20, 28-30,33-34.

51. J. D. Spengler and K. Sexton, "Indoor Air Pollution: A Public Health Perspective," *Science*, 1 July 1983, 9-17.

52. American Lung Association, *Childhood Asthma* (Washington, DC: American Lung Association, 2002), http://www.alaw.org/childhood_asthma/facts_about_asthma/ (accessed 13 May 2004).

53. Office of Air and Reduction, Environmental Protection Agency (EPA), *Healthy Buildings, Healthy Lifestyle* (Washington, DC: EPA, 2001).

54. WHO, *Inheriting the World: The Atlas of Children's Health and the Environment* (Geneva, Switzerland: WHO, 2004), http://www.who.int/ceh/publications/en/atlas.pdf (accessed 27 July 2004).

55. C. J. L. Murray and A. D. Lopez, note 8 above.

56. Food and Agriculture Organization (FAO), *The State of Food Insecurity in the World 2000* (Rome, Italy: FAO, 2000); and *The*

State of Food Insecurity in the World 1999 (Rome, Italy: FAO, 1999).

57. P. J. Taormina, L. R. Beuchat, and L. Slutsker, "Infections Associated with Eating Seed Sprouts: An International Concern," *Emerging Infectious Disease* 5, no. 5 (1999): 626-34, http://www.cdc.gov/ncidod/eid/vol5no5/taornina.htm#table percent201 (accessed 17 April 2004).

58. T. Horimoto and Y. Kawaoka, "Pandemic Threat Posed by Avian Influenza A Viruses," *Clinical Microbiology Review* 14, no. 1 (2001): 129-49; and K. F. Shortridge et al., "Interspecies Transmission of Influenza Viruses: H5N1 Virus and a Hong Kong SAR Perspective," *Veterinary Microbiology*, 74, no. 1-2 (2000): 141-7.

59. R. G. Webster, "Wet Markets—A Continuing Source of Severe Acute Respiratory Syndrome and Influenza?" *The Lancet* 363, no. 9404 (2004): 234-36.

60. N. Eckley and H. Selin, "The Arctic at Risk: *Arctic Pollution 2002*," *Environment*, September 2003, 37-40.

61. R. A. Hites et al., "Global Assessment of Organic Contaminants in Farmed Salmon," *Science*, 9 May 2003, 226-9. For information on the problems of salmon fanning in the Pacific Northwest, see R. L. Naylor, J. Eagle, and W. L. Smith, "Salmon Aquaculture in the Pacific Northwest: A Global Industry with Local Impacts," *Environment*, October 2003, 18-39.

62. T. Colborn, D. Dumanoski, and J. P. Myers, *Our Stolen Future: Are We Threatening Our Fertility, Intelligence, and Survival? A Scientific Detective Story* (New York: Dutton, Penguin Books, 1996).

63. J. Lelieveld et al., "The Indian Ocean Experiment: Widespread Air Pollution from South and Southeast Asia," *Science*, 9 September 2001,1031-36.

64. Commonwealth Scientific & Industrial Research Organization (CSIRO), *Drought: Air Pollution Link Found* (Melbourne, Australia: CSIRO, 2002), http://www.csiro.au/index.asp?type=mediaRelease&id=SahelDrought (accessed 17 April).

65. J. Verrengia, "Famines Linked to Pollution," *Gazette* (Montreal), 20 July 2002.

66. J. Eyles and R. Sharma, *Infectious Diseases and Global Change: Threats To Human Health and Security* (Victoria, BC: AVISO, 2001).

67. J. Laidman, "Lake Erie's Low Oxygen Has Scientists Stumped, Worried," *Pittsburgh Post-Gazette*, 23 June 2002, http://www.post-gazette.com/healthscience/20020623sickerie3.asp (accessed 27 July 2004).

68. P. H. Raven and L. R. Berg, *Environment* (Orlando, FL: Harcourt, 2001).

69. G. W. Evans and E. Kantrowitz, "Socioeconomic Status and Health: The Potential Role of the Environmental Risk Exposure," *Annual Review of Public Health* 23: 303-31.

70. U.S. Centers for Disease Control and Prevention (CDC), *National Report on Human Exposure to Environmental Chemicals*, NCEH pub no. 03-0022 (Atlanta: CDC, 2003).

71. WHO, *Healthy Environments for Children* (Geneva, Switzerland: WHO, 2003), www.who.int/features/2003/04/en/ accessed (25 June 2004).

FLU SHOT FEVER
Vaccine Shortage Leads to Panic

ATLANTA— If you're like most people, getting a shot is something you dread. Just thinking about it is scary: A cold-handed stranger grabs your arm and jabs a long, thin needle into your skin. Ouch!

Still, despite the pain, a lot of people are more than eager to get shots lately—flu shots, that is. Around the nation, lines of people snaked through clinics, pharmacies, and doctors' offices to receive the vaccine.

At some sites in New York City, lines formed at 2:30 in the morning. At one city clinic, police were called to quell a crowd of angry elderly people who were denied the shot after the clinic ran out of the vaccine. "[They] can't do this to people, especially the elderly. It's criminal!" a *New York Times* reporter overheard 77-year-old John Gruen shouting.

In New Jersey, officials told of people in wheelchairs and others carting oxygen tanks waiting for hours to get a shot. In California, two women collapsed in line. A third woman, who had spent hours waiting, hit her head in a fall and died.

In Aurora, Colo., police reported that 620 doses of the vaccine had been stolen from a pediatrician's office. Some pharmacies reported price gouging by distributors. A pharmacist in Wichita, Kan., for example, told reporters that distributors offered to supply a vial of 10 shots of the vaccine for $600. The normal cost is $80.

Flu Shot Freak-Out

Why all the frenzy for a flu shot? On October 5, Chiron—one of two flu vaccine suppliers to the United States—announced that it would be unable to ship the 48 million doses that it promised because of problems at one of its plants. That's almost half the nation's expected supply. Last year, 83.1 million doses were distributed in the United States.

Health and Human Services Secretary Tommy Thompson said that the government is scouring the world for supplies and that an extra 2.6 million doses will be available in January. But with flu season beginning this month, that may be too late for many people who need to get a shot.

The Centers for Disease Control and Prevention (CDC) in Atlanta has advised health-care professionals to dispense the available shots to those most at risk of suffering complications from the flu: people 65 and older, children 6 to 23 months old, people with chronic illnesses, pregnant women, and healthcare workers in contact with patients.

Some towns are getting creative. In Bloomfield, N.J., for example, there's a flu shot lottery for the 300 available doses there. Only high-risk patients are eligible, "We are hoping the public sees this as the most fair and equitable way to do this," Trevor Weigle, Bloomfield's health director, told reporters.

Nothing to Sneeze At

According to the CDC, the flu (short for *influenza*) can be a killer. It kills an average of 36,000 people a year in the United States and puts about 200,000 in the hospital. Most of those people—about 90 percent—are elderly.

The disease is caused by the influenza virus, which infects the respiratory tract (nose, throat, and lungs). Flu season typically runs from November through March. The disease is highly contagious and spreads through droplets when a person coughs or sneezes.

The best way to prevent the flu, of course, is to get the vaccine. But for those unlucky people who can't get flu shots, the CDC recommends that they avoid contact with sick individuals, wash their hands regularly, and do not touch their eyes, nose, or mouth. For the really unlucky people who do contract the flu, the CDC advises: Stay home! Avoid spreading germs.

The good news is that health officials say this will be a milder flu season than once feared. "The Southern Hemisphere [where winter is just ending] saw a moderate year, so we're hoping we will too," said CDC spokesperson Dave Daigle.

However, the flu is unpredictable, warns the CDC. Influenza strains are constantly changing, so it's not unusual for new strains of the influenza virus to emerge at any time of the year.

More good news is that tests indicate that the flu strains now circulating match those in the vaccine. Researchers guess which strains are most likely and develop the vaccine several months before the flu season begins.

Health officials say something needs to be done to prevent a vaccine shortage from happening again. Some say the U.S. government should oversee the nation's flu vaccine supply, rather than relying on private pharmaceutical companies. Others say strict regulations enforced by the Food and Drug Administration (FDA) make it too difficult for companies to produce vaccines. Expensive equipment and strict quality-control requirements make it hard to profit from developing vaccines.

A Shot at the Shot

As health officials debate the best way to prevent future flu shot fallout, people continue to queue up for a chance to get the shot. Although panic might not bring out the best in some people, others find a way to make the best of a bad situation. Cecile Windels, of Stamford Pediatrics in Connecticut, told *The New York Times*. "Some people are being rude and panicking, but there is good in many others. We had a ... woman with four children, two of whom have chronic illnesses. She said, I'll give my two [children] who need it most the shots, and I'd like the other two doses to go to somebody who really needs it.'"

When Does Autism Start?

Scientists are now looking for the earliest signs of the mysterious disorder as desperate parents hunt for treatments that may improve their children's lives.

By Claudia Kalb

It's a winter night in Northbrook, Ill., and brothers David and Jason Craven are on the move. They're watching a "Baby Beethoven" video. They're bouncing on a mattress in their basement playroom. They're climbing up their dad's legs. David, 7, and Jason, 5, with their mops of brown hair, look physically healthy. But both boys are suffering from a devastating developmental disorder: autism. David speaks only about 10 words, still wears diapers at night and sucks on a pacifier. Jason drinks from a baby bottle. Neither one can vocalize his glee as he plays. Neither one can communicate pain or joy in words. Neither one can say "I love you."

Since their sons were diagnosed, both at the age of 2, Barry and Dana Craven have tried a dizzying array of therapies: neurofeedback, music therapy, swimming with dolphins, social-skills therapy, gluten-free diets, vitamins, anti-anxiety pills and steroids. To reduce the boys' exposure to environmental chemicals, which the Cravens believe might aggravate their conditions, the couple replaced their carpeting with toxin-free wood floors and bought a special water-purifying system. They even installed a $3,500 in-home sauna, which they think will help remove metals like mercury and arsenic from the boys' bodies. Warm and loving parents, the Cravens spent $75,000 on treatments last year alone. "I'm willing to try just about anything if it makes sense," says Dana.

In the six decades since autism was identified, modern medicine has exploded: antibiotics cure infections, statins ward off heart disease, artificial joints combat osteoarthritis. And yet autism, a vexing brain disorder, remains largely a mystery. Researchers still don't know what causes it, nor do they know how best to treat a condition that prompts one child to stop speaking and another to memorize movie scripts. With a tenfold spike in numbers over the past 20 years—one in every 166 children is now diagnosed with an Autism Spectrum Disorder (ASD)—researchers, advocacy groups and the government are racing to improve the lives of children and their families, many of them emotionally and financially drained. This year the National Institutes of Health will spend $99 million on autism research, up from $22 million in 1997.

"I haven't been this excited about research in a very long time."
—Wendy Stone, Vanderbilt University

Some of the most exciting new work involves efforts to spot clues of the disorder in infants as young as 6 months. In the complicated world of autism, where controversies reign and frustration festers, a two-word rallying cry is growing louder by the day: early diagnosis. This week the Centers for Disease Control and Prevention launches a $2.5 million autism-awareness campaign, "Learn the Signs. Act Early." The goal: to educate healthcare providers and parents about red flags, to intervene as quickly as possible—and to give kids with autism a shot at productive, satisfying and emotionally connected lives. "This is an urgent public-health concern," says the CDC's Catherine Rice.

Today, most children aren't even seen by specialists until they've passed their 2nd birthdays, and many aren't diagnosed until at least the age of 3. Kids with Asperger's, on the higher-functioning end of ASD, may be overlooked until well into elementary school. "If we had a way of screening for autism at birth and then could begin very early to retrain the brain, that would really be the ticket," says Dr. Thomas Insel, head of the National Institute of Mental Health. Scientists are now attempting to do just that. In a joint effort by the National Alliance for Autism Research and the National Institute of Child Health and Human Development, researchers at 14 sites, from Harvard to the University of Washington, are studying the baby siblings of children with autism, who have a genetic liability for the disorder. By measuring the infants' visual and verbal skills and their social interactions, scientists hope to identify early markers of autism before children turn 1. "I haven't been this excited about research in a very long time," says consortium member Wendy Stone of Vanderbilt University. "Not only are we getting clues about the earliest features of autism, but we're helping these families along the way."

Canadian researchers Dr. Lonnie Zwaigenbaum and Susan Bryson have enrolled 200 siblings, half of whom have been observed to the age of 2. Roughly 10 percent have been diagnosed with autism. Zwaigenbaum, of McMaster University in Ontario, says that signs of the disorder, though at first subtle, are often there from the very beginning. Preliminary data show that 6-month-olds who are later diagnosed with autism generally have good eye contact, but they're often quieter and more passive than their peers. And they may lag behind in motor developments, like sitting up or reaching for objects.

The signs often become more obvious as children reach their 1st birthdays. By then, some show patterns of extreme reactivity, either getting very upset when a new toy or activity is presented or barely noticing at all. Others already exhibit repetitive behaviors characteristic of autism—rocking back and forth or becoming fixated on an object, like a piece of string dangling in front of their eyes. And they're less responsive to playful interactions with others. When a typically developing child plays peekaboo, her face lights up, she looks at the person she's playing with, she makes sounds, she reaches for the peekaboo blanket. Children with autism, by contrast, show little facial expression. They may not look at their playmate, and it can take enormous energy to elicit a reaction. "What's been striking," says Zwaigenbaum, "is the lack of response or the distress that these activities can elicit."

The Baby Sibs consortium is also looking for early physical markers of the disorder, starting with the size of children's heads. A landmark study published in 2003 found that kids with autism experienced unusually rapid head growth between 6 and 14 months. Consortium members want to see if their young siblings do, too. Scientists aren't sure what accounts for the increase, but one theory is that it has to do with an overgrowth of neuronal connections. Normally, the brain clears out biological debris as it forms new circuits. "Little twigs fall off to leave the really strong branches," says University of Michigan researcher Catherine Lord. In kids with autism, however, that pruning process may go awry.

In their hunt for neurological clues, scientists are unveiling the inner workings of the autistic mind. Using eye-tracking technology, Ami Klin, of the Yale Child Study Center, is uncovering fascinating differences in the early socialization skills of children with autism. Klin has found that when affected toddlers view videos of caregivers or babies in a nursery, they focus more on people's mouths—or on objects behind them—than on their eyes. Klin's toddler study echoes findings in adults and adolescents with autism when they watched clips of "Who's Afraid of Virginia Woolf?" "Richard Burton and Elizabeth Taylor were engaged in a passionate kiss, and they're focusing on the light switch," says Klin. "Our goal is to identify these vulnerabilities as early as possible."

Might it be that the autistic brain's operating platform is different, as if it's a Mac in a world of PCs? Functional MRI scans show that the brain's "fusiform face area," the control tower for face recognition, is underactive in people with autism. The more severe the disorder, the more disabled the fusiform. But is it actually dysfunctional? Or is it just not interested in people? In an intriguing early study, Yale's Robert Schultz took brain scans of a child with autism who had trouble distinguishing human faces but loved the cartoon character Digimon. "Lo and behold," says Schultz, "his fusiform showed strong activity." Schultz and James Tanaka at the University of Victoria in Canada are hoping computer games can help kids with autism learn how to engage with human faces and identify emotions. The children follow directions to shoot at smiley faces or click on the guy who looks sad. In "Emotion Maker," they choose features—angry eyes, a scowling mouth—to create their own faces. And in "Who's Looking at Me?" they scan an array of faces to sensitize them to eye contact. So far, says Schultz, the kids appear to be improving. But will it help change the course of their lives? "That's the million-dollar question," he says.

An intellectual thief, autism infiltrates children's brains, stalling or stealing cognitive and social development. In classic autism, babies fail to coo or babble by their 1st birthdays. Or words that do develop ("dada," "up," "toy") inexplicably disappear. One-year-olds don't respond to their names. A child once bursting with potential finds spinning tops more captivating than her mother's smile. Kids with Asperger's may not be as closed off, but they suffer severe social deficits. Many are verbal fanatics, immersing themselves in long-winded monologues about obscure topics, like fat fryers or snakes. Klin recalls a child who bowed and spoke in Shakespearean English, "almost as if I had plucked him from 14th-century Verona." Such oddities can make these children social pariahs. Baffled by human interactions and frustrated by their inability to make friends, some kids spiral into debilitating fits of anxiety and depression. Many children on the autism spectrum will never live independent lives. "We're talking about children who need lifelong care," says NIMH's Insel. "This is an astonishingly devastating disease."

And its current treatment is all over the map. Every day, it seems, there's a new "cure." With no known cause and no clear guidance, parents must navigate a maze of costly therapies, most of which have little hard-core science to prove their effectiveness. Many children now take medications, ranging from anticonvulsants (about one third suffer from seizures) to stimulants like Ritalin to calm hyperactivity. Low doses of antidepressants such as Prozac may help reduce the severity of repetitive behaviors. And risperidone, an anti-psychotic drug, can quell aggression and tantrums, says Dr. Christopher McDougle, of the Indiana University School of Medicine. The drug, whose side effects include weight gain and sedation, is now before the FDA and could become the first medication approved specifically for autism.

"I am willing to try just about anything if it makes sense."

—Dana Craven, mother of two boys with autism

Drugs, however, won't help a child learn to speak. One of the few treatments that just about everyone agrees is critical is behavioral intervention, which uses word repetition, game-playing and specialized exercises to develop a child's language and social skills. At the Lovaas Institute in Los Angeles, senior instructor Sona Gulyan engages Adam Ellis, who turns 4 next month, in language drills known as discrete trials. "Say 'hi'," says Gulyan. Adam, a chubby-cheeked little boy in jeans and a white T shirt, responds with a "k" sound. "No, 'hi'," says Gulyan. After several failed attempts, Gulyan switches the focus. "Do this," she says, pointing to her nose. Adam imitates the gesture and is congratulated. And then it's back to the original task: "Say 'hi'." Finally, success—and an orange balloon as a reward. In 1987, founder Ivar Lovaas reported that children who received an average of 40 hours a week of his intensive one-on-one therapy called Applied Behavior Analysis increased their IQs by 30 points, compared with a control group. Other studies, however, have been mixed, and critics believe the program is too militaristic. But for Adam's mother, Megan, it's progress that matters. "He has mastered so many skills," she says. "It's just amazing."

Things are more relaxed at Cleveland's Achievement Centers for Children, where Lisa and Tim Brogan play with their son, Alex. Alex is learning to communicate through an intervention called Floortime, which focuses on a child's individual strengths and his relationships with others. Kids learn to engage with their parents through "circles of communication." If Alex wants to line up toy cars in a row, his dad will join him, then nudge one out of place. The move prompts Alex to interact with his father—a circle of communication—rather than isolate himself with the toys. "We have come such a very long way," says Lisa.

Children with autism have as many styles and personalities as any group of toddlers. A behavioral intervention that suits one child (or his parent) won't necessarily work for another. Many treatment centers now mix techniques from different approaches, including one of the newest on the block: Relationship Development Intervention, or RDI. Here, parents learn how to use everyday events as teachable moments. A trip to the grocery store, for example, becomes an opportunity for kids to learn to adapt to sensory overload—the chatter of shoppers, 100 different kinds of cereal. In the past, Pam Carroll's son, Morgan, now 9, was fixated on instant oatmeal with blueberries, and he melted down if it wasn't available. Now he roams the aisles in Gainesville, Fla., and helps his mom shop. Linda Andron-Ostrow, a clinical social worker in Los Angeles, likes the way RDI empowers parents and allows for creative thinking. "Life isn't structured," she says.

With autism's medley of symptoms—which can include a heightened sensitivity to sound and picky eating habits—many families search for alternative treatments. Kacy Dolce and her husband, Christopher, recently took their son, Hank, 4, to see Mary Ann Block, an osteopath in Hurst, Texas, for a $2,500 assessment. Block prescribes vitamins and minerals, diets free of wheat and dairy, and a controversial treatment, chelation, which strips the body of metals like mercury. Block believes these toxins could come from vaccines and are at the core of autism. Mainstream doctors, pointing to scientific studies showing no connection, worry that chelation puts children at serious risk. Despite the possibility of dangerous side effects, like liver and kidney problems, the Dolces say they'd consider it. "We don't know enough yet to say no," says Kacy. "I'll do anything to help our child."

What parents really need is a road map. Earlier this month six U.S. medical centers joined forces to launch the Autism Treatment Network, which will evaluate therapies, pool data and, ultimately, create guidelines. "We can't have parents chasing down the latest treatment," says Peter Bell of Cure Autism Now, a research and advocacy group allied with the effort. "We need to understand what works." At the forefront of ATN is Massachusetts General's Ladders program, where Dr. Margaret Bauman is using a multidisciplinary approach. In addition to offering standard regimens like physical therapy and behavioral intervention, Bauman assesses overall health. When she saw a teenager crying and twisting her body, symptoms other doctors attributed to autism, Bauman sent her to a gastroenterologist, who found ulcers in her esophagus. The writhing was caused by pain. A boy's head-banging went away after he was treated for colitis. "We really have to start thinking out of the box," says Bauman.

And thinking early. Today many kids aren't getting treatment until well after their 3rd birthdays. Diagnosing an infant with autism at 6 months or a year—maybe even one day in the delivery room—could mean the difference between baby steps and giant leaps. At the Kennedy Krieger Institute in Baltimore, a handful of 2-year-olds toddle at the next frontier in autism treatment. The children are part of an NIH-funded study run by Rebecca Landa to see if early intervention, before the age of 3, can improve the trajectory of cognitive and social development. As Landa looks on, David Townsend fusses and stamps his feet. Then, he notices his twin sister, Isabel, turning the pages of "Ten Little Ladybugs." David looks at Isabel, watches her hands, then flips a page himself, accomplishing what autism experts call "joint engagement." "That was beautiful," says Landa. A fleeting moment, a developmental milestone—and, if all goes well, a new world of possibilities for a sweet little boy with dimples.

With Karen Springen, Ellise Pierce, Joan Raymond and Jenny Hontz

Index

Index

Test Your Knowledge Form

We encourage you to photocopy and use this page as a tool to assess how the articles in *Annual Editions* expand on the information in your textbook. By reflecting on the articles you will gain enhanced text information. You can also access this useful form on a product's book support Web site at *http://www.mhcls.com/online/*.

NAME: _____   DATE: _____

_____

TITLE AND NUMBER OF ARTICLE:

_____

BRIEFLY STATE THE MAIN IDEA OF THIS ARTICLE:

_____

LIST THREE IMPORTANT FACTS THAT THE AUTHOR USES TO SUPPORT THE MAIN IDEA:

_____

WHAT INFORMATION OR IDEAS DISCUSSED IN THIS ARTICLE ARE ALSO DISCUSSED IN YOUR TEXTBOOK OR OTHER READINGS THAT YOU HAVE DONE? LIST THE TEXTBOOK CHAPTERS AND PAGE NUMBERS:

_____

LIST ANY EXAMPLES OF BIAS OR FAULTY REASONING THAT YOU FOUND IN THE ARTICLE:

_____

LIST ANY NEW TERMS/CONCEPTS THAT WERE DISCUSSED IN THE ARTICLE, AND WRITE A SHORT DEFINITION:

We Want Your Advice

ANNUAL EDITIONS revisions depend on two major opinion sources: one is our Advisory Board, listed in the front of this volume, which works with us in scanning the thousands of articles published in the public press each year; the other is you—the person actually using the book. Please help us and the users of the next edition by completing the prepaid article rating form on this page and returning it to us. Thank you for your help!

ANNUAL EDITIONS: Health 06/07

ARTICLE RATING FORM

Here is an opportunity for you to have direct input into the next revision of this volume.
We would like you to rate each of the articles listed below, using the following scale:

1. **Excellent: should definitely be retained**
2. **Above average: should probably be retained**
3. **Below average: should probably be deleted**
4. **Poor: should definitely be deleted**

Your ratings will play a vital part in the next revision.
Please mail this prepaid form to us as soon as possible.
Thanks for your help!

RATING	ARTICLE
	1. How To Live To Be 100
	2. Putting a Premium on Health
	3. Why the Rich Live Longer
	4. Happier and Healthier?
	5. Enough to Make You Sick?
	6. Are You OK?
	7. Dealing with Demons
	8. Too Young to be Stressed
	9. The Trouble with Trans Fat
	10. 10 Myths That Won't Quit
	11. What Does Science Say You Should Eat?
	12. Sweating Makes You Smart
	13. The Skinny on Popular Diets
	14. The Female Triad
	15. Stretching…Out?
	16. Eat More Weigh Less
	17. Why We're Losing the War Against Obesity
	18. The New Drug War
	19. Sports and Drugs
	20. Just Say No Again: The Old Failures of New and Improved Anti-Drug Education
	21. Dangerous Supplements Still at Large
	22. Sexual Healing
	23. Male Contraception: Search Is On for Options
	24. It's Just Mechanics
	25. Promiscuous Plague
	26. 'Diabesity', a Crisis in an Expanding Country
	27. The Battle Within: Our Anti-Inflammation Diet
	28. Why We're Losing the War on Cancer and How to Win It
	29. The Puzzling Origins of AIDS
	30. The Overtreated American
	31. Stay Safe in the Hospital
	32. A High Dose of Tech
	33. Putting a Value on Health
	34. Doctoring Yourself: When is it Wise?
	35. Making an Informed Decision About Breast Implants
	36. How to Ease Your Pain
	37. Agencies Work to Corral Mad Cow Disease

RATING	ARTICLE
	38. Just Too Loud
	39. What's at Risk?
	40. Flu Shot Fever
	41. When Does Autism Start?

(Continued on next page)

207

BUSINESS REPLY MAIL
FIRST CLASS MAIL PERMIT NO. 551 DUBUQUE IA

POSTAGE WILL BE PAID BY ADDRESEE

McGraw-Hill Contemporary Learning Series
2460 KERPER BLVD
DUBUQUE, IA 52001-9902

NO POSTAGE
NECESSARY
IF MAILED
IN THE
UNITED STATES

ABOUT YOU

Name

Date

Are you a teacher? ☐   A student? ☐
Your school's name

Department

Address   City   State   Zip

School telephone #

YOUR COMMENTS ARE IMPORTANT TO US!

Please fill in the following information:
For which course did you use this book?

Did you use a text with this ANNUAL EDITION? ☐ yes ☐ no
What was the title of the text?

What are your general reactions to the *Annual Editions* concept?

Have you read any pertinent articles recently that you think should be included in the next edition? Explain.

Are there any articles that you feel should be replaced in the next edition? Why?

Are there any World Wide Web sites that you feel should be included in the next edition? Please annotate.

May we contact you for editorial input? ☐ yes ☐ no
May we quote your comments? ☐ yes ☐ no